PSYCHOLOGY RESEARCH PROGRESS

NEW DEVELOPMENTS IN CLINICAL PSYCHOLOGY RESEARCH

Psychology Research Progress

Additional books in this series can be found on Nova's website
under the Series tab.

Additional e-books in this series can be found on Nova's website
under the e-book tab.

PSYCHOLOGY RESEARCH PROGRESS

NEW DEVELOPMENTS IN CLINICAL PSYCHOLOGY RESEARCH

DROZDSTOJ ST. STOYANOV
AND
ROLF-DIETER STIEGLITZ
EDITORS

nova publishers
New York

Library of Congress Cataloging-in-Publication Data

New developments in clinical psychology research / editors, Drozdstoj St. Stoyanov and Rolf-Dieter Stieglitz (Medical University, Plovdiv, Bulgaria, and others).
pages cm. -- (Psychology research progress)
Includes index.
ISBN 978-1-63483-223-6 (hardcover)
1. Clinical psychology--Research. 2. Psychology, Pathological--Research. 3. Clinical psychology--Research. I. Stoyanov, Drozdstoj, editor. II. Stieglitz, Rolf-Dieter, 1952- editor.
RC467.N49 2015
616.89--dc23
2015022479

Published by Nova Science Publishers, Inc. † New York

CONTENTS

INTRODUCTION: CLINICAL PSYCHOLOGY AS A MULTIFACETED DISCIPLINE

Clinical psychology as a discipline has a long tradition, which reaches back till the 19th century. Over the years, it went through manifold developments and is today the most popular discipline in psychology. It focuses especially on psychological disorders and psychological aspects of somatic illnesses by means of etiology, analysis of conditions, classification and diagnostics, prevention, psychotherapy and rehabilitation; in this context, it also applies aspects of epidemiology, health care and evaluation (Baumann and Perrez 2011). Furthermore, clinical psychology has always been open to other disciplinal branches or neighboring subjects. Of special interest amongst the subjects in *psychology* are diagnostic psychology, differential psychology, personality psychology and developmental psychology, as many psychological disorders can only be understood within a framework of time. Moreover, there has always been a strong connection to *psychiatry*, which mainly developed due to the fact that both disciplines are concerned with psychological disorders. This connection affected all relevant areas in clinical psychology, ranging from etiology to pathogenesis, from diagnostics to (psycho-) therapy.

During the last 100 years, the subject of clinical psychology has become more and more expanded and differentiated. Taking into account the complexity of psychological disorders, the cooperation between different disciplines is essential. As a result, methods that were used in only one discipline first have been established in others, such as genetics and imaginary techniques in medicine, or neuropsychology in diagnostic procedures of clinical psychology. Only within this interdisciplinary perspective can a comprehensive description and characterization of a person be possible, which is needed for the complex gain of knowledge essential for doing justice to a psychological disorder.

The first step in meeting these requirements has been the introduction of a *multiaxial system*, which has traditionally been ascribed to DSM-III, but has in fact been conceptualized as early as the 1940s (Stieglitz et al. 1988).The underlying thought of this procedure is that a person with a psychological disorder can only be understood if all aspects are accounted for. This need had not been met with psychiatric disorders, as additional dimensions are necessary (e.g.: a social dimension) in order to account for all clinical relevant aspects.

Putting this critical aspect into practice, a multimethodological or multimodal approach has come into existence (cf. Stieglitz 2003 and Chapter 9).This approach takes a step forward by focussing on a differentiated description of people on the basis of a distinction between the levels of data (e.g.: psychological, biological), the sources of data (e.g.: patient, third-party) and functional areas (e.g.: constructs within the different levels of data). Especially the psychological level of data with its far-reaching differentiations of potential constructs plays an important role, even if only roughly discriminating between experience, behaviour and achievement.

The newest development is represented by the Project Research Domain Criteria (RDoC), which has its origin in a critique of the actual diagnostics and proclaims a new perspective on patients (Cuthbert and Insel 2013). It tries to bridge the gap between psychology/ psychopathology and neurobiology by aiming to discover more valid diagnostic groups of disorders which are, amongst other things, characterized by means of biomarker. The basis for this kind of development are (neuro-) psychological constructs (e.g., motivation, learning, attention, memory), for which one needs to establish reliable and valid assessment tools.

The present book aims to account for these considerations. The main aspects of developmental psychology can be found in Section I (Clinical and Mental Development). The concept of attachment (cf. Chapter 2), which is a central construct of developmental psychology since years, has gained more and more importance in clinical psychology and psychotherapy. Neuropsychological disorders, which play a central role in many other psychological disorders (e.g.: executive functions, learning difficulties, dyslexia), will be addressed in separate chapters (Chapters 3 and 4).

Section II (II. Diagnostic and Clinical Psychology) focuses on different facets of diagnostics, with diagnostic key aspects in clinical psychology. The connection between the construct of attention and mindfulness therapy exemplifies the transfer into concrete therapeutic approaches (cf. Chapter 5). In Chapters 6 and 7, important considerations in connection with differential diagnostics will be addressed by means of two disorders, which have only come into focus during recent years: autistic spectrum disorders and adult ADHD (attention deficit/hyperactivity disorder). Both of them are of special importance when considering developmental aspects. Other important aspects to be aware of are potential comorbidities (cross-sectional or longitudinal) with other disorders, which puts high demand on the diagnostic process, a fact that will also become apparent in Chapter 8 (diagnostics of burn out syndromes). This rather controversial complex of symptoms requires a comprehensive diagnostic assessment, especially for ruling out depressive disorders.

The complexity of clinical psychology shall be illustrated by means of some examples in Section III (Clinical Psychology and Other Disciplines).Chapter 9 provides an overview of the previously outlined possibilities and necessities in integrating methods of neuroscience in clinical psychology (cf. Chapter 8). In the area of clinical psychology (and here especially in psychotherapy), such studies gain more and more importance that they reach beyond sole evidence of efficacy. This has an impact on, for example, studies and theoretical considerations about general effects, placebo effects, or side effects of psychotherapy, pointing towards the fact that there are still many questions unanswered. Also, considerations outside traditional approaches should be taken into account, for example, spirituality (cf. Chapter 10).

In the last chapter, a more practical approach is applied. For the clinical psychologist, the vast amount of empirical studies and clinical relevant results bear the problem of accomplishing them and putting them into practice. Here, a continuous education is essential (cf. Chapter 11).

REFERENCES

Baumann U. and Perrez M. (2011) Grundbegriffe – Einleitung. In: Baumann U. and Perrez M. (eds.) Lehrbuch der Klinischen Psychologie und Psychotherapie. (4th edition). Bern: Huber, 31-51.

Cuthbert BN. and Insel TR. (2013) Toward the future of psychiatric diagnosis: the seven pillars of RDoC. BMC Medicie 11: 126.

Stieglitz, R.-D. (2003). Multimodal assessment (including triangulation). In R. Fernandez-Ballesteros (Ed.), *Encyclopedia of psychological assessment*. London: Sage, 606-610.

Stieglitz, R.-D., Fähndrich, E. & Helmchen, H. (1988). AMDP in multiaxial classification. In J.E. Mezzich & M. v. Cranach (Eds.), *International classification in psychiatry: Unity and diversity*. Cambridge: Cambridge University Press, 180-204.

Stoyanov, D., Machamer, P. K. and Schaffner, K. F. Rendering clinical psychology an evidence-based scientific discipline: a case study. *Journal of Evaluation in Clinical Practice*, 2012; 18: 149–154.

Rolf-Dieter Stieglitz
University of Basel, Switzerland
Email: rolf-dieter.stieglitz@upkbs.ch

Drozdstoj Stoyanov
Medical University, Plovdiv, Bulgaria
Email: dstoyanov@meduniversity-piovdiv.bg

I. Clinical Psychology and Mental Development

In: New Developments in Clinical Psychology Research
Editors: D. St. Stoyanov and R.-D. Stieglitz
ISBN: 978-1-63483-223-6

Chapter 1

ATTACHMENT: THERE AND THEN, HERE AND NOW

Vanya Matanova*, PhD, DSc, CertCBT
Sofia University "St. Clement of Ohrid", Bulgaria

ABSTRACT

Attachment is a deep and stable relation. Its formation is influenced by all components of the human personality – mind, body, emotions, relations, values. Attachment is not something that parents do for their children but rather something that children and parents build together on the basis of mutual and reciprocal interactions. Attachment leads to a world which is safe, warm, welcoming and non-threatening. On the other hand, separation makes the child feel insecure, unsafe, frightened and forgotten. In addition the child experiences the loss, not only of the mother figure, but also a loss of part of himself and the loss of self identity. The loss of the mother and her love creates insecurity and anxiety that the person will experience repeatedly later on in life.

INTRODUCTION

In 1969 Bowlby defined the term attachment as a psychological bond that exists between the human beings. Bowlby (1907- 1990) was a British psychoanalyst who developed a new interpretation of the psychoanalytic understanding of early child development and created his own theory of mother and child attachment that differed from the classic psychoanalytic theories. Bowlby's work is now well known amongst psychologists around the world. It is widely accepted that Bowlby and his close associate Mary Ainsworth were the founders of this new stream of psychology known as attachment theory. Thanks to Bowlby's work, the psychoanalytic understanding of the relationship between the mother and child has been transformed. His work reveals a new meaning in a child's development and awareness and the role that this has on the onset of disorders in the child's early development.

* Email: v_matanova@yahoo.com.

THEORY OF ATTACHMENT

Regardless of the fact that psychoanalysis is the basis of his attachment theory, his ideas are much closer to Darwin's evolutionary theory, than to Freud's theories (Burmenskaya 2003).

Bowlby reinterpreted the psychoanalytic understanding of the early affection relationships from an ethological approach. He viewed the affective connection with the mother as something that is inherited through evolution and as a basic authentic reaction that all children are born with. This connection is pre-programmed through human evolution. Every child has been born with the need to connect with a mother figure and this connection is as important, or even more important than the need to be fed. What the child requires the most from his/her mother is to be protected and emotionally close, especially in threatening situations. In this context; Bowlby defined attachment as "lasting psychological connectedness between human beings. The child needs to be attached in a way that develops and sustains close emotional relationships with their primary care giver. According to Bowlby, those two behaviors, to develop and maintain a close emotional relationship, form – perhaps the strongest emotional relationship in the human's lifetime and it is the prototype for connecting with other people.

His research (1973) suggested that Freud was wrong to think that key to understanding anxiety is that people get anxious because they don't have anybody to love and to dream about. Bowlby postulated that there is no single key to understand what causes anxiety, because people experience anxiety in different conditions. Bowlby's idea was that one of the main factors in getting anxious is to miss somebody who you love or are dreaming about and this specific form of anxiety leads to great suffering.

According to him, the main disadvantage of psychoanalysis is that it focuses too much on the internal fears and phantasms, rather than the real threats that exist in reality and the fear that has been conditioned from real experience.

He suggested that the development follows a few different paths and the final outcome of a humans development depends on a combination of the individuals genetic makeup and the environment that the individual is exposed to.

For a long time, researchers put a lot of effort into studying the form and the sequences of the highly intensive responses that follow separation, loses etc. but later they realized that it is more effective to study the less intensive responses, which can be observed in young children's behavior on a daily basis. For example, when the figure of the mother is responsive to the child's needs, usually the child is satisfied and after it begins walking, the child starts to study its environment with confidence. If the mother is missing, then the infant might get upset and to respond to unknown and unexpected situations with tension and anxiety. In addition if the mother figure is unavailable it is possible that the child will act in a way to try and hold onto her and is extremely anxious if he/she can't achieve this.

In Psychoanalytic studies and theory, there are many different explanations for this behavior by young children. The birth trauma theory developed by Rank (1924, cited by Bowlby 1973) and Freuds signal theory of anxiety (1926 cited by Bowlby 1973), had been explicitly developed to answer the question; why is the young child anxious, when the mother figure is not around? The earliest Freud theory for the transformed libido and M. Klein's theory of persecutory and depressive anxiety (1934, 1935) have been later applied to explain separation anxiety in young children. All these theories are very complex but they exclude the idea that the overriding explanation for the child's anxiety is the simple fact that the mother figure is missing. There are other authors who have developed theories of separation anxiety based on this being a simple response to the child being separated from the mother figure, this is because the child is naturally emotionally attached to the mother figure. Some of these authors are Suttie (1935), Hermann (1936), Fairbairn (1943, 1963) and Winnicott (1952). It is interesting to note, that half a century earlier, William James (1890) stated that the most terrifying experience for a young child is to be left on his/her own.

As an existential point of view, attachment is what is needed to build up the "basic trust". With her presence and her physical touch, the mother reassures the infant that the world is a safe place to be and to build up its trust in itself. In this relationship – between mother and child – the baby builds up its confidence that "all diffuse body experiences and all confusing social messages from the early life experiences are connected and they combine in the internal and external reality". This is the way that the ontological source of faith and hope arises, known as "basic trust" (Erikson 1996). Basic trust is one of the main components of mental health.

Erikson proved that the sense of trust can be sustained, only if the child gets over the feeling that it has been abandoned or deprived. That is why the experience in early life is so important in building up basic trust and it is down to how well the mother looks after the child in terms of satisfying the infant's emotional needs.

Attachment leads to a world which is safe, warm, welcoming and non-threatening. On the other hand, separation makes the child feel insecure, unsafe, frightened and forgotten. In addition the child experiences the loss, not only of the mother figure, but also a loss of part of himself and the loss of self identity. The loss of the mother and her love creates insecurity and anxiety that the person will experience repeatedly later on in life. Love, trust and anxiety are the main components that individuals need to build their identity (Erikson 1996).

The parent's love could be internalized as a sustainable sense of security and trust. In the same way, anxiety could also be internalized as long term feelings of insecurity and mistrust of the world.

Attachment makes the child feel secure and curious to explore the world. The curiosity and the feeling they can trust to the world comes from the "basic trust" and they are confirmed by the mother's positive emotional reactions. The human's ability to learn comes from building up this sense of security which has been provided and guaranteed by the presence of the mother figure.

Separation Stages

In the very beginning of its life, the infant starts to develop a "central emotional position," which would allow the child to understand as Adler said "the main problems of life". After it has been developed, the main central emotional position becomes sustainable and the person comes back to it throughout their lifetime. This position could be used either as a shelter or to be the weakest and most painful part of their mind, in which case the individual might dedicate his entire living to defend himself from the pain that their central emotional position brings.

The bond between the mother and the child has evolutionary meaning. The child was born with basic abilities to survive and to demand the mother figure to look after him. That specific behavior provokes specific behavior from the mother as well and that relation forms the foundation for the child's ego and identity development. This specific behavioral activity between the child and the mother also determines the creation of a secure attachment. When the primary care giver responds in an adequate way to the child's needs, he starts to form a trust in the world around him. This process is known as the "trust cycle". Children that develop their ability to internalize safety and security and are capable to operate with their emotions also can accept and learn from their mistakes and bad experiences.

The child needs to be close to the mother and it needs her when it's upset, insecure, when it explores the world or simply when it wants to share its happiness with her. Bowlby believed that the mother also needs to look after her baby. She has a particular instinct which is part of her biological heritage. All that the child needs is to be looked after and loved, usually the one that gives this is the biological mother but in other cases this may be another care giver. To disrupt the primary relationship between the child and the mother figure may cause severe mental health issues.

The biological mother is the main figure that the child is attached to but this role may be played by someone else. The specific behavioral activity that exists between the mother and the child are a prerequisite to form secure attachment. Different studies suggest that the mothers are tuned to accept and to respond to the child's emotional expression and the children are also tuned to understand the mother's emotions. The quality of the social interaction between the mother and the infant is more important in developing secure attachment, rather than the amount of time spent together. The attachment mechanism is a very strong instinct that starts because the newborn child starts to demand the attention from the primary care giver, but after it is the care giver that must maintain and develop the attachment. Despite the strength of the attachment, the separation from the mother figure or when the care giver changes very often is an obstacle that can corrupt the attachment and lead to severe psychopathology later on in life (Bowlby J. 1958).

In creating his theory, Bowlby had the following assumptions:

- The first 5 years of a child life are crucial for its development. This means that the difficulties that start in childhood will appear in later life.
- The interaction with the mother has a general and important impact on development; the loss or separation from the mother is the main reason for traumatic experiences.

According to the attachment theory; parent's behaviour has a great impact in creating anxious behaviour in children. Bowlby (1973) researched the influence on children who have been threatened by their parents with abandonment or withdrawal of affection. The research revealed that this type of parental behaviour has a huge impact in forming anxiety in childhood. He viewed the main reason for school phobia in this context, as a fear of being separated from the care giver, rather than a real fear of school.

Studies have focused on the interaction between parent and child in families where children experience anxiety disorders; these have shown that one of the factors is that the parent's behaviour is over controlling or negatively controlling. The parent's negative control is defined as intrusive behaviour, over regulation of the child's activities and allowing the child too little autonomy in respect of their age (Grinsburg, Grover, Cord & Lalongo 2006, cited by Feng, Shaw & Silk 2008). The research has shown that the parents of anxious children control too much their children's behaviour and emotions (Hudson & Rapee 2001; Siqueland, Kendall & Steinberg 1996, cited by Feng, Shaw and Silk 2008). For instance, Hudson and Rapee (2001, cited by Feng, Shaw & Silk 2008) discovered that the mothers of children with anxiety disorders have been providing more support to their children to cope with complicated cognitive tasks in more intrusive ways compared to mothers of children without anxiety disorders.

Negative parental control increases the child's dependency, reduces the sense of autonomy and has a negative effect on their adaptation to their environment (Wood et al. 2003, cited by Feng, Shaw & Silk 2008). This type of behaviour reinforces anxiety because it can make the child feel helpless and that events are out of their control (Chorpita & Barlow 1998, cited by Feng, Shaw and Silk 2008). Over controlling parents may regulate the child's exposure to experiences that may be potentially frightening for the child in an attempt to protect the child from unwanted anxiety (Kortlander et al., 1997, cited by Feng, Shaw & Silk 2008). This pattern of behaviour reinforces the child's anxiety because it gives the child the impression that it is unable to cope with its own experiences and with its negative emotions. This is the way that children learn to count on their parents to deal with negative emotional experiences and they slow down or prevent the formation of the ability to self regulate such negative experiences.

Bowlby showed a few negative outcomes as a result of damaged relationships between children and their care givers:

- Potential deviant behaviour in the future;
- Emotional disorders – incapability to have "normal" relationships and feelings for other people;
- Apathy that develops into depression;
- Retarded physical development;
- Retarded speech and cognitive development; (thinking)
- Felling insecure for other people and feeling frustrated with exploring the environment;
- Anxiety and anger.

MECHANISMS OF ATTACHMENT

Bowlby referred to ethology to seek an explanation for the traumatic and perhaps irreparable effects of raising children in institutions.

Bowlby believed that human attachment is imprinting in a similar way to animals. Imprinting – is the process of learning to respond to those stimuli from the environment which trigger their social instincts. This type of behaviour has the function to guarantee the survival of the species. The research of ethologists suggests that the chicks would get attached to any object that is similar to the mother duck. In the beginning, little chicks would follow different moving objects but with time they follow less and less objects and by the time they have imprinted their mother, they follow only her.

Bowlby believed with no doubt that imprinting is playing an important part in building relationships between the child and mother. We can observe a very similar, but much slower process in humans. During the first weeks, children can't actively follow moving objects, but they focus on their social reactions towards other people. They smile, they burble, they grasp adults and cry, all this helps them to keep others close to them. But up to six months, their attachment is limited to a few people and usually mainly one person. This is because the child needs this person to always be close and this is the stage when fear of strangers appears. Bowlby thought that individuals who have been deprived of love in their childhood have been deprived of the opportunity to imprint other humans into their lives and to build up relationships of affection with another person. This point of their development influences their life as an adult. Because of the lack of a chance to develop close relationship in early childhood, as adults they would have shallow relationships with the others (Bowlby 2003).

Bowlby studied in detail 44 children with behavioural disorders and he described the so called "affectionless character." He also discovered that for various reasons, the majority of these children had been separated from their mothers early in their lives and they didn't have any other permanent substitute for their attachment relations (Bowlby 2003).

If the impossibility to develop imprinting explains the negative effects of depravation, then there must be a crucial time after which these effects become irreparable. Therefore children who are missing social relations with others up until a certain age may never be able to develop adequate social behaviour. Most of the researchers struggle to define the exact limit of this critical period.

Bowlby believed that this critical period ends when the reaction of fear starts. Therefore, the end of this critical period is about 8-9 months old because this is the stage when almost all children show fear of being separated from the primary care giver and show fear of strangers. Many researches show that for children who have been deprived of interactions with other people up until this age, it is possible for them to have permanent difficulties vocalising. Social depravation puts children in a "freezer" and slows down their social development and extends the critical or sensitive period. After the sensitive period, the children that have difficulties communicating with other people may never develop normally (Krane 2002).

Bowlby was very interested in incapability to develop imprinting and the impact that this has on the child's development but he was even more focused on the cases where the child has developed attachment and then suffered separation. In 1948 he published an article about how psychotherapy intervention reduces the tension in the family titled "The study and reduction of group tensions in the family"; this article is accepted as the first published work on family psychotherapy. In the meantime he started to study separation by observing the behaviour of children who had been separated from their parents because they had been hospitalised, the observation also included the children's reactions when the mother was visiting and when the children returned home.

After several years study, Bowlby together with John Robertson made a film documentary called "A Two-Year Old Goes to the Hospital". The film showed how deeply the children suffered when they were separated from their mothers. The facts that had been exposed by the documentary provoked a wide social response that reached beyond the medical community. The documentary helped people to realize how important the issue of separation is for early childhood development and the necessity to acknowledge its negative influence when working with upset children.

Both Bowlby and Robertson discovered that there are different stages to the process of separation. Young children are able to experience separation from the age of 6 months and this process goes through 3 stages: Protest, despair and detachment. This pattern of behavior is obvious with children who had a perfectly good relationship with their parents before their hospitalization. From the start, the children that had been separated from their mothers started to protest desperately by crying, panicking, expressing a fear of being left alone, they expected the mother to return, they didn't accept any alternative care givers and showed intense yet frustrated attachment behavior and "anger derived from hope" for when the mother returns.

During this stage the child is very upset by the separation and does everything possible to get their mother back. The child is agitated and is trying to get their mother back by crying, shouting and rejecting any other care giver. After the fear of being left alone is reduced then the anger appears. If the mother comes back during this stage, the child may push her away. How long and how intense the child protests, depends how high quality the relationship with their mother is. In some case, the protest can last a few hours, in other cases it can last for a week. Bowlby believed that for the child, there is no stronger emotion than the anger following the separation. Children may express this anger by refusing to have eye contact with the mother, refusing to give her a smile or refusing to approach her. He assumed that this anger is not only an expression of how angry the child is about the separation but also proves how valuable the relationship with the mother is for the child.

The despair phase follows if nobody answers the child's protests. During this stage the child is less active and gives the impression that it is accepting the separation in a positive way, but their sleep patterns and appetite are affected, the child is sad, is feeling desperation and they can't use their previous experience to support themselves.

Bowlby described this phase as a mental state of deep sorrow. The condition is characterized by withdrawal, weakness and apathy. The child gets depressed and is not active.

If nothing changes for the child, then the next phase is detachment. In this phase, the child shows high interest in objects, but this type of behavior is hiding deep long term mental damage. If the mother comes back, the child doesn't trust her and won't react to her and will give the impression that it doesn't recognize her. Children experience sadness because they hate the person who they actually deeply love and they need the most (J. Bowlby 1952). Even at this stage, if the separation is not for too long and if the mother gradually rebuilds their relationship, the outcome can still be positive for the child.

The detachment is a very deep process; it's hard for the child to get over it and could cause serious mental issues later on. During this stage the child gets more and more interested in their surroundings, in playing and starts to smile. The child develops new defending mechanisms including seeking a new attachment figure. If the mother comes back, the child may seem uninterested in her.

In the end of the despair phase the child meets their returning mother with protest and anger, but it is still easy to rebuild the relationship between them. During the phase of detachment, to rebuild the relationship is extremely difficult, painful and takes a long time (Bowlby 2003).

When the child experiences separation, this experience contains two main emotions: anxiety and anger. The specific type of anxiety is determined by the bond between the mother and child and is known as separation anxiety. Separation anxiety is the very first interpersonal anxiety that the child experiences and is a very deep feeling of loss. The child develops an internal sense of confidence by connecting with other people. Disrupting this connection will make them feel insecure and this is the prototype for existential insecurity.

Separation anxiety is triggered by certain conditions and activates individuals instinct to flee as well as attachment behavior but in this case, the attachment figure is not around. The longer the separation is for, the more severe the mental damage. The anxiety differs from the fear that is caused by being in a threatening environment and from the anger and aggression which appear when the child is separated or pushed away from the primary care giver (Ainsworth M, Bowlby J, 1991).

In contrast to psychoanalysts, Bowlby believed that too much separation anxiety is caused by negative experiences in the family, such as repeated threats of abandonment by the parents and when the child is made to feel responsible for a sibling or parent being ill or dead (Bretherton I, 1992).

To be left alone put people – especially children – in a potentially high risk situation, so that is why, according to Bowlby (1973), that to react with fear when the primary care giver is not around, can be considered as a simple evolutionary adaptation response and is part of human behavioral patterns.

As the cognitive capacity of the child grows, the child develops the ability to predict that certain situations will occur, including threatening situations. From the variety of threatening situations that the adult or child can predict there is nothing more frightening than for the mother figure to be missing, especially when her presence is desired. What Bowlby specified as the mothers presence, is not necessarily to be physically always there, but for the child to have the certainty that she is easily accessible. In addition, the mother figure has to be willing to respond in an appropriate way, which means to be comforting and protective. Only if at the same time the primary care giver is accessible and responsive can they be considered as being available.

Bowlby (1973) made three basic points to support these theories. Firstly, if the individual is confident that the primary care giver will be available when they need them, they will be less vulnerable to tense or permanent fear, than an individual who, for whatever reason doesn't have such confidence.

Secondly, the confidence that the mother figure will be available or unavailable is building up slowly during childhood and adolescence and remains sustainable for the rest of their lifetime.

Thirdly, the different expectations for how accessible and responsive the primary care giver will be develop during the childhood and reflect their real experiences. Bowlby suggested that the most important and sensitive period to develop attachment is between the ages of six months up until five years old. This is the most sensitive period to develop the expectations of how accessible and responsive the attachment figure is, but sensitivity still exists throughout their lifetime.

Children's fears and excessive anxiety in some situations are a natural but maladaptive reaction that comes from the parent-child relationship. When the parent is threatening the child with affection withdrawal to discipline the child or if the child witnesses arguments between the parents it gets anxious because it fears that it may lose the primary care giver. When this type of parent's behavior is repetitive and is part of the child's every day experience then its reaction becomes a sustainable pattern of behavior. This type of parents have developed this pattern of behavior through their own experiences as children and yet the awareness of the mechanisms that play a role in young children's personality development and the awareness of the importance of the bond between the parents and the child might contribute to being able to break this vicious circle.

Attachment, Anxiety and Fear

Both anxiety and fear have a few components, but the difference between fear and anxiety is that with anxiety, its components follow a sequence. The first sign of anxiety is arousal and recognition of the threat. The next component is to realize the physical reactions of the body. This second component of anxiety is mainly cognitive and is what makes anxiety different from fear. According to Bowlby, there are two different stimuli that trigger children's fear, a present danger and/or the absence of the attachment figure. The systems that control the flight instinct and the attachment are part of the behavioral systems that are responsible for reducing stress levels and increase personal security levels.

All psychoanalytic and psychiatric views on anxiety point out that the emotional state of anxiety and the emotional state of fear are very similar. Freud, for example, was constantly comparing the two and demonstrating the contrast between them.

Lewis (1967 cited by Bowlby 1973) reviewed many articles on psychopathology and underlined that very often the term "anxiety" is used to designate "emotional state that can be described as subjective experience of fear or very similar to the fear emotion." Both terms very often are used interchangeably, yet the origin of anxiety is unclear but the nature and origin of fear is considered as simple and easy to understand. In Bowlby's theory (1973), these emotional states are accepted as similar as well. Maybe the most common upstanding is that fear is triggered by something potentially harmful. This raises the question about the nature of the stimuli and objects which we accept as threatening and cause us to retreat from them. We are frightened, not only by the presence or the expected presence, but also from the absence or expected absence of these stimuli.

Cross researches, comparing human and other mammal behavior, show that the conditions that lead us to experience fear and withdrawal are very different from Freud's hypothesis. Very often it may be seen the conditions that lead to fear have a normal but indirect connection with a potentially harmful stimulus. For human, the main stimuli triggering anxiety and withdrawal are sudden noises and moving objects, the unknown, darkness, isolation etc. People associate these stimuli with increased risk of danger, so that is why they are natural marks for a dangerous threat. Ultimately, how sensitive the individual is to these marks may affect the way that individuals develop.

According to Bowlby (1973), the tendency to react to any of these common situations depends on the genetic predisposition of the individual which results into a "readiness to face the real threat." He believed that these tendencies are common for humans as well as for animals and for humans they exist throughout their life time, not only during childhood. Therefore, the fear to be separated from the attachment figure against their will, regardless of which stage of their lives is not a mystery any longer, but can be understood as a natural instinctive response to any of the marks that indicate a high risk.

The patterns of the personality start to develop during the early childhood. How the individuals think, behave, react emotionally, interact and communicate with others depends very much on their earliest interactions. How successfully people function in the adult world, depends on the attachment that individuals have built up during the stages of their development. Infants usually develop multiple attachments, but they have one preferred attachment figure that they rely on in stressful situations.

If the infant gets an adequate response from the primary care giver to its signals, then the baby develops "internal working models" which are mental representations for understanding the world, self and others (Bowlby 1969, 1973). A baby with a mother that responds quickly in a sensitive way to its signals develops a "working model" of itself as loved and deserving of attention. Thus the baby starts to expect a positive reaction to its needs from other people, when it requires something.

The infant builds up self confidence and belief that it has the ability and strength to make things happen. Internal working models of attachment develop patterns for different types of relationships and the outcome is a child that is knowledgeable in many different activities.

To develop the internal model depends on how much the child believes that the primary care giver is responding to their needs. The internal working model is based on the perception of:

1. How responsive the main care giver is to the child's needs and
2. whether the child has a self perception of deserving the care givers attention (Bowlby 1973). The internal model depends on the experience that the child has with the care giver. Once formed the model becomes unconscious, remains relatively sustainable throughout the lifetime and could be changed, only if it is consciously identified, challenged and determined.

ATTACHMENT AND WORKING MODELS

According to attachment theory, each individual develops working models to understand the world and self and these models help them to perceive events, to anticipate the future and to plan. The key in building this working model is how accepted or unaccepted the individual feels from the attachment figure. The individual continues to build these working models through experience and by interacting with their environment. That is why children are able to cope with new types of social relationships.

Bowlby used the theory of information to explain the stability of the internal models and their distortion by the defending mechanisms. Their stability derives from:

- The models of connecting are becoming unconscious and automatic with time and
- Double sided models of connecting are more difficult to change than single models because of the duel expectations.

The individual prognosis for how easily accessible and responsive the figure of attachment will be is based on the structure of the working models.

The predisposition that an individual has to respond with fear and anxiety when facing any type of potentially anxious situations is closely connected to the prognosis that he has about how accessible and responsive is the attachment figure.

The real presence or absence of the attachment figure is a variable, which determines whether an individual would or would not experience anxiety in potentially anxious situations. That is also connected to another variable – the individual's confidence that the attachment figure is accessible and responsive. The younger the individual is, the stronger the influence of the first variable. Up to three years old, the first variable is the dominant one (Bowlby 1973).

The individual's confidence that the attachment figure is possible to be responsive is determined also by two variables:

- Whether the individual assesses that the attachment figure is responding to their needs of protection and support.
- Whether the individual assesses themselves as a person that other people and especially the attachment figure respond to in an adequate and favorable way.

The outcome is that the attachment figure model and the working model for the self develop as supplementary and mutually confirming. Thus a child that is unwanted, will possibly feel unwanted, not only by the parents, but by all people. The opposite is that a child that is truly loved, will feel confident not only in the parents love but would be confident that others will consider them as deserving of love and would believe that the things they desire can be possible. Bowlby thought that those general principles are hard to prove but they are commonly seen in reality.

Since the working models are mental representations, it is hard to be studied in young children. We can't ask very young children what they think or how they feel but after three years old, it is possible to assess them. Cassidy (1990) discovered that three year old children can complete stories that are related to attachment. Children that have developed secure attachment will, at the end of the story describe their parents as caring and helpful.

M. Rutter (1979) studied children that had been separated from their mothers and who have grown up to be well adapted adults. Rutter discovered that if children, who suffered from separation, later rebuild their relationship with the attachment figure then they cease to suffer. Rutter noted that there is a big difference between the disruption of the relationship and to be deprived of such a relationship. For individuals that have been deprived of a relationship with an attachment figure, they are likely to suffer from desperation, alienation, guilt, lack of moral values and to have an inability to connect with others. He stated that individuals with emotional disorders would recover more or less successfully depending on the quality of their primary relationship.

The real situations of separation that a child experiences are highly traumatic and may lead to anxiety later on in life. Bowlby (1973) stated that such traumatic experiences are far beyond the child's ability to cope with, so the child becomes excessively sensitive about future separations or losses. If the child has experienced a traumatic separation, any prediction that this could occur again leads to a strong feeling of anxiety. This may lead to inadequate activation of attachment behaviors of which the purpose is to keep the attachment figure near in a way to avoid another traumatic situation.

According to attachment theory, a mature personality is a result of the relationships of the individual with key figures during childhood, especially with the attachment figures. Thus an individual who has been raised by caring parents and knowing people who are available and able to offer support, such an individual would be confident that in a difficult situation, they could seek help and support from others.

The parent's attachment behaviors have an impact on their style of parenting. It is expected for the parent to be responsive to the full spectrum of the child's needs, but some parents misinterpret the signals coming from the child and respond in a selective way to their needs. These types of parents neglect and/or reject the child's needs and comfort seeking behaviors which leads to an impersonal relationship. This type of parent, considers the child's emotions to be unnecessary. As a response to the child's distress, the parent remains firm and indifferent, this encourages the child to be independent, but in an over stimulating and over controlling way.

The child becomes emotionally distant and it becomes more independent than is appropriate for their age and demonstrates excessive politeness to their parents. The child looks unimpressed when separated from their parents, but at the same time they are aggressive toward their peers.

Very often, the reason for many parents to be responsive in a insensitive way to children's attention seeking is their own deep confusion. This model of parenting increases children's comfort seeking behaviors and keeps the parents focused on their own needs. This type of parents have either excessively positive or excessively negative opinions on their children, either way, their judgment is not realistic. These types of parents are discouraging their child to be independent. The interactions between the parents and the child are tense and highly emotional in tone, which shows affection and/or emotional conflict. The parents are unnecessarily focused on the child's attachment behaviors even when the child does not show distress. When the child shows distress then the parents have the opposite reaction, they ignore the child's signals, or respond too late or inadequately which instead of reducing, it increases the child's anxiety. The children of these type of parents are emotionally immature and highly strung.

Traumatized parents are either scared by their child or they in turn scare their child. This makes the child frightened that their parent will use physical violence against them as is in the case of abusive parents. The research shows that there is a high correlation between past traumatic experience and psychiatric diagnosis in adults such as depression, anxiety and borderline personality disorder. Traumatized parents often would describe their child as "out of control," as "their best friend" or they consider the child to be responsible to care for them. To discipline the child, they use severe punishment, maltreatment, they shout, threaten or they have sudden and intense outbursts of anger. Traumatized parents are so frightened and lack confidence in their parenting ability that they often abdicate their role as parent and switch roles with the child. The result of this is that three year old children, in this situation, are very controlling because they have taken control of the relationship from their parents. Parent's behaviors have a direct impact on the child's behavior and eventually determine the type of attachment the child has (Berlin & Cassidy 2001).

Some people never had caring and supporting figures in their lives and their experiences have always been determined by insecurity. As adults these types of people lack confidence that the people they are close to will be around or can be relied on. They have mental representations of the world being joyless, unpredictable and that real life situations are a struggle and that no one can be relied on to support them. The result of this is that they either accept their life as being a battle between themselves and the rest of the world, or they withdraw from the world.

Between these two situations of either having traumatized parents, or being without any attachment figures there are many different possible variations. In some cases the attachment figures are responsive in an appropriate way only when they are invited to so. Because of this, their children believe that everyone functions in this way. In other cases, the individuals have learned from their experience of discipline as a child, that they can only get a positive response from people by following certain rules. For example, if the rules have been reasonable and sanctions have been moderate and predictable, the child develops the belief that it will get support when it needs it. When the rules have been very rigid and difficult to fulfill for the child and the sanctions have been harsh and unpredictable, the child loses faith that they can find support. Some of the sanctions that parents use for discipline are very damaging for the child's mental health, such as when the child seeks affection and support but the parent rejects them or when the parent threatens the child with eviction from the home. When such threats have been used many times or rarely but in an highly emotionally charged way they have a distorting effect on the child's development. Such threats may intensify the child's fears of being abandoned and the child's predisposition to react with fear and anxiety in various circumstances.

Parents with an unresolved trauma feel scared by the child or scare the child. This makes the child be afraid of physical violence as in the case of abusive parents. Studies report that the category with unresolved trauma correlates with that of psychiatric diagnoses in adults – depression, anxiety or borderline personality disorder. Main topics in the interactions are fear, protection and hierarchy in relationships accompanied by inadequacy, helplessness and loss of control. The parent with unresolved trauma can describe his child as "out of control" or as a "best friend" or as the one taking care of the parent. Such parents use severe punishments, maltreatment, yelling, threats or have sudden and intense outbursts of anger. The parent with unresolved trauma is often so afraid that he abdicates completely the parental position heading toward role reversal and disorganization of the usual hierarchy. Parental behavior toward the child directly influences the behavior of the child and ultimately ensures the type of attachment to the parent (Berlin & Cassidy 2001).

For other children, the existence of caring and supporting figures is unknown and unexperienced and experiences were always accompanied by a state of insecurity. As adults these individuals do not have the confidence that caregivers will be available to them and they can be trusted. The world through their eyes is joyless and unpredictable, presenting difficult situations to overcome without being able to rely on other people. The answer is either a fight with others and the world or shrinking into one's shell.

Between these two extremes there are many other possibilities. Sometimes caregivers respond in a soothing way only when they are invited to do so. Such children grow up with the conviction that others function in a similar way. Using their experience others have learned that the desired response can be received only when following certain rules. In case the rules are moderate and the sanctions mild and predictable the child gradually begins to believe that support will always be present when he needs it. When rules are too strict or hard to follow and when sanctions for lack of adherence are cruel and unpredictable, the conviction that support will always be present fades away.

There are punishments that lead to damaging consequences like refusal to respond to the attempts of the child for closeness, threats for leaving or threats for sending the child away from home. When they are used frequently or rarely but with high intensity, they can have detrimental effects on the developing person. Such threats can intensify the fears of the child that he is going to be abandoned as well as his predisposition to respond to different situations with fear and anxiety.

According to Bowlby a secure attachment is crucial for the development of fear and anxiety regulation in threatening and difficult situations (Bowlby 1973; Thompson 2001, Feng, Shaw & Silk 2008).

An insecure attachment style is considered one of the main reasons for anxiety because in this case the child lacks security in regard of the presence of the caregiver and his vigilance in controlling the environment. Some studies report a direct link between an insecure attachment and later problems related to anxiety (Cassidy & Berlin). Many studies prove the association between childhood anxiety and type of insecure attachment (Warren, Huston, Wgeland & Stroufe 1997), and between anxiety and disorganized attachment style (Shaw, Keenan, Vondra, Delliquadri & Giovanelli 1997). Bradley (2000) claims that the insecure attachment – avoidant type can lead to anxiety disorders due to its connection to rejecting parenting in distressful situations.

Bowlby assumes the existence of an innate ability or predisposition to develop attachment. In the first months after birth there are a couple of specific behavioral activities on the part of the baby that provoke certain actions on the part of the mother. These interactions are the basis for the development of the ego and identity of the child. The specific behavioral activity on the part of the child and the mother are a prerequisite for the formation of a secure attachment. The first object relation of the child – that with his mother, can be observed at the end of the first year and consists of "a certain number of instinctive reactions which in the beginning are relatively independent of one another." These reactions occur at different times during the first year of the life of the child. Some of them are sucking, grabbing, tracing, crying, smiling etc. They are aimed to stimulate the behavior of the mother. When the child is insecure and upset, exploring the world or wanting to share his joy, he needs the closeness of his mother. In order to attract and keep her closeness the baby uses the so called "innate signals." In the developmental process the instinctive reactions are integrated in more complex behavioral patterns and form the foundation for the "attachment behavior". They are activated by different external or internal stimuli. Reactions to those stimuli are associated with food intake and closeness with the mother as well as with activating the behavior of the mother and influencing it by crying and smiling. None of these reactions is primary to the rest. In that regard Bowlby distinguishes between "attachment" and "dependence." There is dependence when the child seeks the mother only as a source of food.

According to Winnicott the good mother is the one providing the child with the opportunity to explore and build new ideas. The vitality of the mother and her ability to see the world through the eyes of her child, to understand what he feels, makes the newborn sense the human in her. She is the person who creates a comfortable environment for the baby where he lives and grows. For that reason he needs to feel that the mother is in the situation, part of it. She is the one who provides an adequate environment which she and the baby feel comfortable in. Crying is an important aspect of the mother-child interactions. It is not caused only by the need for food but by other stimuli as well – kinesthetic and tactile. When the child is crying, he is asking the mother for help. By crying he expresses internal states and induces responsiveness of those who take care of him and tries to take control over them. The baby takes the same pleasure in crying as he does in exercising any other bodily function. Any new accomplishment is interesting for him. Crying is very valuable for him because it brings reassurance and confidence when he feels anxious and insecure. When crying is squeaky and shrill, the mother knows that the baby feels pain. This pain may be caused by different things, it may not be physical but be a result of emerging concerns. When the baby gets acquainted with the world he realizes that in some cases he may expect pain. When the baby is disappointed with the mother he might experience a state of anger. He screams, yells, shakes, bites and scratches intending to destroy everything and everyone including himself. When he cries because he is angry, he still believes his mother and hopes he can change her. The furious baby knows what he wants, how to get it and never stops hoping. When the baby cries because he is sad, he has gone a long way in terms of emotional development. Sad cry is musical, the baby experiments with different tones until sleep comes or he is able to drown his sorrows. This cry is a sign that the baby has won his place in the world and has started taking responsibility for the surroundings. He does not simply react to the circumstances any more, but feels responsible for them. The sad baby has the need to know that he is being loved and wants to be left to recover spontaneously from his sadness and guilt. Smiling is a very important element of the mother-child interaction as well. It is the essential means for maintaining reciprocity, response to foreign presence, expression of a positive attitude. It appears early in childhood development – usually around the sixth week. First smiles are responses to inner states but they gradually become replies to external events. This is a movement from internality to externality when to the physiological component a cognitive, emotional, and social one are added as well. This means a gradual development of the ability to recognize and interpret external stimuli. The child forms his attachment according to the care he receives. When caregivers are responsive, attentive and consistent, he develops a respective style of attachment. Attachment quality creates the basis on which the child builds his feeling toward himself which determines his later relationships. Attachment behavior is caused by perceptions of pain, exhaustion, absence of a mother figure, fright or stressful events in early childhood.

ATTACHMENT TYPES

M. Ainsworth discovers four attachment types: secure, reliable attachment and three types of insecure attachment: avoidant, ambivalent and disorganized.

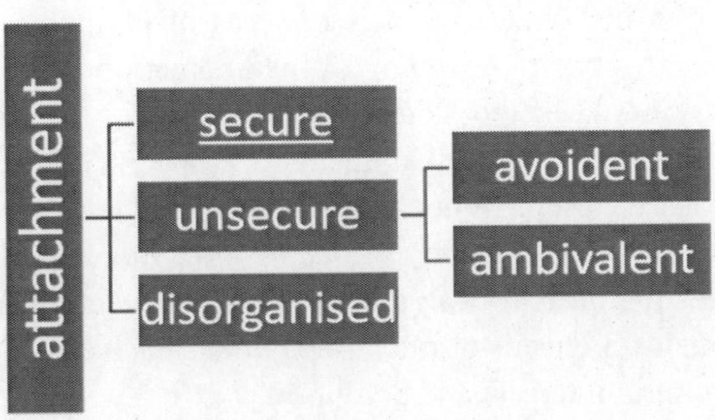

Figure 1. Types of attachment.

In experiments with children with secure attachment they actively explore the surrounding environment, moving freely in the entire space, using mothers as a secure base for their explorations. Children played and often went back to their mothers to assure in their presence. When mothers left, children felt upset and ended their activity. When mothers came back, children greeted them with warmth, felt joy and tried to restore physical contact with the mother. The basic functions of a secure attachment for the child are:

1. To acquire basic trust and to respond in a reciprocal way – the basis for future emotional relations.
2. To explore the environment with feelings of security and safety – leading to full cognitive and social development.
3. To develop his abilities for self-regulation that leads to effective management of impulses and emotions.
4. To create the basis for identity formation including a sense of competence, of self-value and a balance between dependence and autonomy.
5. To establish prosocial moral frames which bring empathy, compassion and conscience.
6. To generate an essential system of convictions, consisting of cognitive evaluations about oneself, others and life as a whole.
7. To develop defenses against stress and trauma and to form resources.

M. Ainsworth determines that mothers of such children are sensitive and responsive to the needs of the child. They have always been there and have shown their love when their children needed to be soothed. The consistent responsiveness of the mothers made the children feel secure and perceive the mother as their protector. The only thing that gives children bravery in an "unfamiliar situation" and makes it possible for them to explore the surroundings is the presence of the mother. At the same time the reactions of children when their mothers left as well as when they returned demonstrate a strong need for closeness with the mother.

One of the factors that are indicative for the formation of a secure attachment is attachment to non-social objects. Winnicott calls them "transitional objects." These are toys, objects helping the child to separate from the mother. The child puts his thumb or a toy in his mouth receiving gratification for his arousal but also expressing his feelings of attachment. This object becomes very important for the baby because it is the first thing in the world that belongs to the baby and at the same time it is not part of his body. Through attachment to non-social objects the child sets the beginning of his interactions with the world. Transitional objects are the boundary between the state of symbiosis with the mother and the state of building a relationship with her. The attachment to a specific object is very important in situations when the mother is absent. When she is not there, it represents the internal image of the mother. In that way the baby handles the separation more easily. Interaction with the transitional object creates the basis for the play abilities of the child. With time these objects fade away but there remains a cluster of phenomena that reach beyond the scope of children play, namely those of cultural interests and activities.

The baby has several behavioral activities through which he seeks and creates contact with his mother. Sucking is a way not only to receive food but also to develop attachment. It is a direct way to achieve touch. Touching is a way of survival and skin contact facilitates attachment formation. When the baby is sucking he feels warmth, love and tranquility. The mother also experiences calmness, strength and confidence that she can provide her child with what he needs.

According to Bowlby only when the baby and the mother are constantly together a secure attachment can be formed. Emotional security for the baby at these first levels of his development is provided by the touch with the mother. Three groups of factors are important for the theory of attachment:

- Physical
- Emotional, and
- Social.

The first group relates more to physiological factors and is represented by the features of the central nervous system and the hormonal development.

One of the important roles of emotions in attachment formation is to play a role in the assessment and evaluation of the inner world and the external environment of the child.

The main goal in the process of forming an adequate attachment is establishing successful social interactions. Only when someone can understand the affective state of the other can he be successful in his social interactions.

Attachment is a result of the process of forming a relationship which is accomplished between a child and a mother or a primary caregiver during the first year of the life of the child. This is the year of needs – the need for touch, contact, movement, smile, food. When the baby has certain needs, he announces those needs and in the process of interaction through multiple repetitions the child learns that the world is a safe place and develops trust toward others and the world itself. Formation of emotional bonds makes the child feel free of his environment and confident that he can explore it effectively. Attachment is a reciprocal process in which a child and a mother together create a deep and caring relationship. In case of secure attachment the child is upset when his mother leaves the room but his distress is not excessive. There are signs of warmth when they are reunited. The child is easily soothed and readily goes back to playing.

Attachment is the foundation for the development of mental abilities and emotionality of the child and plays an important role for the emotional, cognitive and social functioning throughout the life of the person.

The sensitive parent satisfies the basic needs of his child which alleviates the discomfort and arousal of the child. Children with an adequately formed attachment trust others and believe their needs are valid. The ones who do not succeed at forming a secure attachment are at high risk for developing:

1. Low self-esteem
2. Needy, clingy and pseudo-independent behavior
3. Decompensation in times of stress
4. Loss of control
5. Inability to initiate and maintain friendships
6. Separation and oppositional attitude to parents
7. Antisocial behavior

8. Aggression and violence
9. Inability for trust and intimacy
10. Unreliable and pessimistic attitude toward oneself, family and society.
11. Lack of empathy, compassion and guilt.
12. Behavioral and learning problems.

In case of an insecure avoidant attachment children remain aloof. They make the impression of ones who are confident in themselves. In their explorations they do not use their mothers as a secure base, they do not look for contact with their mothers in a "strange situation". It seems like they do not even notice their mothers. In case of separation they do not show an apparent distress and when the mother returns they ignore her. When mothers tried to pick them up children tried to avoid that by tearing themselves away from the arms of the mother or averted their gaze in another direction. Since these children manifested independence in the "strange situation" it seemed like they are entirely healthy. But when M. Ainsworth noticed their avoidant behavior she assumed that these children feel certain emotional difficulties. Their detachment reminded her of children who had experienced traumatic separations. Domestic observations confirm her hypothesis. Studies show that these children are ignored or even deliberately rejected. Experts describe the confidence of these children as a defense strategy. According to M. Ainsworth when children are placed in the "strange situation" they are afraid that they cannot count on the support of their mothers and this provokes their defensive behavior. They use aloof, restrained behavior to protect themselves. They had been rejected so frequently in the past that they tried to forget their need of their mother in order to avoid new disappointments. When the mother came back after separation episodes they did not want to look at her as if rejecting any feelings toward her. In case of an insecure avoidant attachment the child shows little or no distress when the mother leaves the room and actively avoids or ignores the mother when she comes back. The mother also avoids the child and observes him from a distance. These children act as if they want to say "Who are you? Do I need to respect you? – the one who would not help me when I needed it." (Ainsworth 1978).

Bowlby believes that this defensive behavior can turn into a fixated and an all-embracing part of the personality of the child. The child grows into an adult who is overly confident and detached into someone who can never trust others to such a degree so that he can build close relationships with them (Crane 2002).

An ambivalent attachment makes children insecure and resisting in the "strange situation". They stay close to their mothers and worry for them and practically do not explore the environment. They react intensely to the departure of the mother but after her return they show an expressed ambivalence toward her. On one side, protest and anger are observed, but on the other – a weak desire to establish a contact with the mother. Observations show that mothers of children with ambivalent attachment are inconsistent in their behavior, they react inconsistently to the signals of the child – sometimes tender and kind, other times rejecting and neglecting. The conflict is between the desire for a close contact with the mother and the anger caused by the fact that she responds inconsistently to his signals. In case of an ambivalent-resistant attachment the child experiences extreme distress in case of separation, clinging and staying close to his mother and to the door, and crying. He looks for contact after the reunion but pushes his mother away angrily because he cannot afford it.

Insecure disorganized attachment reflects the highest insecurity of the child in the reactions of his parents. After the return of the mother the behavior of the child is controversial. In many of these children an indication of their internal disorganization is their facial expression. The attempts of the child to resume contact with his mother may be interrupted by conflicting behavior. There is a tendency that such children are constantly hypersensitive and difficult to soothe. Mothers of such children have an unresolved trauma from their childhood – death of a parent, maltreatment, abuse etc. Children are scared by the fear and anxiety of the parent. A large number of these children are subject to violence. Bipolar disorder or alcoholism in parents is a prerequisite for an extremely controversial behavior toward the child. The reactions of these children to separation and encounter reflect not only the history of the parent-child interactions but also the parental style and psychosocial functioning of the child (Bretherton 1985).

There is one more category of children that is characterized by a loss of coherence. These children are classified as disorganized-disoriented. Their behavior is characterized by 7 types of reactions (Main, Solomon 1990).

1. Consecutive manifestation of controversial models of behavior: extreme attachment behavior or angry behavior followed by withdrawal and coldness.
2. Simultaneous manifestation of a controversial type of behavior. The child demonstrates seeking behavior and withdrawing at the same time.
3. Incomplete or interrupted movements and/or expression.
4. Stereotypical, persevering, asymmetrical, untimely movements and strange poses.
5. Frozen, quiet, slow movements and expressions.
6. Manifestation of responsiveness to and validation of the parents. They often show extreme fears as a response to the attitude of the parent – cover their faces with hands, run away when parents return or come closer to them.
7. Such children directly show disorientation and disorganization. There is a rapid change between affects – laughter-cry. Their disoriented expression is noticeable when they approach the parents.

15% of children with two parents show models of disorganized attachment (Van Ijzendoorn 1995). These percentages reach 82% when the family has a high risk of maltreatment, use of psychoactive drugs, depression of the mother, neglect of the child, adolescent parenting etc. (Lyons-Ruth 1991).

Children with disorganized attachment are labeled as indecisive, fearful, traumatized. They do not complain about losses and are afraid to admit past traumas (Main 1994). They actively and contemptuously devalue attachment and often abuse or neglect other children (Lyons-Ruth 1991). Mothers of such children often have a history of family violence or abuse. Such mothers are not responsive to the needs of their children and give inaccurate, inadequate and controversial signals to their children (Lyons-Ruth 1994). They show high levels of negative affect toward their children and low levels of tenderness (DeMulder, Radke-Yarrow 1991). Often parents coming from abusive families transfer their fears and indecisiveness to their children. They act as insensitive, abusive, depressive, without showing love and attachment. Children of such parents are placed in a paradoxical situation: closeness to parents increases their fears while at the same time they need a soothing contact and support. This situation provokes fears in them related to security and comfort.

The vicious circle of development of the parent-child relationship has 4 main components:

1. The child does not respond with comfort and relaxation to the efforts of the parent to soothe and calm him down.
2. The parent becomes anxious, angry, insecure, and starts losing his confidence that he provides an adequate care.
3. Each one of the parent-child dyad withdraws and starts becoming more and more intrusive and/or punishing.
4. Unresponsiveness increases stress and anxiety, negative cues and signals bring insecurity for the child.

Early traumas related to attachment can have one of the most detrimental effects related to child development because of the long-term effects on the developing abilities of the child for emotional and behavioral regulation of his behavior.

Attachment Disorders

Attachment disorders are not identical with individual differences in attachment styles established by the "strange situation" of M. Ainsworth. These disorders are deep and all-encompassing impairments in the formation of a sense of security and safety in the child. These children do not look for comfort and do not engage in reciprocal emotional relations with the caregiver. Their reaction usually is a result of a failure to develop an adequate attachment or of a separation with the object of attachment. Therefore, when the attachment behavior exhibited by the child is not successful at providing support and relation with the object of attachment, the child is forced to "develop defense mechanisms, that would throw the painful information away from the mind" (Solomon & George 1999). These defense mechanisms can include deactivation and disconnection of affect and cognitions related to the experiences in the process of attachment formation. "The degree of disconnection is usually associated with the intensity and duration of the experiences that a child has with a parent who is able or unable to provide protection and care" (Solomon & George 1999).

Children who have experienced a profound early deprivation and/or abuse in the process of developing a primary relationship with the caregiver, often show an especially disorganized system of attachment. In behavior of those children highly expressed are:

- active repression/suppression or "blocking" of attachment behavior and posing
- attachment behavior that is outside of context and control, ostentation and posing; or
- alternation between the previous two conditions (Solomon & George 1999).

Their coping strategies include setting barriers in front of establishing relationships. They often use the so called strategy "compulsive self-reliance" which means that they do not perceive others as a source of help, care and kindness (Bowlby 1973). Their diminished ability for empathy can be due to the perception of others as objects that can be manipulated.

Many studies follow to what extent the behavior of children in the "strange situation" would influence their future development. Since the results from the "strange situation" show fundamental differences between children, it should be able to determine differences in their future behavior as well. Children with secure attachment continue to maintain this type of behavior in adolescence. In cognitive task execution they distinguish themselves with persistence and self-reliance. In social situations they receive higher evaluations on friendliness and leadership. These results confirm Ainsworth's point of view that children with secure attachment show the healthiest forms of development (Crane 2002).

To establish differences in behavior at later stages in children with avoidant and ambivalent attachment is more difficult. Children with ambivalent attachment continue to exhibit anxiety and dependence. However, the ones with avoidant attachment often show dependence as well. Ainsworth claims that a secure attachment appears as a result of the sensitivity of the mother to the signals of the child. This discovery is theoretically significant since ethologists believe that children have inherent gestures that need to be considered in order for development to proceed in an adequate way (Crane 2002).

In adults certain thoughts and feelings regarding attachment and attachment attitudes are formed which later influences what type of parents they themselves would be. Main et al. (Main, Kaplan & Cassidy 1985) in an interview called Adult Attachment Interview asks mothers and fathers questions about their own early memories. Concentrating on openness and flexibility of the answers of the parents, Main designs a typology that positively correlates with the classification of children in the "strange situation" (Crane 2002).

With the help of the Adult Attachment Interview (AAI) designed by M. Main the internal working model of the parent is measured. Using the interview the goal is to reach sensitive topics from childhood – "surprising the unconscious" as M. Main says (Fonagy 2001). Main, Kaplan, Fonagy and Cassidy note that attachment experience of the parent can determine the attachment model of the child in 76% of the participants (Karen 1990). There are 4 types of working models in mothers. Mothers with a secure working model value the attachment relations with their parents as well as their present interactions. They describe them in a balanced realistic way, not idealistic, expressing positive as well as negative feelings toward them. Mothers who are avoidant ignore and devalue the importance of relations with their parents, do not remember much about those relations and deny their influence. Those mothers have a higher chance to reproduce avoidant attachment in their children. Mothers who exhibit a model of preoccupation with their parents and actively try to live according to their standards, usually also idealize them and worry about their current relations. They have the tendency to talk about their childhood experience with anger, however, they do not have a well-organized picture of their early relations. Parents with an unresolved trauma from childhood – psychological or physical continue to be afraid of loss and have irrational views regarding experience with their parents. They do not realize the contradictions in their own statements and defensively idealize the parent. The types described by Main are: Confident story-tellers who talk about their early experience openly and freely. Children of such parents in general form a secure attachment towards them. Apparently the acceptance of the parent of his own feelings is tightly connected to the acceptance of the signals and needs of his children.

Denying story-tellers talk about their experiences as if they are very insignificant. Such parents as a rule have insecure and avoidant children. They denied their own experience in the same way that they denied the need and strive of their children for closeness.

In a separate group are the preoccupied story-tellers. The interview allows to hypothesize that they still make attempts to conquer the love and approval of their parents. Most likely parental needs get in the way of reacting consistently to the needs of their children.

Insecure working models prevent the mother from perceiving the signals of the baby by tuning them to her own model (Fonagy 2001). Main, Kaplan, Fonagy and Cassidy conclude that it is more important how we see our childhood than what actually happened. In 75% of the cases precisely the parental perceptions of this experience determined their behavior. In a stressful and insecure environment there is a tendency to invest more in finding a partner than in parenting which increases the risk of neglecting the children. According to Scarr (1992), however, even "super parenting" is not enough to successfully bring up a child. Children may tolerate a wide range of parental styles and still manage to grow up successfully (Bjorklund, D. & Pellegrini, D. 2000).

The understanding that attachment models of newly born babies are placed on a continuum and are not so categorically divided becomes stronger although the styles described by Ainsworth are actually useful in practice. E. Waters notes that the attachment theory on its own does not require or suggest separate attachment models. Different studies of Grossmann, K.E., Grossmann, K., Huber, F., & Wartner, U. (1981), Takahashi, K. (1986), and Sagi, Miyake (1985) show cultural differences in category distribution such that in Northern Germany children with avoidant and in Japan and kibbutzim in Israel children with ambivalent attachment constitute a bigger percentage of the population. There are cultural differences in attachment organization and upbringing practices.

A study by D. Robertson makes Bowlby modify his understanding of traumatic consequences following separation where not enough attention is being paid to the influence of professional care by a known substitute. In 1984 Skuse also criticizes Bowlby basing his argument on the work of A. Freud who shows in the description of her cases that children can develop in a relatively normal way in the presence of adequate care despite severe deprivation in early years. After the observation of development of children with similar experiences from Romania, Rutter concludes that separation from the caregiver is only one of the factors that contribute to the quality of development. Pearce JW, Pezzot-Pearce TD (2007) note that 70% of children who are adopted late do not show attachment disorders. Rutter points out that other deprivations in institutional care or family disagreement could also be important reasons for negative outcome. He calls mother deprivation a "vulnerability factor", and not so much a causing agent, with many different influences. In regard to the fear of a stranger Allison Clarke-Stewart adds that it subsides if the interaction of the mother and the stranger is perceived as pleasant and positive by the child. It cannot be claimed that this fear is universal (Gardner, H. 1979). Although the critical period is transformed to a sensitive period with wider boundaries some authors point out that even small children adopted from institutions form attachment to their foster parents although the quality of attachment is put into question since often there are atypical insecure and disorganized models (Boris, N. & Zeanah, C. 2005). New studies in the theory of mind and attachment claim that unlike Bowlby who uses Piaget's theory of child cognitive development, contemporary scientists use the theory of mind, autobiographical memory and social representations for a more complete explanation. P. Fonagy and M. Target look at the attachment theory and psychoanalysis from the point of view of the theory of mind according to which children with an insecure attachment experience difficulties developing abilities to recognize thoughts, emotions and intentions of other people. Attachment history in part determines the strength of these abilities in different individuals (Fonagy, P. 2001).

Some studies show that when parents are interviewed before the birth of their child the classification derived from the interview positively correlates with the type of attachment of their children when they are placed in the "strange situation". Fonagy establishes that if in the prenatal interview the mother distinguishes with confidence and independence and the father with negation/denial, the child in the "strange situation" acted confidently with his mother and avoided his father. A series of similar research has shown that the classification of parents and their children coincide in 70% of the cases (Main 1995).

Behavior in adulthood is formed under the influence of dysfunctional beliefs, established in early experience from the interactions with the primary caregiver. Information processing is influenced greatly by the role of the mechanism of "imprinting." Traumatic events in early childhood form negative elements in representations about the world, others and oneself which can be in a latent state and other positive, active and functional parts can be "built" above them. Under the influence of traumatic events that resemble the ones experienced in childhood or a critical incident as a precipitating factor in a vulnerability situation those negative dysfunctional beliefs become active and determine the non-adaptive behavior of the individual.

In ICD 10, in the group of disorders of social functioning (F94) is described the attachment disorder in childhood, reactive type (F94.1). This disorder is characterized by abnormalities in the structure of the social interactions of the child that are related to emotional disability and are reactive to changes in the conditions of the environment. The etiology of the reactive disorder of development is associated with a consistent neglect of the basic physical needs of the child, repetitive intentional injuries, maltreatment and bad upbringing. A key feature is the abnormal style of interactions with the caregivers which develops before the age of five and includes non-adaptive features that are usually not encountered in normal children. This style is stable but can be influenced by changes in the way of upbringing that are prominent enough (ICD 10, 2003). A main feature of the reactive attachment disorder is the presence of a "negative attachment cycle" in the family. The child has a marked negative behavior that cannot be neglected and which parents react to emotionally creating an intense but unsatisfactory relation. As a result of this both the parent and the child withdraw from one another and their relation is destroyed.

There are situations and experiences which put the child into a high risk of developing a reactive attachment disorder. Those can be initiated both by the parent but also by the child or his surroundings. On the side of the parent risk factors are: maltreatment, neglect of physiological and emotional needs, ineffective caring, depression, severe mental disorders, adolescent parenting, substance abuse, prolonged absence, integrative difficulties etc.

Depression in mothers has a profound and long-lasting effect on the baby. 10-12% of pregnant women have chronic depression which influences the condition of the fetus. Such children are irritable, inconsolable, exhibit some delay in motor development (Abrams 1995). 40-70% of women suffer from postpartum depression as a result of a radical change in hormonal levels. Around 30% have a prolonged and severe posttraumatic depression. Such mothers find it difficult to provide quality care for their children as a result of their depressive symptomatology but also of their lack of sensitivity to the signals of their children. If depression continues during the first six months after giving birth, delay in childhood development will affect locomotion, weight gain and social responsiveness. When depression in the mother continues throughout the entire first year of the life of the child, he shows a profile of behavioral and physiological dysregulation, which may result in behavioral problems or aggression in preschool (Field 1995).

There are studies that show that children with depressive mothers have a stronger sensitivity and sense of responsiveness to distress in another person. 2, 3-year-old children of mothers with depression are much more likely to be upset and overly engaged when there is conflict or distress and receive more gratification from play with children own age (Zahn-Waxler 1984). These children show more care and conformity toward their mothers. It is possible that depressive mothers expose their children to distress, show more disappointment from their children, and use a strategy to impute guilt in order to regulate the behavior of the child.

There are some risk factors on the side of the child as well. They are usually associated with neurobiological problems that interfere with the ability to receive food, non-subsiding pain, colic pain, aborted fetus, extensive hospitalization etc. Some children are physically or emotionally unresponsive to their parents. This may be a result of the influence of several factors: temperamental characteristics, drug effects, non-subsiding pain, prenatal or postnatal stress, genetic disability or impairment. Often such cycle is formed in children with prolonged pain or colic pain. Mothers of such children are more anxious and experimenting. 80% of parents that physically abuse their children report excessive crying as the reason for the maltreatment (Weston 1986). Some believe that prolonged colic pains are a result of ineffective care, while others, that ineffective care is due to the physiological condition of the child.

The social environment and others also might be an etiological factor for developing a reactive attachment disorder. Sudden separation with the primary caregiver, being a victim and/or witness of abuse, lack of support, constant moving “out of home,” lack of stimulation, marital conflicts, disorganization and chaos in the family further increase the risk for such a disorder.

In ICD 10, in disorders of social functioning (F94) the attachment disorder in childhood, disinhibited type is also included (F94.2). This syndrome is characterized by unusual diffusion in selective attachment during the first five years of life combined with clinging behavior in infancy and/or behavior seeking attention in early or mid childhood. This is a peculiar style of abnormal social functioning which shows a tendency for persisting behavior even in the face of marked changes in the environment. At the age of two it is usually expressed with clinging, diffusive and random attachment behavior. At the age of four the diffusive attachment remains but clinging behavior starts being substituted by strive for attracting the attention of others and undifferentiated friendly behavior; in mid and late childhood children can develop or not selective attachment but often there is a persisting tendency to seek attention. The syndrome is most clearly identified in children brought up in institutions in early childhood but may be encountered in other situations as well. It is believed that it is due to the lack of the possibility to develop selective attachment which is a result of exceedingly frequent change of the people taking care of the child.

Attachment disorders do not lead solely to emotional and social problems but also result in biochemical dysfunctions of the developing brain. Children growing up without love and security have extremely high levels of stress hormones which may impair brain and body growth and development (Perry,1994, van der Kolk,1996). The neurobiological consequences of emotional neglect may lead to behavioral impairments, apathy, depression, learning problems or chronic somatic illnesses. Adolescents with an attachment disorder are three times more likely to commit a criminal act (Raine 1993). It has also been observed the so called "pyramidal effect" – children who have not formed secure attachment grow up to be parents who are incapable of building basic attachment in their children.

One of the most detrimental consequences of abuse and neglect of the child is his chronic inability to modulate his emotions, behavioral models and impulses. Attachment plays an important role in mastering self-control for the child. "The first function of parents is to help the child modulate his arousal through timely distributed means of play, feelings, comfort, touch, gaze etc.; in short by training the child in skills that would help him modulate his own arousal in the future" (van der Kolk 1996). This modulation is achieved by the parents through balancing the regulation – stimulation or soothing. Parents incapable of that form either chronic high arousal or the opposite – insufficient levels of arousal. It is known that more than 80% of children who were abused develop disoriented-disorganized models of attachment resulting in a wide range of symptoms.

Emotional and behavioral regulation is an essential element of mental health that is built in the process of interaction between a parent and a child. Signals of the child like – gazes, screams, coos etc, increase emotional reactions in the parent. Depressive, abusive or neglecting parents cannot respond to the emotions and needs of the child and because of that the child grows up without the necessary external regulating support (Robinson, Geaves 1996). This results in three main reactions:

1. Disorders of the emotions about oneself – feelings of alienation and loneliness, impaired representation of one's own body.
2. Inability to control impulses – physical and sexual aggression, self-disfigurement.
3. Lack of trust and intimacy. Others are perceived as threatening (Cole, Putnam 1992).

Attachment can be formed only in a context of relations that include care, unimpaired power, eye contact, smile, positive affect and need for execution. Communication transferred through touch is the most powerful way to create human attitude. Attachment brings love and caring touch the same way sensitivity does in appropriate quantities. Without touch children can die and aggressive touch leads to developing severe biopsychosocial problems.

Secure attachment formation assumes the presence of several fundamental stages in parent-child relations:

1. Stage of homeostatic control – 7-10 days after birth. There is control over the internal and external systems and motor activity. The caregiver needs to possess a deep sense of empathy in order to be in line with the needs of the child.
2. Stage of extension of the duration of attention and interactions (1-8 weeks). The child uses his capacity in order to keep the attention of the parent – the child uses smile, vocalization, and facial expression which are indicative of receptivity of the child to cues and signals. The child gradually learns to synchronize his interactions. This suggests high sensitivity on the side of the parent in capturing cues and needs for support.
3. Stage of boundaries testing (3-4 months). The parent and the child test the boundaries of the child as they mutually learn more about each other.

4. Stage of autonomy emergence (4-5 months). The baby begins to look for and respond to social cues, develops imitative abilities, and wants to play with objects. His sense of autonomy develops as well as his voluntary control over the environment and his sense of competence. Cognitive development is characterized by the acquisition of new knowledge about sounds, surfaces, lights etc. He seeks attention and responds with cry to displays of inattention toward him. Gradually he realizes that objects have constant characteristics, he looks for them when they are outside of his visual field. In this period parents need to be tolerant to the need of attachment and autonomy.

According to R. Karen, Clarke & Clarke fundamental changes in attachment behavior can occur after the suggested sensitive period as well. Age, cognitive development and social experience develop and complicate the internal working model. Behavior related to attachment is age specific as in preschool age it includes the use of negotiation. A four-year old child is not stressed out by a separation if it has been negotiated beforehand. At the age of 6 most children develop partner-like attitude toward their parents in which any new partner is ready to compromise in order to maintain a satisfying relationship. In mid childhood (7-11 years) there is transference to mutual co-regulation of secure relations as the child assumes higher levels of independence. A unified general model of attachment relations begins to develop usually in adolescence although it may appear in mid childhood as well. The parent-child relationship might influence the interactions with coevals; in mid childhood coevals cannot become attachment figures although if parents are unavailable children may direct attachment behavior also to coevals.

Attachment is a deep and stable relation. Its formation is influenced by all components of the human personality – mind, body, emotions, relations, values. Attachment is not something that parents do for their children but rather something that children and parents build together on the basis of mutual and reciprocal interactions. Attachment to e protective and loving parent who foresees, manages and supports is a basic human need rooted in the million years of evolution of the humankind. Humans possess an instinct to attach – the baby instinctively reaches with his hand toward the caregiver for security and protection. Parents instinctively protect and raise their offspring. Attachment is a physiological, emotional, cognitive and social phenomenon. The social trigger of instinctive attachment is activated in the baby by cues and signals of the parent. The process of attachment is defined as a "mutually regulating system" in which the baby and the parent influence each other.

Attachment accompanies us throughout our whole life on Earth – from then and there when we helplessly waited to be loved and cared for, until here and now, when we actively build romantic relationships and professional realization and again to then and there in the future which awaits us in order to leave worthily this world.

REFERENCES

[1] Ainsworth, M. (1993). Attachment as related to mother-infant interaction. *Advances in Infancy Research,* 8.

[2] Ainsworth, M. (1985). Patterns of attachment. *Clinical Psychologist, 38,* 27-29.

[3] Bowlby, J. (1983). Attachment and loss: Retrospect and prospect. *American Journal of Orthopsychiatry,* 52.

[4] Bowlby, J. (1978). Attachment theory and its therapeutic implications. *Adolescent Psychiatry,* 6.

[5] Bowlby, J. (1958). The nature of the child's tie to his mother. The International Journal of Psychoanalysis, 39.

[6] Brodie, R. (2008). Mary Ainsworth and Attachment Theory. *Child Development Media.* Retrieved from: http://www.childdevelopmentmedia.com/mary-ainsworth-and attachment-theory.html

[7] DeWall, C. N., Lambert, N. M., Slotter, E. B., Pond, R. S., Deckman, T., Finkel, E. J., Luchies, L. B., & Finchman, F. D. (2011). So far away from one's partner, yet so close to romantic alternatives: Avoidant attachment, interest in alternatives, and infidelity. *Journal of Personality and Social Psychology, 101.*

[8] Harms, P. D. (2011). Adult attachment styles in the workplace. *Human Resource Management Review, 21.*

[9] Main, M., & Goldwyn, R. (1994). Adult Attachment Rating and Classification System, Manual in Draft, Version 6.0. Unpublished manuscript: University of California at Berkeley.

[10] Main, M., Kaplan, N., & Cassidy, J. (1985). Security in infancy, childhood and adulthood: A move to the level of representation. In I. Bretherton & E. Waters (Eds.), Growing Points of Attachment Theory and Research. Monographs of the Society for Research in Child Development (Vol. 50). Chicago: Chicago University Press.

[11] Mcleod, S. (2007). Bowlby Attachment Theory. *Simply Psychology.* Retrieved from:http://www.simplypsychology.org/bowlby.html.

[12] Mcleod, S. (2008). Mary Ainsworth-Strange Situation. *Simply Psychology.* Retrieved from: http://www.simplypsychology.org/mary-ainsworth.html.

[13] Mcleod, S. (2009). Attachment. *Simply Psychology.* Retrieved from: http://www. simplypsychology.org/bowlby.html.

[14] Natarajan, G., Somasundaram, C. P., & Sundaram, K. R. (2011). Relationship between attachment security and rejection sensitivity in early adolescence. *Psychological Studies,* 56.

[15] Slough, N. M., & Greenberg, M. T. (1990). 5-year-olds' representations of separations from parents: Responses from the perspective of self and other. New Directions for Child Development, 48.

[16] Solomon, J., George, C., & Dejong, A. (1995). Children classified as controlling at age six: Evidence of disorganized representational strategies and aggression at home and at school. Development and Psychopathology, 7.

[17] Sroufe, L. A., Fox, N., & Pancake, V. (1983). Attachment and dependency in developmental perspective. Child Development, 54.

[18] Wright, J. C., Binney, V., & Smith, P. K. (1995). Security of attachment in 8-22 year olds: A revised version of the Separation Anxiety Test, its psychometric properties and clinical interpretation. Journal of Child Psychology and Psychiatry, 36.

[19] Schultheis, E. (2009). Attachment Security: Born or Made?. *Psychology Today.* Retrieved from: http://www.psychologytoday.com/blog/family-affair/200901/ attachment security-born-or-made.

[20] Zlatka, C. (2011). Relation between children's attachment to kindergarten teachers, personality characteristics and play activities. Early Child Development and Care, 18.

In: New Developments in Clinical Psychology Research
Editors: D. St. Stoyanov and R.-D. Stieglitz
ISBN: 978-1-63483-223-6

Chapter 2

EXECUTIVE FUNCTION DISORDERS, LEARNING DIFFICULTIES AND DEVELOPMENTAL DYSLEXIA: THEORETICAL UNDERPINNINGS

Vanya Matanova*[1*]*, PhD, DSc, CertCBT,
and Ekaterina Todorova*[2]*, PhD
[1]Sofia University "St. Clement of Ohrid," Bulgaria
[2]New Bulgarian University, Bulgaria

ABSTRACT

Executive function plays a crucial role in the initial mastery of new skills, before the skills become automated.developmentally motivated attempt in this direction. When kids have issues with executive functioning, any task that requires planning, organization, memory, time management and flexible thinking becomes a challengeExecutive functions consist of several mental skills that help the brain organize and act on information. These skills enable people to plan, organize, remember things, prioritize, pay attention and get started oExecutive functions allow people to plan, organize, and determine priorities, to concentrate on performing a particular task, to They also help people use information and experiences from the past to solve current pruse information and past experience in order to solve current problems. When there are problems with executive functions, any task which requires planning, organization, memory, time management, and flexibility of thought represents a challenge to the individual. The more you know about the challenges, the better you'll be able to help your child build her executive skills and manage the difficulties. Impediments to executive functions are common in children with ADHD and developmental dyslexia. Executive function disorders cause a wide range of symptoms linked to the mental and social functioning of children. These symptoms could be observed in different nosological units, which poses a challenge to the differential diagnosis of developmental disorders.

* Email: v_matanova@yahoo.com.

INTRODUCTION: THEORY OF FUNCTIONAL SYSTEMS

The brain is not only the main structural unit of the nervous system, but it is also one of the most important organs in the human body. It plays a vital role for the organism, and as a substrate for mental processes, it is a complete system of its own, consisting of various differentiated sections, playing different parts in the performance of mental functions.

The concept of the functional systems was formulated by P. K. Anokhin. He developed the concept of the functional system as an integration unit for the whole organism, constructed dynamically in order to achieve adaptation, always based on cyclic relationships and selective unification of central-peripheral structures.

Between 1955 and 1974 Anokhin formulated fully the basic ideas behind the theory of functional systems, including the following basic mechanisms in a dynamic sequence: afferent synthesis, decision-making stage, action result acceptor, action program, result of the action, reverse afferentation of the result of the action. Based on the theory of functional systems, he developed a theory of systemogenesis proposing a new definition for the role of reticular formation in the mechanisms of sleep, alertness, pain, selective action of narcotic substances, and a hypothesis for the integrative activity of neurons.

Each function results from integrated brain activity. Complex mental processes occur through the cooperation of entire systems of organs, i.e., within a complete functional system. Even relatively simple random movements are the product of complex functional systems, comprising an entire group of afferent and efferent impulses. Efferent stimuli lead to a certain action and through reverse afferentation the brain receives integrated information about the results of the action. The principles of functional organization of the central nervous system were established by A. R. Luria. According to this concept, the CNS is comprised of three main units, each performing its function in the organization of mental activity, and each higher mental activity is performed with the simultaneous participation of all three functional units of the brain.

The three functional units of the brain represent its structural-functional organization, defining the general rules for its work as one whole and provide a basis to explain its integrative capability. Such a model allows for the differentiation of three basic structural-functional units:

I. Energetic unit – regulating tone and alertness;
II. Unit for obtaining, processing, analyzing, and storing information arriving from the external and internal environment;
III. Unit for programming, regulating, and controlling complex functions and mental activity.

The functional unit regulating the tone and alertness is comprised of nonspecific structures on various levels: reticular structure in the brain stem, nonspecific structures of the midbrain, diencephalic regions, limbic system, mediobasal segments.

The significance of the first functional unit in ensuring the mental functions lies in its role in regulating the activation process, maintaining the general tone of the CNS, necessary for any mental activity. This brain unit perceives and processes interoceptive information about the internal state of the organism and regulates these states with the help of neurohumoral biochemical mechanisms. According to A. R. Luria, the energetic unit receives signals from internal organs and sensors, detecting events from the outside world. It processes these signals, which activate the cerebral cortex.

In this way, the first unit of the brain plays different roles and participates in each mental activity, and particularly in processes involving attention, memory, basic emotional states, motivation, and consciousness as a whole.

Alertness is taken to mean a state of the nervous system, which allows the the directed interaction of the organism with the surrounding environment. The most significant indication for the condition of sleep is the loss of a directed reactivity of the organism to changes in the surrounding environment. It is accompanied by an increase of sensory thresholds, reduction of excitability of the prevalent number of reflex arcs, and reduction of muscle tone. It has been determined that there is a certain link between the state of alertness and sleep.

In case of disturbances in tone and alertness, the following three phases are observed:

- equalizing – during which reactions to weak and strong irritants are equalized;
- paradoxical – during which the reaction to a weak irritant is more severe than to a strong one;
- ultraparadoxical – during this phase there is a severe reaction to a weak irritant and no reaction to a strong one.

The second functional unit obtains, processes, analyzes, and stores information arriving from the external environment. It includes the posterior regions of the cortex, i.e., the parietal region and unlike the first functional unit it is modular-specific. It consists of three sections – visual (occipital), auditory (temporal), and general sensory (parietal). Each of these sections has primary, secondary, and tertiary zones. Primary or projection zones have a dual connection with the subcortex, where impulses are received from the periphery and sent to the periphery. Here, the initial analysis of the irritants is performed, i.e., the incoming information is separated into its components. The secondary zones summarize these signs and react to a group of modal-specific irritants. The tertiary zones integrate the information from the various sensory inputs. These facilitate the performance of complex mental activities requiring the combined participation of many zones. In patients with damage to these cortex regions, complex actions are hindered. When distinguishing between individual objects and sounds, patients experience difficulties with spatial awareness, losing direction, have trouble comprehending complex grammatical structures, and complex logical operations.

The third functional unit is tasked with programming, regulating, and controlling complex mental activity. It is responsible for planning and organizing behavior, transitioning from one operation to another, monitors the performance of the program, compares the product of the activity to the initial intention, corrects mistakes, etc.

This unit is comprised predominantly of tertiary cortical zones. It plans activities and monitors their performance. The unit includes motor, premotor and prefrontal cortical zones in the frontal brain sections. Frontal sections are characterized by complex structures and multiple two-way connections with various cortical and subcortical structures. On one hand, these provide the ability to process and integrate afferentation, and on the other - other types of regulatory influences.

The research of A. R. Luria and his students show that bilateral damage to the frontal sections leads to inability to store complex programs and action goals, resulting in discrepant program impulses, as well as inability to achieve sustained concentration on the task at hand. Behavior is then regulated not by internal goals but by all kinds of random outside impulses, the ability to critically assess one's own actions is lost, as well as that to realize and correct mistakes. Frontal sections play an important role in programming, regulating, and self-regulating behavior.

The anatomical structure of the third functional unit of the brain determines its leading role in programming and controlling mental functions, in constructing concepts and goals of mental activity, as well as seeking means to execute and control changes to the plan. It corrects mistakes in execution and regulates, and controls the outcomes of various actions, activities, and behavior as a whole, comparing the results with the original target leading to the experience of pleasure or displeasure from the achieved goal.

Mental activity is carried out with all three functional units of the brain working together, each unit contributing to its performance. The functional units of the brain are characterized by certain structural peculiarities, physiological principles which underly their work, and the role they play in executing mental functions.

Brain Functioning and Executive Functions

Any conscious mental activity is performed with the mandatory participation of the three functional units of the brain. Damage to one of these affects mental activities since it disturbs the respective stage of its execution.

Each brain unit has a hierarchical structure which creates a structural and functional subordination between the three types of cortical areas - primary, secondary, and tertiary. The central zones of the analyzers include the primary and secondary areas, and the periphery - tertiary areas.

Primary sensory zones are characterized by topical organization according to which each section of the receptor surface corresponds to a certain section of the primary cortex thus giving us reason to call the primary cortex - projective. The size of the zones in the primary cortex depends on the functional significance of the respective section. These receive information from receptors or sensory organs forming cortical projections of sensory stimulation, thereby starting efferent paths - the ability to see, hear, perceive but without processing. Neurons in this zone are highly specialized for certain sensory modalities, they perform initial analysis of various physical parameters of stimuli with certain modality and synthesize sensory information. What is more, detector cells of primary areas react to the respective stumilus by type and do not show indications of a weaker response, if the stimulus is repeated.

Secondary cortex areas are characterized by the presence of cells, which transfer afferent impulses from the fourth layer to the pyramidal cells in the third layer, where cortical associative links stem from. This type of transformation is called "secondary projection-associative neuron complex." These cortex areas process the obtained information or the respective behavioral program is prepared for execution. Secondary cortex areas carry out perceptive processing through analysis and break-up of incoming sensory information, determining significant features, and forming a model-perception, which is used as a comparative basis. In other words, secondary cortex areas receive more complex processed information from the periphery than the primary ones.

Tertiary cortex areas of the posterior regions in the large hemispheres are outside the "central zones" of the analyzers. The tertiary areas of the cortex are characterized by a "tertiary associative complex," i.e., the transfer of impulses from the astrocytes in the second layer to the cells in the third layer. Tertiary areas are directly linked to the periphery and connected to other zones in the cortex. They participate in the most complex abovemodal types of mental activity – symbolic, linguistic, intellectual. They are responsible for the cooperation between different cortex zones. It is considered that these zones are structures typical for humans, related to cognitive activities, symbols, abstract notions, logical structuring for spatial processing of information. Any damage to these zones causes inability to formulate action programs, follow instructions, creates difficulties with arithmetic operations, impairs thinking, etc. This vertically hierarchical, cosubordinated, structurally-functional organization of the cortex is the result of progressive evolutionary differentiation of the cortex, clearly manifested in humans. This organization continues beyond the boundaries of the analysis systems to include the respective analyzers, action programs and mental, somatic, and vegetative behavioral control systems. According to the law of hierarchical organization of the cortex, underdevelopment of primary areas limits the development of secondary and tertiary ones. Hierarchical subordination is top-down and in fact tertiary areas are dominant in the performance of cortex functions. According to another principle for the reduction of specificity from lower to higher zones, it is considered that primary areas have a high specificity to various sensory modalities, secondary areas have limited specificity, and tertiary areas overlap different sensory modalities and behavioral integration of excitation processes and construction of abstract notions. The third principle refers to the progressive lateralization of functions, i.e., primary cortical zones are identical for both brain hemispheres, while for the secondary and especially for the tertiary ones, progressive lateralization can be observed. This is reflected in the behavioral functions of the organism – right-handedness, left-handedness, dominance of centers which control speech, emotional status, etc. As it is known, according to modern psychological notions, every mental activity has a particular structure, that begins with the phase of motives, intentions, and concepts, which in turn are transformed into a specific activity program, including an image of the result and perceptions of the methods for implementing the program, followed by a program performance phase supported by certain operations. Mental activity is concluded by a phase of merging the obtained results with the initial perception. In case of discrepancy between these data, mental activity continues until the desired result is achieved. This design and structure of mental activity has been described many times in the works of numerous psychologists in accordance with the model of the three functional units. During the first stage of forming motives for any conscious mental activity, the first functional unit of the brain plays a predominant part. It provides the optimal total level of brain activity and selective forms of activity, necessary to perform the specific type of mental action. The first functional unit of the brain is primarily responsible for the emotional support of mental activity, i.e., experiencing success or failure. The stage of formulating the goal and program as well as the program control and performance stage are primarily associated with the work of the third functional unit of the brain. The operational stage is primarily carried out with the help of the second functional unit of the brain.

Although there is no generally accepted definition of EF. Although there is no generally-accepted definition of the executive functions, most researchers agree that these include inhibitory control, attention characteristics, and information updating (Miyake et al. 2000).

Especially during early ontogenesis, the ability to actively maintain an abstract goal in the working memory is one of the most important aspects of executive functions (Munakata et al. 2012). This aspect Individual differences in executive functions have important consequences in everyday life. For example, they are a powerful predictor for maturity and achievements in school. Direct effects are especially noticeable when it comes to learning to read, write, and do calculations. (Bull et al. 20112011, Lee et al. 2009), individual differences in EF are Lee et al. 2009;, Gathercole 2006). However, their examination is a particularly difficult problem for researchers, mainlyFriedman 2012). due to the large number of individual variations.Moreover, when studying EF in children, the problem is exacerbated (Huizinga et al. 2006; Hughes et al. 2010; Hughes et al. 2010; Wiebe et al. 2008). Wiebe et al. 2008). Executive functions and cognitive processes are linked with the so-calledIn order to deal with this problem and to appropri-The concept of *metacognition* is also broadly and mostly vaguely defined in the literature, meta-knowledge. It is defined as higher-order cognitive processes, which process and regulate information (Schneider 2011).).In any of the different models of self-regulated Meta-cognitive processes are activated in certain situations and can be classified as procedural meta-knowledge and declarative meta-knowledge. In this connection, a two-way relationship is sought between cognitive and affective-motivational factors. It is assumed that meta-cognitive functions are developed through chains of reverse connections during various activities or the so-called meta-cognitive experience. Skills are initially implicit but gradually become accessible to the consciousness and explicit. Some behavioral patterns are related to the routine behavior which includes automated responses that require significantly less conscious processing. Other behavioral patterns are highly adaptive reactions to unknown and/or complex situations. "Executive functions" is a summary term used to describe the processes occurring during these adaptive reactions. These are related to acquiring new skills, planning and making a decision, correcting mistakes in activity processes, initiating new actions, managing difficulties, conscious behavioral control, coping with impulsive reactions, etc. Interrelations between EF, Self-Concept (SC), and metacognition.Therapists and Other SpecialYour Child's School (RTI): Some schools use this program to find students who are falling behind and give them extra help.Make checklists. Listing the steps involved in a task will make it easier for your child to see how to get started.Set time limits. Your child may struggle to budget time for an activity and also for each step of that activity.

- Use planners and calendars. Not all planners have to be on paper, which is a good thing if your child has trouble keeping track of items;
- Explain yourself. Children who are inflexible thinkers or who have difficulty with emotional control don't always take feedback well or see the point of learning new ways to do things.

The learning of new skills, planning and decision making, error correction, initiating novel actions sequences; danger or technical difficulty conscious control of behavior need to overcome strong habitual responses. The development of executive functions research until recently and most of the twentieth century, was focused almost entirely on adults. This was mainly because the prefrontal cortex was thought to become functionally mature only late in development, around adolescence (Luria 1973) A. R. Luria/1973/ considers that the maturity of the prefrontal cortex is reached during adolescence, which is refuted by more recent research. It is now clear that the development of executive functions begins and ends much earlier than assumed. Some components of executive function are already developing in preschool children, and play a much greater role in early child development than previously thoughtSome components of executive functions develop in preschool children and play a much more important role in a child's development than it was believed until now.Behavioral and emotional regulation is an extension of fundamental abilities for executive control. It is known that cognitive functioning is lateralized in the prefrontal parietal cortex, premotor and supplemental motor region. Part of the anterior cingulate cortex is activated when dealing with problems which involve making a choice choice when faced with conflicting information, as well as detecting multiple targets and tasks related to working memory. (Banfield, Wyland, Macrae 2004). The dorsal region is involved in attention modulation, executive functions and working memory; it is also activated during the performance of cognitive tasks (Bush et al. 2000). The component of executive control is not necessary for all cognitive processes but it is stimulated under circumstances which require inhibition of the first possible answer, monitoring and correction of mistakes, decision-making, and planning (Diamond 2005). This is related to the work of the third functional unit of the brain.

Modern psychology assumes that executive functions are linked to:

- Abstract thinking (for example, classification of objects according to external characteristics);
- Allocation of attention and redirection to current phenomena;
- Decision-making;
- Action-planning. Disturbances in this function lead to disorganization in actions (inability to form a daily action plan);
- Social functioning. Underdevelopment of this function leads to deficits in empathy, anxiety, non-conformity to social norms;
- Suppression processes – signs of inhibitory impairment include aggression, impulsiveness, perseverances, etc.

One particularly important aspect in children's development is the progressive organization of behavior and acquiring experience related to the ability to inhibit reactions to various stimuli. The world is immensely diverse and nature has gifted us with senses which can capture this diversity. In order to adequately process these stimuli during development, the child constructs the so-called sensory filter, which blocks out signal based on their inappropriateness, insignificance, etc. requiring inhibition of reactions to these signals. If this sensory filter is not functioning, there are difficulties in inhibiting the so-called surpassing stimulus and the child's behavior becomes chaotic, inconsistent, and inadequate. These surpassing stimuli vary in different situations and require flexibility of behavior patterns. Externalized behavior is characterized by outward style and does not express itself as aggression, impulsiveness, violence or insubordination. Internalized patterns are described as directed inward and find expression as withdrawal, loneliness, depressiveness, anxiety. Activity: The richness of the sensor The ability to inhibit reactions to a stronger stimulus is a prerequisite for planned, intelligent actions. The development of inhibitory control begins in early childhood and continues into school age. It is assumed that with regard to inhibitory control, differences between adults and children are eliminated around the age of 10.

Executive function plays a crucial role in the early stages of mastering new skills. Executive functions play a decisive role in the early stages of acquiring new skills. When a child is learning to read, the executive demands of the activity are high. When a child is learning to read and write, the requirements towards the executive functions are very high. A great deal of conscious effort is required on the part of the novice reader simply to decode the written symbols into words. The more the skill is perfected, the lesser the role of executive functions - the action becomes automated. Executive functions play a decisive role in the initial mastering of new skills when they are still not automated. developmentally motivated attempt in this direction.On the other hand. As executive function develops, so children's abilities to learn new skills improve, and they are increasingly able to behave in a planned, strategic and organized manner. with the development of executive functions, children's abilities to acquire new skills are improved and they learn to do this in a directed, organized, and planned manner. They become more flexible in their ability to control their thinking and behavior. Inhibitory control is only one component of development but it is crucial. One way to assess this importance is to look at the implications for child development of a failure to develop typical levels of inhibitory control. One way to assess its significance is to consider the consequences for the child's development resulting from the inability to develop the typical levels of inhibitory control.

EXECUTIVE FUNCTIONS DISORDERS

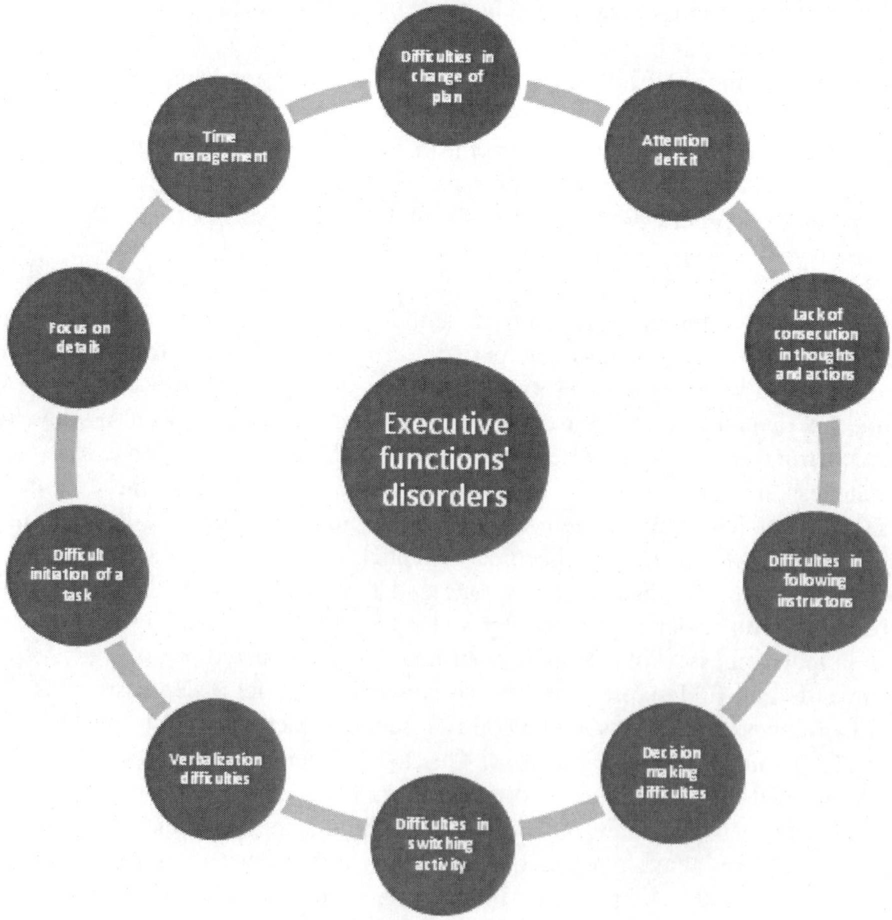

Figure 1. Executive functions disorders.

Attention Deficit and Hyperactivity Disorder (ADHD) in Childhood and Adolescence

Executive function plays a crucial role in the initial mastery of new skills, before the skills become automated.developmentally motivated attempt in this direction. When kids have issues with executive functioning, any task that requires planning, organization, memory, time management and flexible thinking becomes a challengeExecutive functions consist of several mental skills that help the brain organize and act on information.These skills enable people to plan, organize, remember things, prioritize, pay attention and get started oExecutive functions allow people to plan, organize, and determine priorities, to concentrate on performing a particular task, to They also help people use information and experiences from the past to solve current pruse information and past experience in order to solve current problems. When there are problems with executive functions, any task which requires planning, organization, memory, time management, and flexibility of thought represents a challenge to the individual. The more you know about the challenges, the better you'll be able to help your child build her executive skills and manage the difficulties. Impediments to executive functions are common in children with ADHD and developmental dyslexia.

ADHD is defined as a behavioral disorder in children characterized by undirected motor anxiety leading to difficulties with attention concentration and causing significant problems in performing structured tasks.

It was only established during this century that ADHD is a behavioral disorder, which affects learning processes, although there is also the opinion that this is an artifact conditioned by the changing concepts of learning. ADHD includes a group of heterogeneous conditions with different etiology.

Nowadays, ADHD is considered to have an array of symptoms, with the most prominent being motor anxiety, inability to concentrate, impulsiveness, and emotional instability. Many hyperactive children demonstrate clumsiness and dyspraxias. Some develop compensating limiting behavior. Reactions to pain stimuli are lowered, they are unable to preplan their activities, often demonstrate outbursts of rage and irritability. Difficulties in transferring information from one sensory modality to another are also typical.

ADHD is one of the most common development disorders. It is believed to affect 3 to 7% of children in early school ages. The peak of expression is between 6 and 7 years of age. The syndrome is 3-4 times more common in boys. Left without treatment, this disorder often persists into adolescence and adulthood, exposing the individual to substantial risk from a number of abnormalities in personal development and social functioning.

Hereditary factors may affect brain functions in zones responsible for behavior inhibition and modulation. Hyperactivity is an innate characteristic of temperament with biochemical parameters and low reactivity of the central nervous system. This explains the disturbances in brain inhibitors, in the reticular formation, with the latter conditioned by the delay in maturing.

According to one of the most popular genetic theories, the root of ADHD can be traced to problems in the functioning of the Reticular formation of the first functional unit of the brain. At its most basic, the pathogenesis is caused by disruptions in the activating system of the reticular formation, in the limbic system, in the prefrontal sections of the cortex, and in the inhibitory mechanisms.

The reticular activating system is a coordinating center. It has a coordinating function with respect to learning and memory, processing, and allocating incoming information and active attention. The reticular formation has a leading role in activating the cortex and participates actively in the sleep - wake cycle, as well as in activating higher cortex functions and other cognitive processes. Activating the reticular formation also leads to increased activity in the brain cortex and thus conditions the gnostic recognition and classification of information, building models of activity, thinking, and development of all mental processes of importance for the child. This activation is non-specific - i.e., the cortex does not receive specific information to process. The cortex simply "awakes" and receives sufficient energy to begin "work." The activation of the cortex leads to corrective suppression. In this manner, the cortex and the reticular formation exercise mutual control on the basis of the so-called corrective feedback principle.

It is considered that the reticular formation of children with ADHD is less active and its effect on the cortex is weaker, i.e., the activation by the reticular formation is limited and insufficient. Exactly because of this, children with ADHD constantly seek specific external stimuli, usually motor ones, which send information to the cortex in order to maintain the necessary state of functional activity. This theory is supported by numerous studies with EEGs, as well as by the effects of some medication used to treat the syndrome. It is known that applying medication which suppress the activity of cortical processes leads to intensification of ADHD symptoms, while the application of stimulants provides good results. The assumption is that this decreased activity of the reticular formation is genetically conditioned and is passed down generations as a mode of functioning for a certain brain structure which under specific conditions is manifested as ADHD. According to other researchers, this "weakness" of the reticular formation may be the result of discrete brain damage.

New discoveries in the field of neurobiology postulate the idea for the movement of specific neurons from the interior of the brain to certain areas in the cortex. If this movement process changes, slows down or does not occur, the normal development of the basic cognitive processes, the sexual orientation of the individual, and emotionally-behavioral reactions are impeded. According to these theories, ADHD can be included under the heading "minor brain injuries" or "minor brain dysfunctions."

Although some brain injuries can account for certain deficits in some cognitive processes, there are few supporters of this explanation. It can only explain some clinical cases or separate symptoms. It is certainly not always the case that each child in this category has in their medical history complications during birth, head trauma or severe diseases.

ADHD is very often accompanied by disorders of organic nature such as mild dysarthria, developmental dysphasia, developmental dyspraxia and others. Therefore, the assumption that minimal brain dysfunction can be one of the reasons for ADHD should not be dismissed without serious objective arguments.

Actually, the etiological theories about ADHD can be provisionally divided into four groups:

- Neurobiological - there is a mediator (catecholamines, serotonin, etc.) that affects mobility and influences behavior;

- Neuropsychological theories are associated with deficiency in the mechanism of inhibition which is the reason for lack of control over the functioning of the hippocampus;
- Neuroanatomical theories compare the behavior of hyperactive children to that of children with damaged lobes but modern diagnostic tools (CT) do not provide sufficient reasons for it.

Despite all disagreements, three main clusters of symptoms are unanimously adopted: attention deficit, hyperactivity and impulsivity. Some researchers believe that there are two other main characteristics: problems with following rules and instructions as well as extreme variability in responses to situations.

However, according to Barkley, one of the most prominent researchers of this disorder, these characteristics of hyperkinetic disorder are symptoms that arise from the primary problem which is a deficit in the ability to suppress behavior, i.e., the primary problem with this disorder is impaired inhibitory control.

The etiological factors leading to impairment of executive functions are still vague. Nevertheless, some assumptions could be made with respect to heredity, differences in brain function, brain lesions, etc.

Different types of executive dysfunction manifest through a wide range of symptoms such as:

- Difficulty in modulation of a task;
- Focusing on details or on the whole, but not simultaneously on both;
- Inability to determine the time for performing the task;
- Inability to change the plan, even if it is clear that it is not adequate;
- Inability to concentrate and easy distraction;
- Lack of consistency of thought and action when interrupted;
- The need for instructions being repeated;
- Problems with decision-making;
- Difficulty in switching from one activity to another;
- Difficulties in verbalizing and others.

There are several key skills involved in executive function - impulse control, emotional control, flexibility of thought and action, working memory, self-control, planning and prioritizing, modulation, organization and others.

Control, defined as the ability to inhibit a dominant response in order to realize a subdominant one and the ability to identify mistakes and engage in planning, is the main form of self-regulation. Using effortful control, people adopt flexible approaches to situations and inhibit activities which they fear or which they feel are undesirable. The efficiency of control, however, will depend on the strength of the emotional processes against which effort is exerted (Rothbart, Derryberry 2000). Children high in control show higher levels of empathy, guilt, shame and lower levels of aggression (Rothbart, Ahadi, Hershey 1994). Guilt and shame are positively related to control and negative affectivity. Negative affectivity may contribute to guilt by providing strong internal cues of discomfort, increasing the likelihood that the cause of these feelings will be attributed to an internal conscience rather than external reward or coercion (Rothbart, et al. 1994). Effortful control may also contribute by providing the cognitive and attentional flexibility needed to notice these feelings and relate them to feelings of responsibility of one's own specific actions and their negative consequences. Bad impulse control often underlies aggression. Control is gradually formed with the development of physiological regulation, attention and emotional self-regulation, especially self-soothing or seeking help when one is upset. In this period, the capacity for self-regulation can be enhanced by increasing cognitive competence or worsened by cognitive difficulties (Posner, Rothbart 2000). Emotional and impulse controls are closely related. Children who have problems with emotional control often cannot accept negative feedback and get angry at small injustices. Developmental changes in emotional regulation are manifested when the child reaches independent emotional self-regulation from the total dependence on the adult who takes care of the regulation of their emotions, i.e., co-regulation gives way to self-regulation (Keane, Calkins, (2004). Early emotional regulation is mainly influenced by internal physiological mechanisms. It starts when the child is about 3 months old and it is related to attempts for deliberate excitement control which builds up to the end of the first year in relation to motor skills and language. During the second year, the child uses their language skills to develop better impulse control. This promotes the transition from passive to active methods of emotional regulation. This emotional self-control is completely developed between 3 and 4 years of age. Changes in self-regulation that are present in 3-4-year-olds are related to the development of the executive control system (Rothbart, Derryberry 2000). An important skill is the flexibility of thought and actions that is associated with the ability to take a new approach in case of failure of the plan. When there is no such flexibility, thinking is concrete, there are no alternative solutions, etc. This is the ability of the child to analyze the basic idea, to determine the importance of the task, to plan the steps to achieve the objective, and the ability to start a task, which in turn is related to planning and prioritization.When planning and prioritization are impaired, children act chaotically. They take up too many tasks and concentrate only on the more easily manageable parts of a task, thus missing the main idea. Working memory and organizational skills play an important role in information processes because they relate to the ability to hold information necessary to complete a task. In cases of working memory disorders, difficulties in the implementation of multi-step tasks occur due to loss of the ability to track information and process operation. Children suffering from such disorders often lose or misplace their belongings. They cannot get organized, even when there are negative consequences of their actions, and this relates to self-control or the ability to monitor and assess the implementation of the task. Children who have self-control problems lack awareness of strategies and do not check their effectiveness.

Executive function disorders occur significantly more frequently in different nosologies and conditions, which is one of the challenges for differential diagnosis. ADHD, for example, affects attention, impulsivity and activity levels, which often influence the process of studying. Impaired executive functions are a significant part of the symptoms of ADHD. Mood disorders such as depression, anxiety and the like may affect executive functioning. Executive functions are also impacted by states such as Fetal Alcohol Syndrome (FAS), which affects reading, working memory and other executive functions. The most commonly discussed nosological entity characterized by impaired executive functions is developmental dyslexia. Most professionals will also want to see for themselves the way your child interacts with people and the world around her. Step 3: Put it all together. After collecting all the information, the professionals will look at all the results and go over them with you. What conditions are related to executive functioning issues Attention-deficit hyperactivity disorder (ADHD): This is one of the most common childhood brain-based disorders. It affects attention, impulse control and activity

DEVELOPMENTAL DYSLEXIA

Developmental dyslexia is one of the most dynamically developing fields of modern clinical psychology and neuropsychology. Psychologists, doctors, teachers and parents of children suffering from this condition continue their efforts to fully understand the nature of developmental dyslexia and offer different methods to improve the learning and social skills of these children. Many theories and therapeutic strategies emerged in past few years. Some of them did not pass the test of therapeutic practice and were gradually forgotten.

The term developmental dyslexia covers a whole group of disorders, the sufferers from which have problems in one area of learning or in areas that relate to it. Some of the disorders can occur in isolated pure form or in combinations with one another.

The various terms used to describe the different forms of dyslexia cause certain misunderstandings. Even more so, the same terms are used to describe different disorders. This is because dyslexia is a subject of interest to a wide range of specialists - doctors, psychologists, speech therapists, linguists and others - who interpret different aspects of this disorder.

In recent years, there has been a great focus on dyslexia for several reasons. Nowadays, more than ever, learning skills and qualification are extremely important factors for the self-realization of the individual. More and more children attend school worldwide and are interested in their own progress. Knowledge and academic skills are important even in developing countries. Severe childhood diseases have been reduced globally and it is already possible the attention to be focused on non-life-threatening disorders such as developmental dyslexia. Moreover, there is plenty of evidence that many emotional and behavioral problems in adolescence and adulthood are related to specific learning problems in childhood.

For the past 20 years, there has been a steady increase in the number of individuals who experience difficulties in mastering basic learning skills. The reason for this can be found both in the increased diagnostic capabilities and in the evolved understanding that intellectual development determines school achievements. This trend increases the interest in the search for early identification criteria in order to prevent this kind of disorders.

The scientific explanation of developmental dyslexia is related to research in written language disorders. In 1917, the French physician Hinshelwood presented the first publication describing the etiology and interventions of written language disorders. He defined 'word blindness' as a 'condition in which an individual with normal visual acuity for letters and words has no ability to integrate them into written text.' This disability may be due to brain defects in specific brain areas leading to impaired visual memory for letters and words.

In 1930, Orton found that there is probably a lack of hemispheric dominance in children suffering from language disorders who do not have brain damage. Many of the children Orton studied had cross or poor hand, eye and foot dominance. He believed that cross dominance can be hereditary and the location of the brain damage is significantly more important that its amount.

In recent years, there has been a steady tendency to use the terms 'specific learning disorders' and 'developmental dyslexia' interchangeably.

Many authors believe that since the term 'developmental dyslexia' is used very loosely, it is better to adopt the more pragmatically useful term 'specific learning disorders'. It can describe the problems of a group of children whose abilities in reading, writing and arithmetic are significantly below the standards for their age, but their abilities in other areas give reason to expect more from them. Specific learning disorders are related to difficulties in processing information which affect the process of literacy development and are characterized by differences and discrepancies between tasks and their execution /Moray House Centre for Specific Learning Difficulties 1993/. This definition implies that children can exhibit different types of difficulties and demonstrate varying degrees of these difficulties. They are associated with differing-from-standard characteristics of auditory, phonological, visual, motor and cognitive processes. The interpretations of the two concepts 'specific learning disorders' and 'developmental dyslexia' are becoming more and more similar. The broadening of the two definitions warrants the two terms to be interchangeable. Regardless of how the terms 'specific learning disorders' and 'developmental dyslexia' are perceived, defined and understood, it is evident that children suffering from such disorders have special educational needs and require special care in training and the use of alternative educational programs, especially in terms of literacy. This condition can be diagnosed in the absence of intellectual deficit, hearing disability, impaired vision as well as severe emotional and motor disorders.

The term 'developmental dyslexia' continues to exist as a separate nosological unit. Developmental dyslexia does not necessarily form the basis of specific learning disorders. Dyslexia is a combination of many symptoms, which affect learning reading, writing, verbal expression, spatial and temporal orientation and each symptom alone cannot account for the problem. All these symptoms are viewed as a result of brain dysfunction due to developmental disorders of higher cortical functions. The occurrence of one symptom triggers another and the combination of them characterizes the dyslexic syndrome.

Neuropsychological deficits in dyslexia are so compelling that a large part of etiological theories are actually neuropsychological. It was Orton in 1937 who proposed the theory that dyslexia is associated with the lack of hemispheric dominance, which impedes the specialization of the left hemisphere as the one controlling speech. The lack of a dominant hemisphere also explains the different brain structure in these subjects, demonstrated by the emergence of mirror images of the stimuli they have been submitted to. In recent years, however, it has been strongly suggested that this theory should not be accepted unreservedly. After the time of Orton, a new neuropsychological model for explaining developmental dyslexia appeared - minimal brain dysfunction. In 1962, an international team of child neurologists suggested the term. Pathology of writing is viewed as non-specific disorder directly dependent on various neurological disorders. In the 80s and 90s, this pathology was finally considered to be specific and 'is not necessarily related to minimal brain dysfunction' and 'does not depend on intellectual, cultural and emotional reasons' /Thomson 1990/. Being initially universally approved and raising hopes, later on this theory began to lose its upholders mostly due to the vagueness of the concept, the impossibility to prove neurological deficit /except by the presence of soft neurological signs/ and the excessive broadening of this term.

The term 'specific developmental disorders of scholastic skills' is used in ICD-10, code F-81. The normal ways of acquiring skills are impaired in the early stages of development in these disorders. The impairment is not a simple consequence of the lack of opportunity to learn and it is not due to any form of a suffered brain injury or disease. The disorders are considered to be caused by abnormalities in cognitive function resulting from some type of biological dysfunction. This term refers to:

- specific reading disorder,
- specific spelling disorder,
- specific disorder of arithmetic skills and
- Mixed disorder of scholastic skills.

Disorders can be diagnosed when the achievements in these areas measured by means of individual standardized tests are considerably below the ones expected at a certain age. This discrepancy significantly affects academic achievements or activity of daily living.

In written expression, the structure of communicative tasks is related to synchronization of three types of brain activity:

- Reading - receptive activity characterized by visual or tactile /in cases of visual impairment/perception of graphic signs.
- Writing - motor activity characterized by the spelling of a graphic symbol, corresponding to the rules of the language system that is used for written communication.
- Memory activity in relation to the storage of a grapheme code into the long-term memory buffer.

The three types of brain activity cannot be clearly distinguished from one another. From psychophysiological, psychological and linguistic point of view, reading is analogous to auditory perception of messages. The brain structures that perform this process are typically similar to the areas of auditory perception of spoken language.

Writing is a function of the frontal lobe. The written word forms syntagmatic and paradigmatic clusters by means of which 'communication of relations' and 'communication messages' are carried out. Writing is syntagmatically and semantically performed through the process of motivation - thought - idea - inner speech on a deeper level and through graphical realization in linear order on a superficial level.

Written language develops later in childhood than spoken language. In different language systems, the age for forming the ability to perceive, process and comprehend the use of graphemes is approximately the same /5 to 7/. This is the period when brain maturity and psychophysiological readiness for using another sign system occur. Unlike spoken language, writing performance runs parallel with writing competency. In written language, there is no prosody or the so-called third element of high semantic value. There are no paralinguistic elements in written language, although this is partially compensated for by punctuation. Reading and writing skills are acquired almost simultaneously resulting from education and training.

From a psychophysiological and neuropsychological point of view, three channels are involved in mastering written expression: visual, auditory and kinesthetic. Mastering reading and writing goes through the same stages. Both forms of written language are carried out in certain anatomical and physiological areas of the cortex.

According to A. R. Luria, the processes of reading and writing are reversed.

Writing flows from thought to word and reading flows from word to thought. Writing is thought verbalization, transmission of a message, while reading is message reception.

In 1985, Frith identified three main stages of the development of the reading process:

- Logographic stage - words are recognized holistically as visual models but are not always reproduced correctly. This model explains the phenomenon of how young children read without spelling, and vice versa, which indicates that they use two different strategies.
- Alphabetic stage - there is correspondence between letters and sounds; i. e. reading is carried out by means of grapheme-phonemic transfer. Perhaps the difficulties of dyslexic children are linked to stage. Beginning readers use visual strategies for reading and phonological skills for spelling.
- Orthographic stage - automated knowledge of the associations between the elements of graphemes and phonemes, syntax and semantics. The structure and the meaning of the sound-letter relationship are comprehended. Context comes into play and it is understood. The orthographic units are recognized as words.

According to Marsh (1981), reading acquisition goes through four stages:

1. Glance and guess stage. It includes automated learning of high-frequency words, while unknown words are recognized by guessing their meaning in a certain context.
2. Discrimination net guessing stage. It relates to the child's ability to engage in visual processing in order to recognize different words.
3. Sequential decoding stage. Children are supposed to decode unknown words using simple grapheme to phoneme correspondences. At this stage, the child can only use words with simple syllabic construction.
4. The fourth stage is an intermediate stage between the alphabetic and the orthographic stages. At this stage, rules for decoding context as well as analogical strategic reasoning are necessary.

Lexical skills include 'interpretation' of the word from a visual concept into a semantic one. The processes at this stage are defined as lexical. Lexical processing is associated with reading familiar and high frequency words but it is not used for reading unknown words and pseudowords that require sublexical processing. The top-down model is based on the word and the reader's experience; the reader predicts certain words and phrases, recognizes the words and letters and considers context.

Sublexical skills relate to coding graphemes and phonemes by means of grapheme-phonemic correspondence. This is due to abilities, which affect the skills for phonemic analysis, phonemic synthesis, coding within lexical analysis, coding in working memory. Mastering these skills develops metalinguistic knowledge, which improves reading. The debate on the overall analysis of sublexical processing is focused on children's ability to read unknown words and pseudo-words based on different correspondence mechanisms: grapheme to phoneme, a sequence of graphemes to a sequence to phonemes, morphemes to phonological codes.

The bottom-up model includes segmentation, mapping and synthesis of the received information. In regard to reading, the process is described as strengthening the links between the corresponding aspects of the words. These aspects include information about the orthography, phonology, meaning, morphology and articulation of a word. The main difference between lexical and sublexical processes is that an experienced reader identifies familiar words by means of a lexical process and decodes less familiar words using a sublexical process. In cases of reading disorders, both processes can be affected. Difficulties with the alphabet are linked to sublexical processing, while orthographic problems are liked to lexical processing.

Writing is a complex process, which is one aspect of written language. Unlike spoken language, writing requires a higher level of functioning, since it is produced in the absence of a direct interlocutor, it requires a precise selection of the content and is a more conscious and comprehensive activity.

The acquisition of literacy requires the comprehension of written language as a system of signs, which allows the transmission of information through graphic elements, and acceptance of the constancy of the character composition that is to be correlated to the other form of a sign system - spoken language.

The formation of writing skills is a continuous and consistent process that develops as a conscious activity. Depending on the degree of control, it changes from conscious to automatic level of operation. In essence, writing has a sensory, motor, speech and language level.

The sensory level is related to the ability of visual and auditory perceptions and the associated visual and verbal memory. The ability of visual perceptions provides the fine descrimination between graphically similar letters and it is connected with visual memory in terms of memorizing visual symbols and learning the correct position of letters. As to auditory perception, it promotes the ability to differentiate between acoustically similar sounds and it has a constructive function for the phonemic analysis and synthesis and phoneme-grapheme mapping, and they are in turn connected with the parameters of verbal memory.

The motor level is associated with repeating the character code by means of fine praxis programs, which are also related to the ability to switch the motor pattern. During this process both visual and motor controls are performed. On the other hand, in the course of spontaneous writing the motor level upgrades the phonological, lexical, grammatical and semantic part of the language system.

The speech level is related to the so-called internal articulation in writing. The production of writing is always supported by verbal speech. When articulation is impaired, this reflects back on writing dictations and spontaneous self-writing and the errors in writing are identical with the errors in articulation.

The linguistic level is associated with the development of a language system, which plays a fundamental role in reading and writing processes. Writing could be learned provided that the language system has been mastered. This process takes into account the language structure rules, especially with respect to self-writing. In order to construct a written expression, a certain concept program is necessary in which the sequence of thoughts and cogitations are to be structured. This program must comply with the grammatical rules of language – formation, coordination and organization of words in a sentence, correct sentence structure, the ability to create a structural entity of a sentence. In the process of spontaneous writing, ability to keep the order of the sentences is necessary, controlling the part of the text already written and the one to be written. Each sentence is comprised of separate words, which in the process of their graphical representation are divided by certain delimitation. The next step is the complex process of phoneme analysis of the word, determination of its phonological structure, associated with sound context and order, phoneme-grapheme mapping and motor execution.

Language development deficiency is expressed in various errors, concerning:

- Disrupted word structure – reductions in consonant clusters, graphic elisions of vowels and syllables, literal inversions of letters and syllables;
- Poor spelling performance;
- Errors in writing prepositions, conjunctions, particles, prefixes and suffixes, resulting in omission, substitution, contamination (merging) in the preceeding or the forthcoming word;
- Predominant use of certain parts of speech compensating for the lack of others or their incorrect use;
- Substitutions and/or omissions of words;
- Disturbed word order in a sentence;
- Peculiar syntactic forms deviating from the standard sentence structure norms;
- Poor descriptive expression, lack of primary or secondary parts of the sentence;
- Difficulties in setting grammatical relations between objects and between actions;
- Inaccurate coordination due to dificulties in morphological analysis;
- Errors in constructing complex sentences;
- Difficulties in establishing logical and linguistic connections between separate sentences.

Writing cannot be defined as an isolated process since its formation is determined by other aspects of development: the ability of visual and auditory processing, spatial orientation, visual-motor coordination, building up writing praxis, the ability of phoneme-grapheme transfer, well-developed language system parameters, development of verbal and visual memories, development of abstract thought and metacognitive abilities. Deficiency in any or several of these aspects could cause writing impairments often displayed as specific errors indicative of dyslexic behaviour.

Etiological theories of developmental dyslexia can be divided into two large groups - neuropsychological and cognitive. Neurological theories correlate with neuropsychological theories regarding information processing in different brain structures. Cognitive deficiency combined with delayed maturation of the left-brain hemisphere affect linguistic functions and written language learing mechanisms. These processes of immaturity are difficult to assess, but their importance should not be underestimated. Orton's theory about the lack of hemispheric dominance, which has been widely popular for a long time, is now confirmed by some of the recent research, proving that crossover dominance is more common in developmental dyslexia cases. However, there is a growing body of opinion that this theory should not be accepted without any reservations, as the lack of hemispheric dominance cannot be the sole reason for the occurrence of developmental dyslexia.

And yet, the reason for developmental dyslexia is probably the late maturation of brain structures and delayed specialization of the left hemisphere in terms of speech development in right-handed people, which is manifested as perceptive, motor and language deficiency. This hypothesis is also a subject to criticism because of the proven fact that in cases of early damage to the left hemisphere the right hemisphere compensates for this damage by taking up its language functions

A large number of authors believe that the main cause of developmental dyslexia is the functional disintegration between auditory and visual processing of verbal stimuli. Visual and language components of information are stored and processed in different brain structures. Visual information is bilateralized, which creates difficulties in grapheme – phoneme mapping and in the mechanisms of perceptual and linguistic coding.

Cognitive theories about the etiology of developmental dyslexia are related to characteristic features in perceiving, memorizing and processing information. This is also a neuropsychological aspect, in a sense, associated with the activities of the second functional unit of the brain. Information processing is associated with perceptual identification of essential signs, correlating with the previous experience and cognitive development of the individual.

Another part of developmental dyslexia etiological theories are associated with emotional problems, which in a large number of cases appear to be a trigger. We cannot renounce the assumption which argues that these children are hypersensitive and all these impairments have affective nature. Volkova /1989/ for example, considers dyslexic errors as projective resulting from conflict situations, which have negative effect on the emotional state of the child, resulting in poor integration of cognitive functions. However, whether emotional problems are background preconditions for development of dyslexia or they occur as a result of it, is a question still unanswered.

Hamblin /1996/ believes that the environment may be "orthogenic", i.e., it helps the child to acquire pro-normal patterns and pathogenic, which makes the child quit normal patterns, encourages withdrawal and development of deviating patterns. Emotional disorders and behavioral deviations occur as a consequence. Emotional reactions could be demonstrated in a variety of manifestations - deliberate refusal to learn, overt hostility, negative attitudes toward school, proneness to addiction, disobedience, hyper distraction, withdrawal into private world and others. Due to the pressure to improve school achievement, the child begins to avoid anything that is connected with preparation for school. The child seeks to attract the attention of peers and teachers by manifesting indiscipline, clownish or hyperkinetic behavior, indifference, etc. The child develops low self-esteem, and becomes quarrelsome, conflict-seeking, aggressive, shows hypersensitivity to remarks. Their overall mental functioning is marked by a sense of inferiority, indifference, emotional instability. According to a research by Coie, Dodge & Coppotelli /1982/ the sociometric status of these students could be one of the following categories: popular, controversial, neglected, rejected. This research shows that the status categories of these children are connected with their characteristic social perceptions and behaviour.

Developmental dyslexia is a complex disorder which affects the development of personality and overall mental and social functioning. Difficulties are not restricted to reading, writing and arithmetic, but they are related to impairment of executive functions, reflecting in emotional and/or behavioral disorders. It was found out that emotional disorders are characteristic for early school years, behavior disorders - for medium and delinquent disorders - for high school education.

Developmental dyslexia manifestations could be divided into two groups: general and specific. The general ones are connected with psychomotor development, behavior, dominance characteristics and lateralization of functions and cognitive development. The specific manifestations of developmental dyslexia include the developmental charcteristics of executive functions and higher cortical functions.

Developmental dyslexia problems are not restricted to acquiring school skills. The social environment also has an emotional effect on the student, which reflects on their performance at school. Acquisition of social skills comprises the vital part of learning. Social skills deficiency correlates with other types of failure in school performance, though, social incompetence is not inherent to all individuals with dyslexia. Social skills deficiency is usually focused in three main spheres: lack of adequate evaluation of other people's attitudes and mindsets, which is related to mentalization abilities, difficult adaptation to the atmosphere in a specific social situation, which leads to pragmatic deficiency and display of unacceptable behavior patterns.

Development of social perception, in some aspects, is similar to development and command of scholastic skills. In both cases, feedback ability is particularly important, which implies prediction, planning, forecasting, comparison of the result of an act with the initial intention, error correction, etc.; all these are related to the work of the third functional unit of the brain.

Children suffering from dyslexia face difficulties in understanding and adaptation to others' emotions. They are likely to demonstrate inadequate behavior due to their inability to realize the emotional state of others, or their assessments and preferences. They are indifferent to the emotional atmosphere of the social situation. Such children are prone to low self-esteem and susceptible to sense of guilt, attention deficiency, aggression, hyperkinetic behaviour and increased excitability.

Recurring failure creates a sense of insecurity and self-perception based on lack of identity. These children experience failure a lot more often than other children do. This failure is due to the fact that children suffering from dyslexia cannot meet the expectations of others in terms of adopting scholastic skills and behavior. They do not arouse others' content, approval, acceptance and affection, as they do not show the adequate progress expected at their age. The immediate environment and other people usually burden them with their negative evaluations, rejection, criticism social isolation and rudeness. Recurring failure or lack of achievements engender negative attitude and suspicion toward any kind of relationships and activities. Their emotional reaction could be demonstrated in various forms – deliberate refusal to learn, overt hostility, negative attitudes toward school, proneness to addiction, disobedience, hyper distraction, withdrawal into private world and others.

Due to the pressure to improve school achievement, the child begins to avoid anything that is connected with their functional role at school. As a result, from the recurring failures, the child seeks to attract the attention of peers and teachers by manifesting indiscipline, clownish or hyperkinetic behavior, indifference, etc. The child develops low self-esteem, and becomes quarrelsome, conflict-seeking, aggressive, shows hypersensitivity to remarks. Their overall mental functioning is marked by a sense of inferiority, indifference, emotional instability, despite their high intelelctual potential, which remains unrevealed and unutilized in cases where no adequate treatment, attitude and undestranding are provided.

Regarding the specific manifestations of developmental dyslexia certain impairments in the development of higher cortical functions are observed. According to A.R. Luria these functions have social origin, mediated structure, and are voluntary in terms of functioning, which gives us reasons to assume gnosis, praxis and speech are higher cortical functions. Their adequate development is in direct connection with the personality and intelectual functioning.

The research of A. R. Luria and his students showed that bilateral damage to the frontal sections leads to inability to store complex programs and action goals, resulting in discrepant program impulses, as well as inability to achieve sustained concentration on the task at hand. Behavior is then regulated not by internal goals but by all kinds of random outside impulses, the ability to critically assess one's own actions is lost, as well as that to realize and correct mistakes. Frontal sections play an important role in programming, regulating, and self-regulating behavior.

Individuals suffering from developmental dislexia experience dificulties in finding, recognizing, identification and discrimination of stimuli perceived through a specific sensory channel. When visual gnosis is impaired the difficulties are connected with categorization of essential and constant characteristics of objects and the inability to recognize them again with the help of memory mechanisms. This affects their ability to differentiate between similar stimuli, which results in deficiency of fine discrimination. This is most obvious in the perception of language stimuli. The mechanisms of grapheme-phoneme coding-decoding and grapheme-phoneme mapping are affected. The inability to discriminate between similar visual stimuli leads to difficulties in distingushing between graphemes, which have similar graphical visualization. These difficulties are most probably connected with impairments in visual memory, which is evident from the difficulties in memorizing visual symbols, difficulties in learning the correct positions of letters, which leads to inability to correctly recognize whole words.

Auditory perception impairments affect similar parameters, related to perception of stimuli through the auditory channel. These impairments affect the abilities to differentiate between sounds simmilar in their acoustic characteristics and the phonemic analysis and synthesis. In this type of impairment, the child cannot connect the word with its meaning, i.e., there are difficulties in transferring visual language symbols into acoustic. These difficulties cause semantic errors as the words are usually interpreted as morphologic units due to hindered sound synthesis and word analysis. This is most clearly observed in reading new words and pseudowords, while words, whose graphic form is connected with their meaning, are read easily.

Based on the neuropsychological deficiencies the following types of developmental dyslexia are observed:

1. The individual shows satisfactory development of visual-spatial functions and visual-motor coordination. Their sensory abilities are on a physiological level, as well as their ability of abstract thinking and concept creation. However, the ability of immediate memorizing of general information, the ability of verbal expression and verbal memory are impaired.

2. Sensory-motor, visual-spatial, and elementary mathematical skills that are displayed non-verbally are preserved. Immediate memorizing of sequences of order and information preservation are impaired. The stereognosis and visual-spatial memory are severely affected.
3. Minor impairment of stereognosis, visual-motor coordination and abstract thinking is observed. In this case, however, there are more severe disturbances in verbal expression and verbal memory. Especially, the ability to form concepts is highly impaired.

The group sharing Rourke's theory /1996/ conclude that the dysfunction in the first type of dyslexia is located in the left temporal area of the cortex; in the second type – the left temporal, parietal-occipital area. In the third case the damage is located in the left frontal area of the cortex.

A number of studies have proven the presence of impairments in the stereognosis and time-space perception in individuals with developmental dyslexia The impairment in time-space perception affect the visual-spatial, time and rhythm gnosis. These agnosias reflect on the ability to perceive and assess the spatial dimensions of objects – shape, size and position in space. There are impairments observed in the simultaneous gnosis, which is problably connected with the fact that this gnosis is part of the system of spatial relations. The same relation probably explains the impairments of somatogenesis and prosopgnosis. The ability to perform spatial trials and spatial decoding of the actions of another person are impaired. The listed agnosias affect the cognition and the use of words denoting spatial relations, directions and left-right orientation. Disturbed spatial perception in individuals with developmental dyslexia reflects on their orientation in time. The aspects of time dimensions are perceived distorted, especially those that are connected with ordered sequences in time and have periodic nature. The verbal time perception is also disturbed, leading to difficulties in understanding and reproducing words denoting time aspects.

Rhythm gnosis is connected with the perception of rhythm structures and affects the ability to perceive, produce and program them. These imapirments cause difficulties in perception of melodies, pace and tact combinations. The disturbed perception of rhythm structures reflects on intonation and stress in verbal speech and punctuation in written language.

Impairments of space and time perceptions lead to a large range of linguistic errors, connected especially with the perception of order and sequence of graphemes, the perception of a grapheme as a spatial sign and the coherent perception of graphemes within whole syntactic structures. Space and time perception also affects the accurate cognition and use of separate lexical units – prepositions; logical-grammatical structures; tenses, etc.

Difficulties in visual-motor coordination are manifested as problems in the perception of visual constructs produced by painting, drawing and writing. This production is characterized by size disparity with the stimulus, excentric percetual visual space, separate elements persevering, simplification, distortion, etc. Difficulties that are especially significant are those in fine visual-motor differentiations, as they take essential part in the writing-reading learninig process.

Impairment of basic psychological process in cases of developmental dyslexia cause a number of arguments between scientists. The major part, though, describe the deficiency of attention as a specific characteristic in this nosologic unit. Many cases of poor school performance are contributed only to attention deficiency. The clinical etimology of most dyslexia cases include attention deficiency, especially in terms of concentration and keeping it. There is no clear evidence, though, that attention deficiency causes developmental dyslexia, or it results from dyslexia. However, students demonstrating attention deficiency are inactive, meet difficulties in the identification of essential signs, which affects the selective attention. Attention is known to be a determinant factor in learning a language system and the related skills for reading and writing.

Regarding memory problems observed in children suffering from dyslexia, most of the researchers keep the focus on their inability to code information, their difficult preservation of information and low level of motivation for this type of activities. Particularly common are the impairments of short-term memory and preservation of visual-spatial information. These problems correlate with the impairments in grapheme coding and grapheme-phoneme mapping. Long-term and lexical-semantic memories are also disturbed in some aspects. These memory disorders determine difficulties in language processing which affects language functions. A certain inconsistency between the slow-paced internal flow of speech and the fast-paced articulated speech is observed. This affects the understanding and rationalization of visually perceived verbal material.

The combined actions of the three functional brain units provide conscious and rationalized mental activity. The front sections of the brain represent the material substrate of executive functions, which start their development in preschool and reach maturity at the age of 10. Executive function disorders cause a wide range of symptoms linked to the mental and social functioning of children. These symptoms could be observed in different nosological units, which poses a challenge to the differential diagnosis of developmental disorders.

REFERENCES

Ainsworth, M. (1985). Patterns of attachment. *Clinical Psychologist, 38,* 27-29.

Ainsworth, M. (1993). Attachment as related to mother-infant interaction. *Advances in Infancy Research,* 8.

Bowlby, J. (1958). The nature of the child's tie to his mother. *The International Journal of Psychoanalysis*, 39.

Bowlby, J. (1978). Attachment theory and its therapeutic implications. *Adolescent Psychiatry,* 6.

Bowlby, J. (1983). Attachment and loss: Retrospect and prospect. *American Journal of Orthopsychiatry, 52*.

Brodie, R. (2008). Mary Ainsworth and Attachment Theory. *Child Development Media.* Retrieved from: http://www.childdevelopmentmedia.com/mary-ainsworth-and attachment-theory.html

DeWall, C. N., Lambert, N. M., Slotter, E. B., Pond, R. S., Deckman, T., Finkel, E. J., Luchies, L. B., & Finchman, F. D. (2011). So far away from one's partner, yet so close to romantic alternatives: Avoidant attachment, interest in alternatives, and infidelity. *Journal of Personality and Social Psychology, 101*.

Harms, P. D. (2011). Adult attachment styles in the workplace. *Human Resource Management Review, 21*.Main, M., & Goldwyn, R. (1994). Adult Attachment Rating and

Classification System, Manual in Draft, Version 6.0. Unpublished manuscript: University of California at Berkeley.

Main, M., Kaplan, N., & Cassidy, J. (1985). Security in infancy, childhood and adulthood: A move to the level of representation. In I. Bretherton & E. Waters (Eds.), Growing Points of Attachment Theory and Research. Monographs of the Society for Research in Child Development (Vol. 50). Chicago: Chicago University Press.

Mcleod, S. (2007). Bowlby Attachment Theory. *Simply Psychology.* Retrieved from: http://www.simplypsychology.org/bowlby.html

Mcleod, S. (2008). Mary Ainsworth-Strange Situation. *Simply Psychology.* Retrieved from: http://www.simplypsychology.org/mary-ainsworth.html

Mcleod, S. (2009). Attachment. *Simply Psychology.* Retrieved from: http://www. simplypsychology.org/bowlby.html

Natarajan, G., Somasundaram, C. P., & Sundaram, K. R. (2011). Relationship between attachment security and rejection sensitivity in early adolescence. *Psychological Studies,* 56.

Schultheis, E. (2009). Attachment Security: Born or Made?. *Psychology Today.* Retrie-ved from: http://www.psychologytoday.com/blog/family-affair/200901/attachment security-born-or-made

Slough, N. M., & Greenberg, M. T. (1990). 5-year-olds' representations of separations from parents: Responses from the perspective of self and other. *New Directions for Child Development*, 48.

Solomon, J., George, C., & Dejong, A. (1995). Children classified as controlling at age six: Evidence of disorganized representational strategies and aggression at home and at school. *Development and Psychopathology*, 7.

Sroufe, L. A., Fox, N., & Pancake, V. (1983). Attachment and dependency in developmental perspective. *Child Development*, 54.

Wright, J. C., Binney, V., & Smith, P. K. (1995). Security of attachment in 8-22 year olds: A revised version of the Separation Anxiety Test, its psychometric properties and clinical interpretation. *Journal of Child Psychology and Psychiatry,* 36.

Zlatka, C. (2011). Relation between children's attachment to kindergarten teachers, personality characteristics and play activities. *Early Child Development and Care*, 18.

In: New Developments in Clinical Psychology Research
Editors: D. St. Stoyanov and R.-D. Stieglitz
ISBN: 978-1-63483-223-6

Chapter 3

EXECUTIVE FUNCTION DISORDERS, LEARNING DIFFICULTIES AND DEVELOPMENTAL DYSLEXIA: EMPIRICAL RESEARCH

Vanya Matanova[1*], PhD, DSc, CertCBT, and Ekaterina Todorova[2], PhD
[1]Sofia University "St. Clement of Ohrid," Bulgaria
[2]New Bulgarian University, Bulgaria

ABSTRACT

65 children at the age of 9 to 11 years participated in this research. The children were divided into two groups: children with dyslexia (15) and children without dyslexia (50).

The design of the current empirical study uses both independent and dependent variables. It is of interest whether the characteristics of attention as a cognitive process differ for children with and without dyslexia. A battery of tests was used to assess the basic characteristics of attention. A multivariate analysis of variance was conducted to establish the effect of the factor status of the participants on all variables simultaneously. There has also been evaluated the psychosocial functioning of the two groups of participants.

INTRODUCTION

In this research participated 65 children at the age of 9 to 11 years. The children were divided in two groups:

- children with dyslexia – 15
- children without dyslexia - 50

* Email: v_matanova@yahoo.com.

The data was analyzed using following statistical methods:

1. One-way Multivariate Analysis of Variance, MANOVA. This analysis includes one independent variable and five dependent.
2. Unequal N HSD - statistical post-hoc test - Unequal N HSD test by Tukey for testing hypotheses on uneven number of respondents in the different groups.
3. Correlation analysis for testing the hypothesis of no relationship between the characteristics of attention measured by verbal and non-verbal tests.
4. One-way Multivariate Analysis of Variance, MANOVA.

The design of the current empirical study uses both independent and dependent variables. In this analysis there are two independent variables and thirteen dependent variables. It is of interest whether the characteristics of attention as a cognitive process differ for children with and without dyslexia. A battery of tests was used to assess the basic characteristics of attention - range, switching, stability, distribution and concentration. A multivariate analysis of variance was conducted to establish the effect of the factor status of the participants on all variables simultaneously. It is also important the assessment of the psychosocial functioning of the two groups of participants.

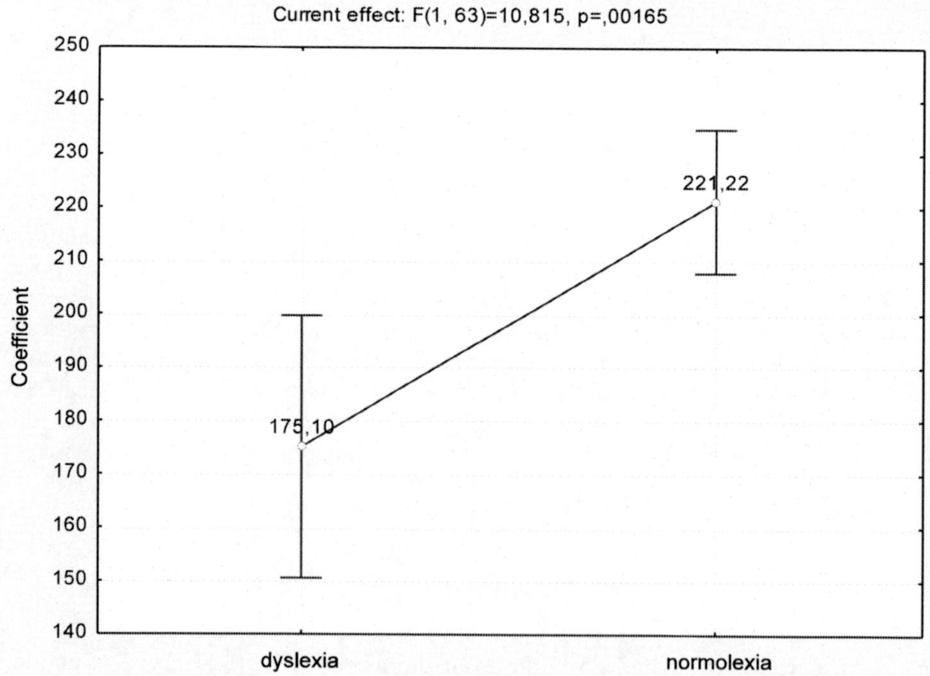

Figure 1. Attention range[1].

[1] Left on the diagram is coefficient in dyslexia, to the right is normolexia. This applies to all figures in this chapter (Editor's note).

RESULTS

The data was entered in a table of the program Statistica and the coefficients for range, switching, concentration and stability of attention were calculated for each of the participants.

For the variable attention range there is a statistically significant difference regarding the average score of the coefficients of the two groups of participants, respectively for the ones with dyslexia it is X = 175,10 and for the normal group – X = 221,22. The test of Tukey yielded a p = 0,002. The score of $p = 0.001$ at a critical level of significance $\alpha = 0{,}05$ shows that there is a statistically significant difference between the participants from the two groups – with and without dyslexia. This means that the two groups differ in their range of attention, assessed by this specific measure.

Attention switching was assessed with a two-letter proofreading sample which requires simultaneous tracking and crossing of two different letters in a different way. The results are shown on Figure 2.

For this variable a statistically significant difference between the average scores for the two groups is observed as well. For the children with dyslexia the score is 398,80, and for the children in the normal group – 605,81. The result for p for the post-hoc test by Tukey is 0,000. The score of $p = 0.000$ at a critical level of significance $\alpha = 0{,}05$ shows that there is a statistically significant difference between the participants from the two groups. It is concluded that the participants with and without dyslexia differ significantly on attention switching assessed with this specific measure.

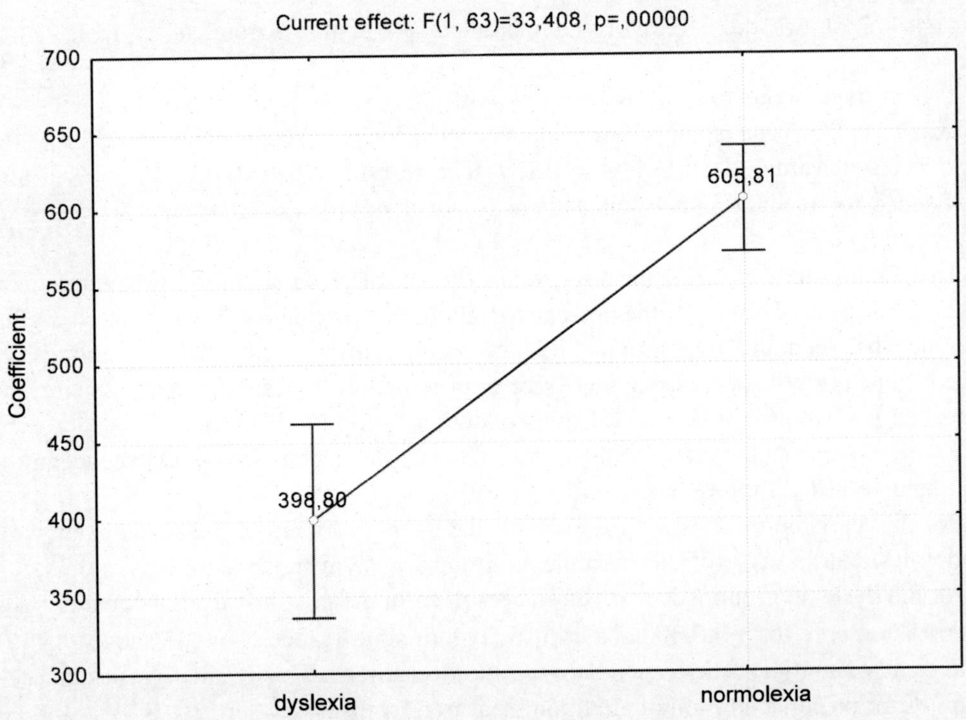

Figure 2. Attention switching.

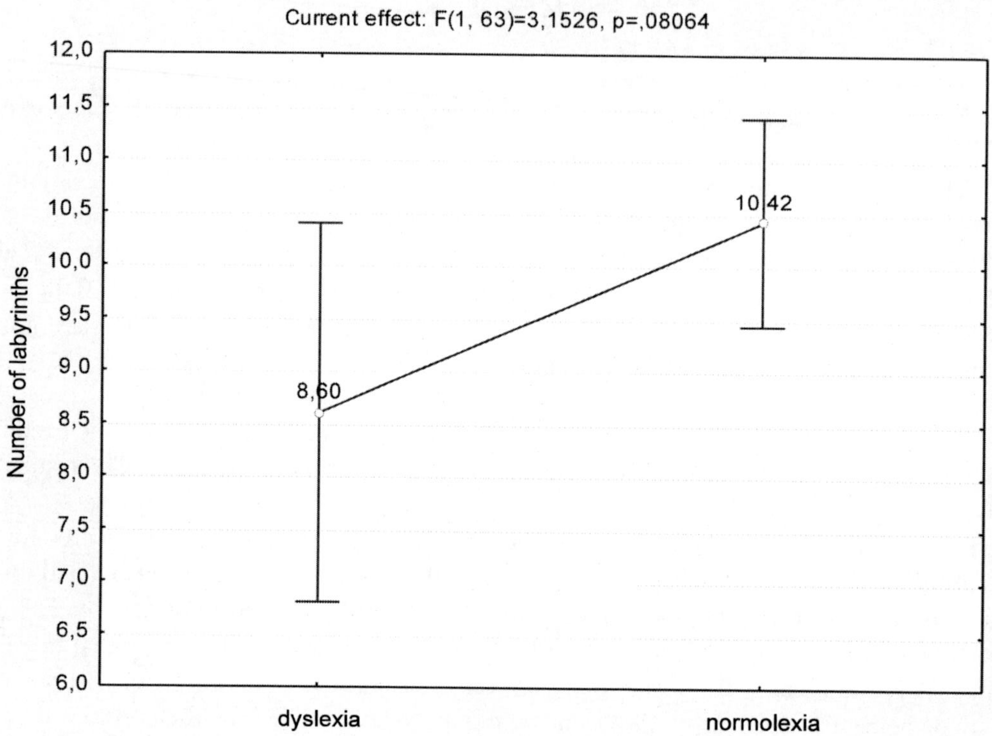

Figure 3. Attention distribution.

Figure 3 shows the effect of the factor status on the dependent variable "attention distribution".

The average score for the participants with dyslexia is 8,60 and for the ones without dyslexia – 10,42. These results show relatively close average scores. The result for p after the post-hoc test Unequal N HSD is p = 0,157. The result for p = 0.081 at a critical level of significance for $\alpha = 0{,}05$ shows that there is not a significant difference between the two groups.

This finding indicates that the two groups do not differ on attention distribution assessed with this measure. However, the results for attention distribution do not show significant difference between the two groups. By comparing the two groups, it is noticeable that dyslexic and normolexic participants have approximately the same average scores, which means that the two groups did not differ on attention distribution.

Figure 4 presents the effect of the factor status on the dependent variable concentration of attention assessed with the Toulouse-Pieron test.

For this variable there is a difference for the average scores of the participants with and without dyslexia in favor of the normolexic group whose average score is X = 0,25, and the one for the dyslexic group is X = 0,16. The result from the post-hoc test Unequal N HSD is p = 0,000. The score for $p = 0.000$ at a critical level of significance $\alpha = 0{,}05$ shows that there is a statistically significant difference between the two groups. This result signifies that the two groups differ on concentration of attention measured by this test.

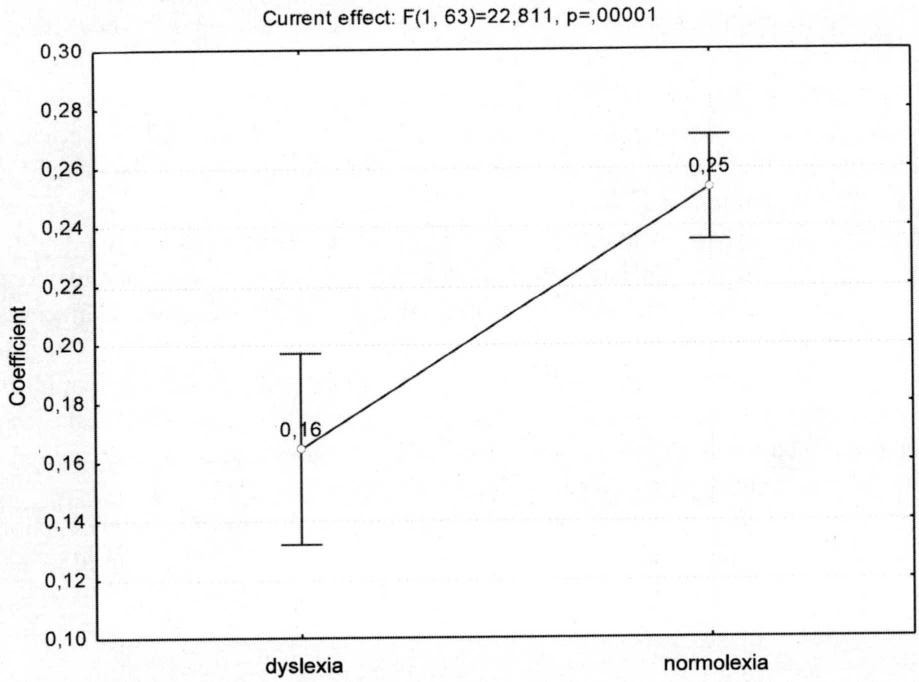

Figure 4. Concentration of attention.

Figure 5 presents the effect of the factor status on the dependent variable attention stability.

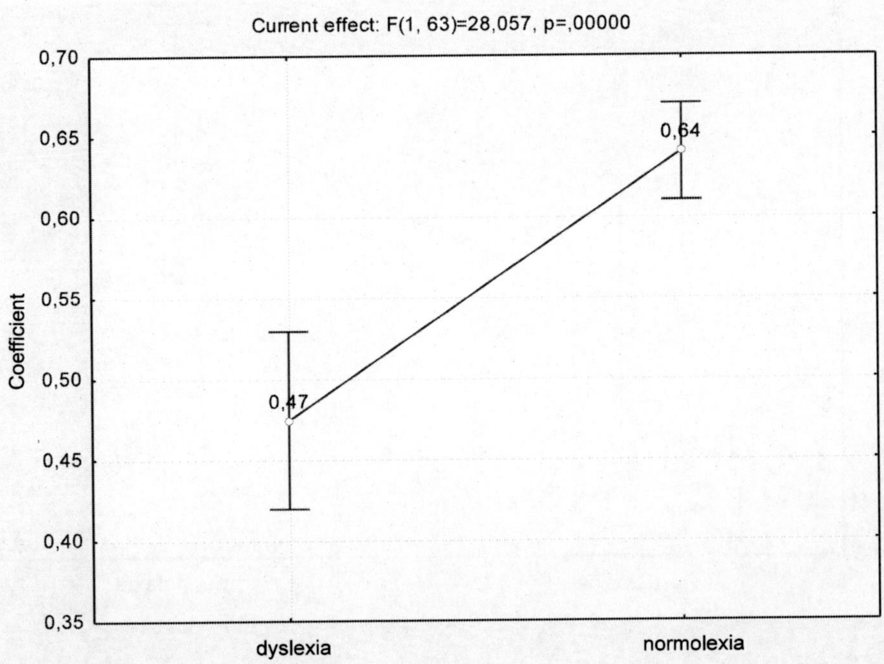

Figure 5. Attention stability.

For this variable the difference in the average scores of the coefficients can be easily noticed, as for the control group it is 0,64 and for the experimental – 0,47. These results show that the participants from the normal group performed better on this test. The score for p on the post-hoc test by Tukey is 0,000 at $\alpha = 0{,}05$. The result for $p = 0.000$ at a critical level of significance $\alpha = 0{,}05$ signifies that there is a statistically significant difference between the experimental and the control group. This means that the participants with and without dyslexia differ on attention stability.

In order to establish the strength of the correlation between the two verbal and the three non-verbal tests, a correlation analysis was conducted. This was necessary to identify the relationship between the verbal and non-verbal stimuli assessing the five characteristics of attention.

All coefficients are positive which indicates that there is a positive correlation between the different characteristics of attention measured with verbal and nonverbal tests. Therefore, it can be concluded that for children with dyslexia there exists a positive correlation between the levels of attention measured by verbal and nonverbal tests.

We tested the hypothesis that there is a difference in the psychosocial functioning of children with and without dyslexia. A multivariate analysis of variance was used to assess the effect of the factor status of the participants on all variables simultaneously. The effect of the independent variable status of a participant was checked against each of the scales of the methodology by Renee Jill i.e., against each of the independent variables.

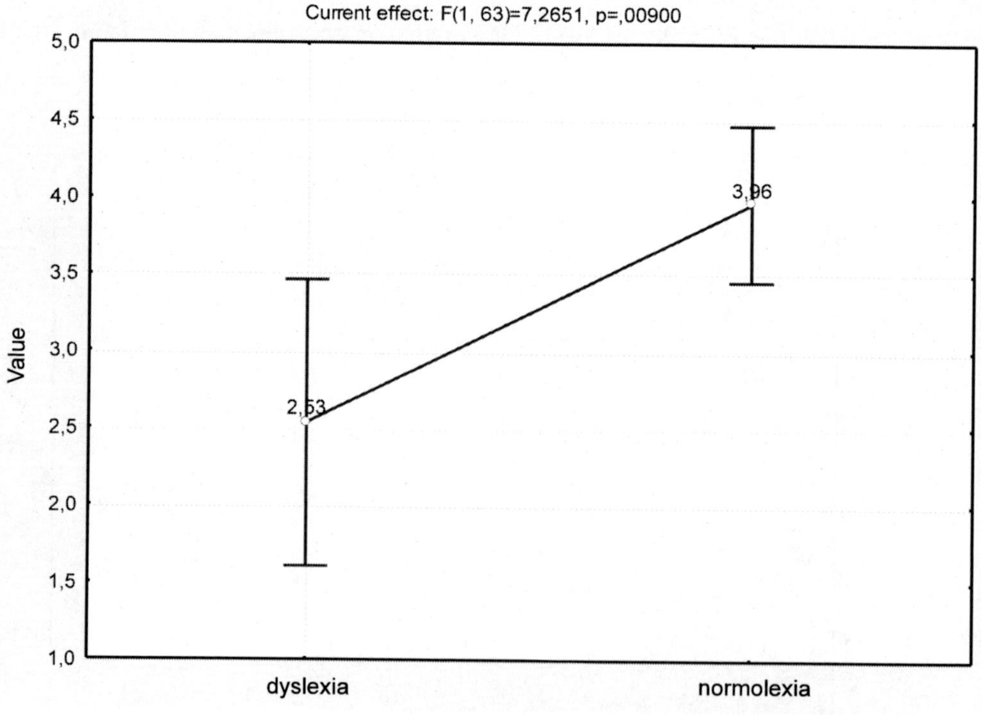

Figure 6. Attitude to family.

The acquired result shows a statistical significance $p = 0{,}002 < \alpha = 0{,}05$, which means that there is a difference between the two groups of participants regarding the investigated variables. Therefore the status of the participants has an effect on the emotional and social functioning of the individual.

The results of the two groups on “attitude to family” are presented on Figure 6.

There is a statistically significant difference between the average scores of the two groups, for participants with dyslexia X = 2.53 and for participants without dyslexia – X = 3.96. The result for $p = 0.009$ at a critical level of significance $\alpha = 0{,}05$, shows that there is a statistically significant difference between dyslexics and normolexics. Thus, it has been established that the acquired results on the control variable give grounds not to reject the hypothesis that there is a difference between the two groups of participants on “attitude to family.”

The following Figure 7 presents the results for the two groups on “attitude to sibling”.

For that variable no significant difference between the average scores of the two groups is observed, as for participants with dyslexia the score is X = 3.27, and for normal participants – X = 2.66. The result for p is 0.539 at a critical level of significance $\alpha = 0{,}05$ which shows that there is not a statistically significant difference between the groups with and without dyslexia. Thus, it has been established that the acquired scores on the control variable give reason to reject the hypothesis for an existing difference between the two groups of participants on the variable “attitude to sibling.”

Figure 8 presents the dependent variable “attitude to friends.”

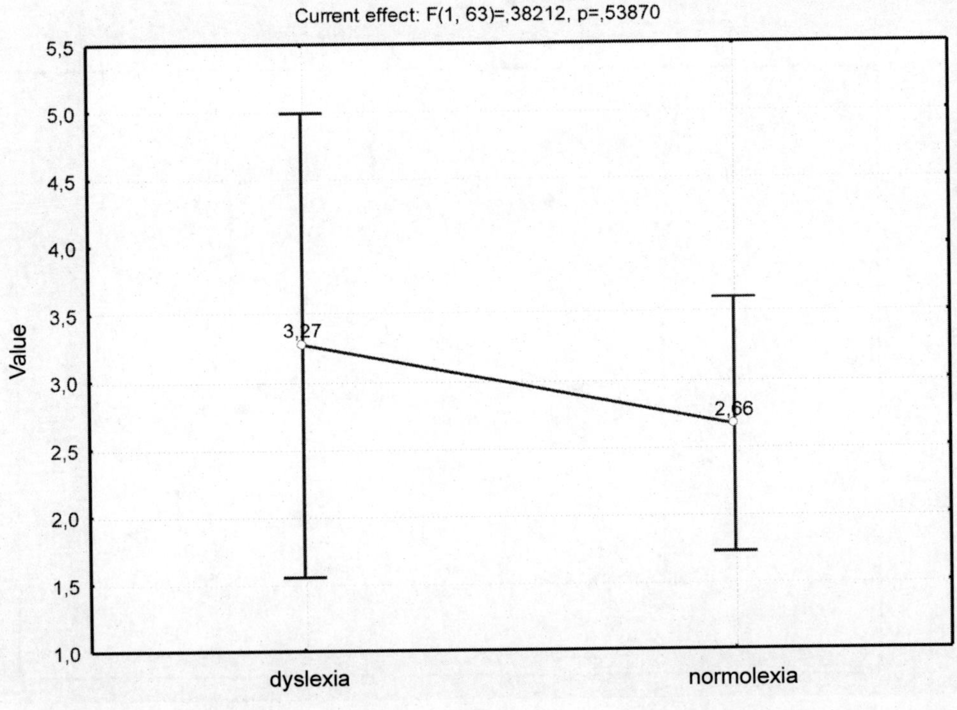

Figure 7. Attitude to sibling.

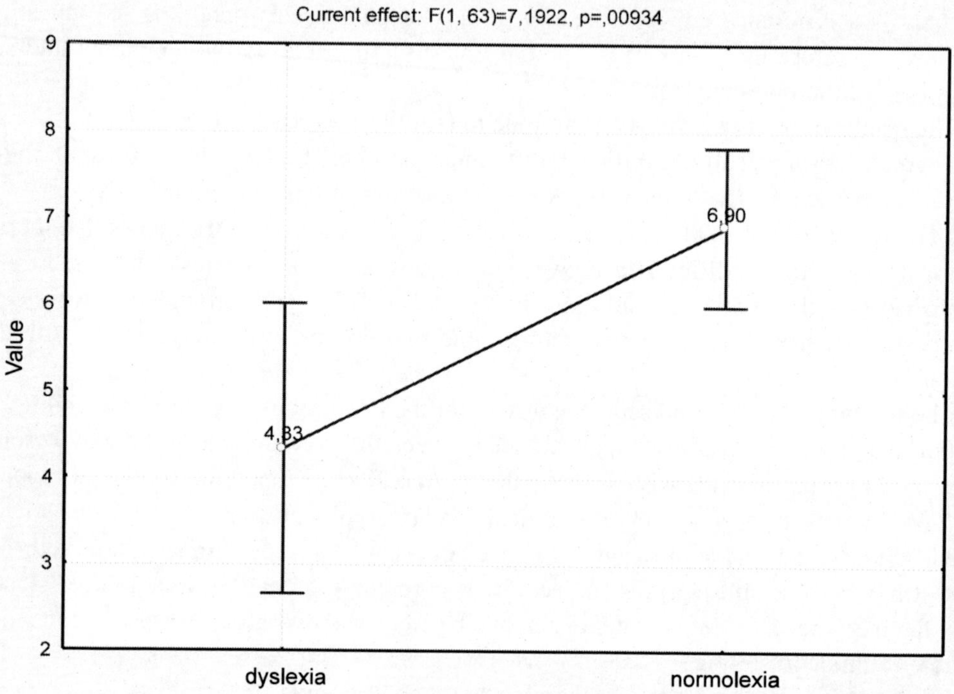

Figure 8. Attitude to friends.

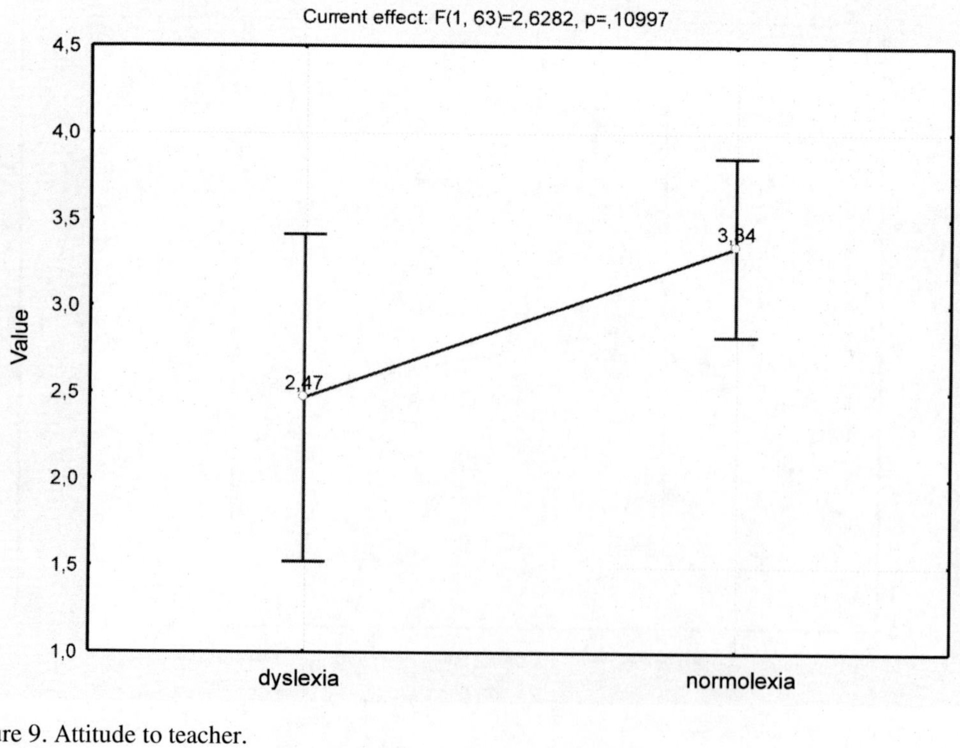

Figure 9. Attitude to teacher.

For this variable there is a statistically significant difference $p = 0.009$ at a critical level of significance $\alpha = 0{,}05$. The average scores for the two groups differ significantly and they are respectively for dyslexics X = 4.33 and for normolexics – X = 6.90. This result gives reasons to believe that a person with dyslexia is more distant and detached in regard to friends compared to someone without the disorder.

For that variable there is no significant difference regarding the average scores of the two groups as for dyslexics the score is X = 2.47 and for normolexics - X = 3.34. The score for $p = 0.11$ at a critical level of significance $\alpha = 0{,}05$ shows that there is no statistically significant difference between the groups with and without dyslexia. In that way it has been established that the results for the control variable give evidence to reject the hypothesis that there is a difference on attitude to teacher between the two groups.

After analyzing the results on the scale curiosity, no statistically significant difference ($p = 0{,}22$) was established between the two variables. It can clearly be noticed the insignificant difference between the average scores of the two groups, for participants with dyslexia X = 5,07 and for normal participants X = 4,36.

On the next Figure 11 the results for the variable "dominance" are presented.

Like the previous variable, this one does not show statistically significant difference between the results for the two groups of participants. Since $p = 0{,}86$, therefore, no significant difference is observed between the average scores of the group with dyslexia (X = 1.47) and the normal group (X = 1.52).

The next Figure 12 presents the results on the scale "sociability" for the two groups of participants.

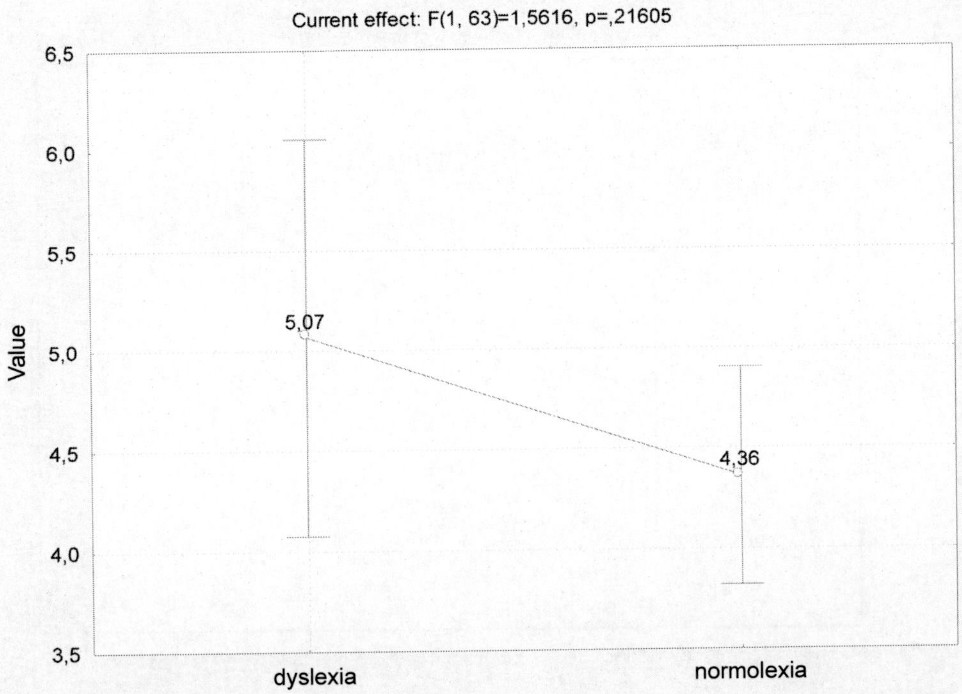

Figure 10. Curiosity.

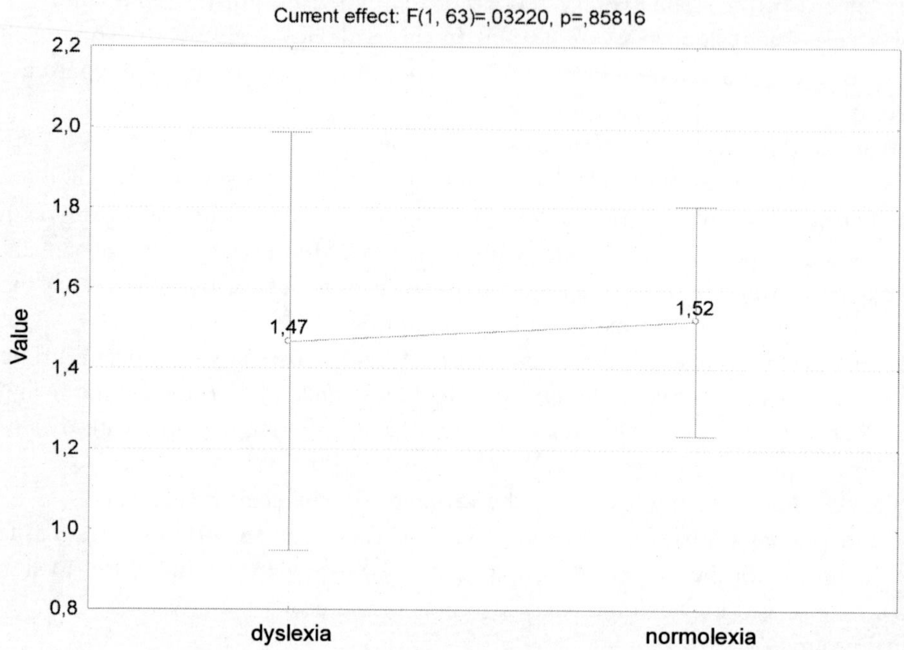

Figure 11. Dominance.

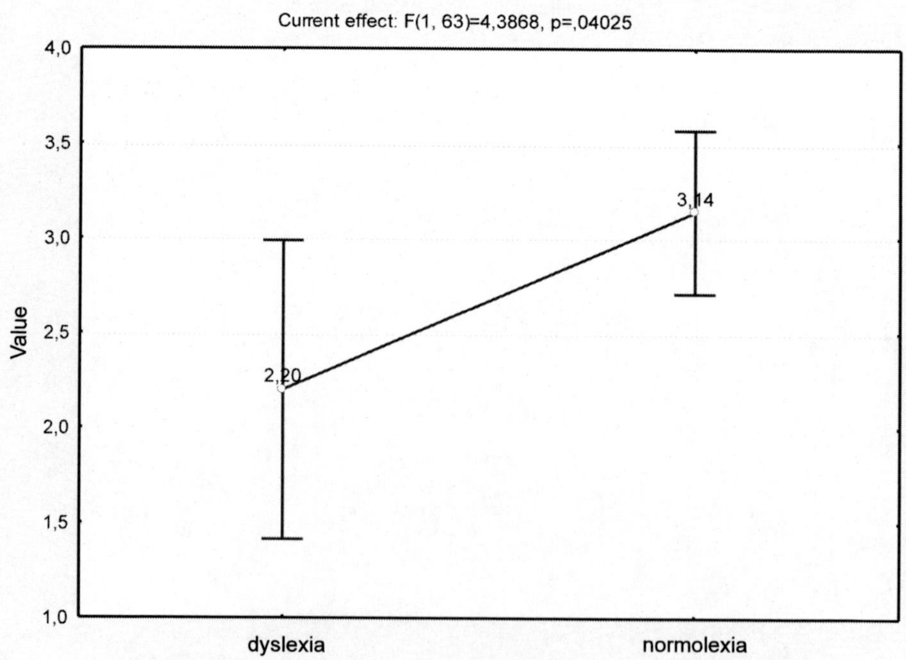

Figure 12. Sociability.

For this variable there is a difference regarding the average scores of the two groups of participants, as for dyslexics it is X = 2,20 and for normolexics it is X = 3,14. The resulting value to test the statistical significance is $p = 0{,}04$ at a critical level of significance $\alpha = 0{,}05$. This score supports the hypothesis that children with dyslexia experience problems when they communicate with peers.

The next Figure 13 presents the results for the two groups on the scale "detachment."

For the scale "detachment" there is a difference in the results of the two groups.

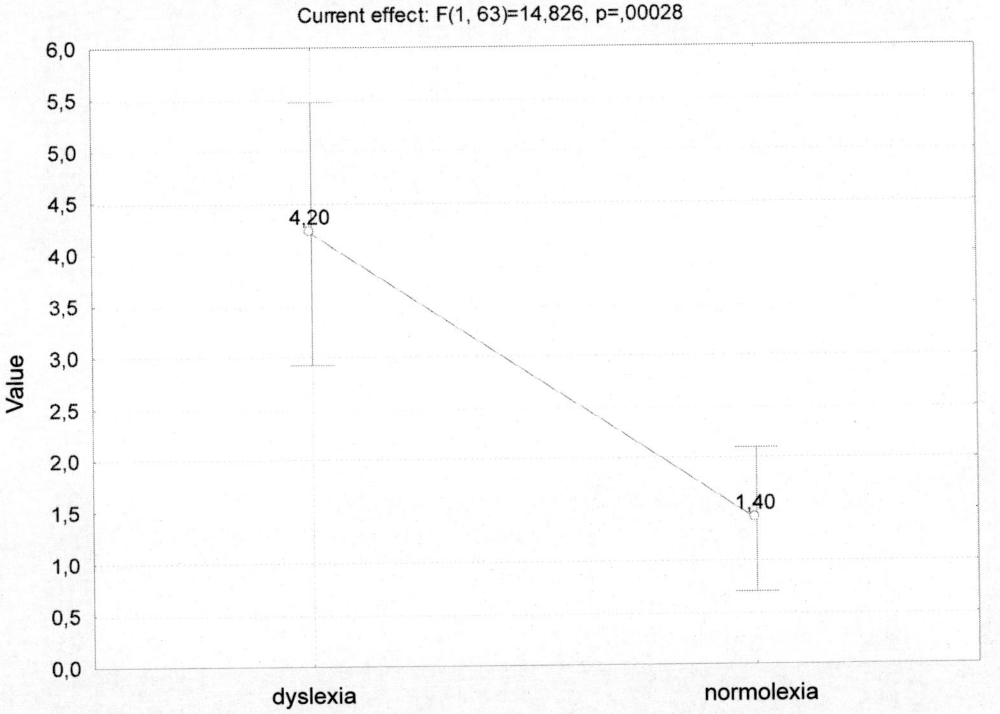

Figure 13. Detachment.

The average score of the participants with dyslexia is X = 4,20 and for the participants without dyslexia – X = 1,40, $p = 0{,}000$. It is evident that the group with dyslexia extends to higher values than the control group. This result can be interpreted in the light that the experimental group shows a tendency for detachment compared to the control group.

Here are the results on the scale "social adequacy".

As it was assumed this variable shows statistically significant difference between the results of the two groups with $p = 0{,}005$. There is a significant difference between the average scores for dyslexics and normolexics, the obtained score is respectively – 3,20 and 5,28. This difference shows that the participants with dyslexia experience difficulties in their social adaptation compared to the normal participants.

Figure 15 presents the results on the scale "Aggression."

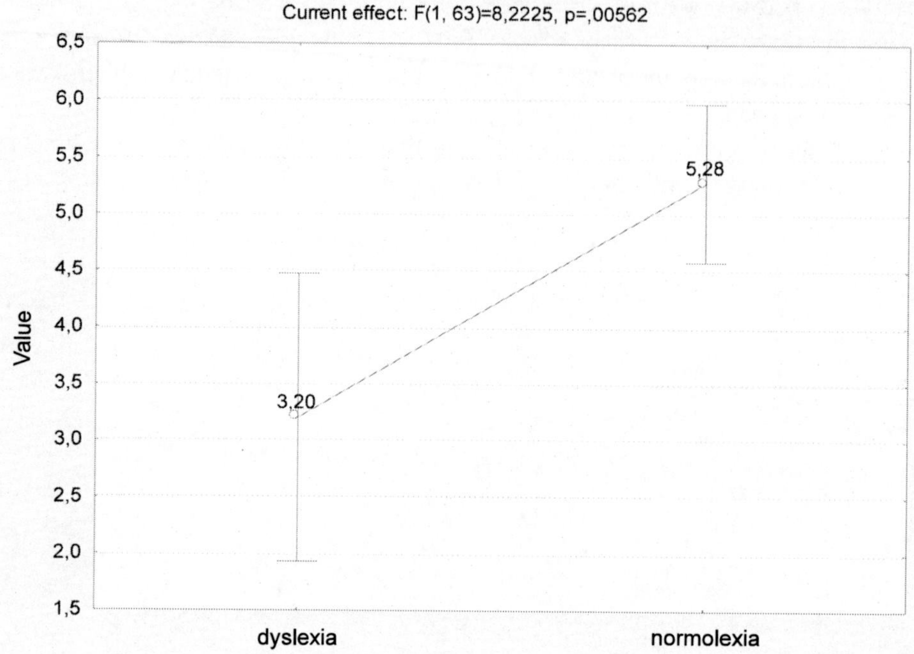

Figure 14. Social adequacy.

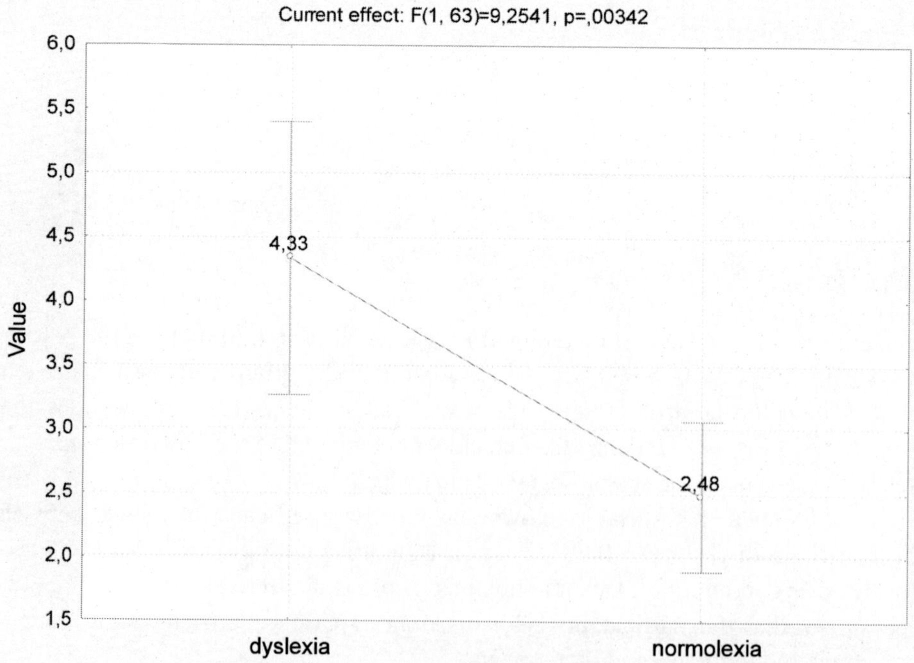

Figure 15. Aggression.

After an analysis of the variable "Aggression" statistically significant differences between the results of the two groups were established. Interesting about Figure 15 is the fact that the score of the participants with dyslexia is significantly higher than the one of the normal group. This means that dyslexics demonstrate a higher level of aggression compared to normolexics. This result is also confirmed by the average scores of the two groups. For participants with dyslexia it is 4,33, and for the control group – 2,48, $p = 0{,}003$.

After analyzing the results of the participants using the methodology by Renee Jill two independent variables were identified – family and personality characteristics in children with and without dyslexia.

The results for the scale "family" are presented on Figure 16.

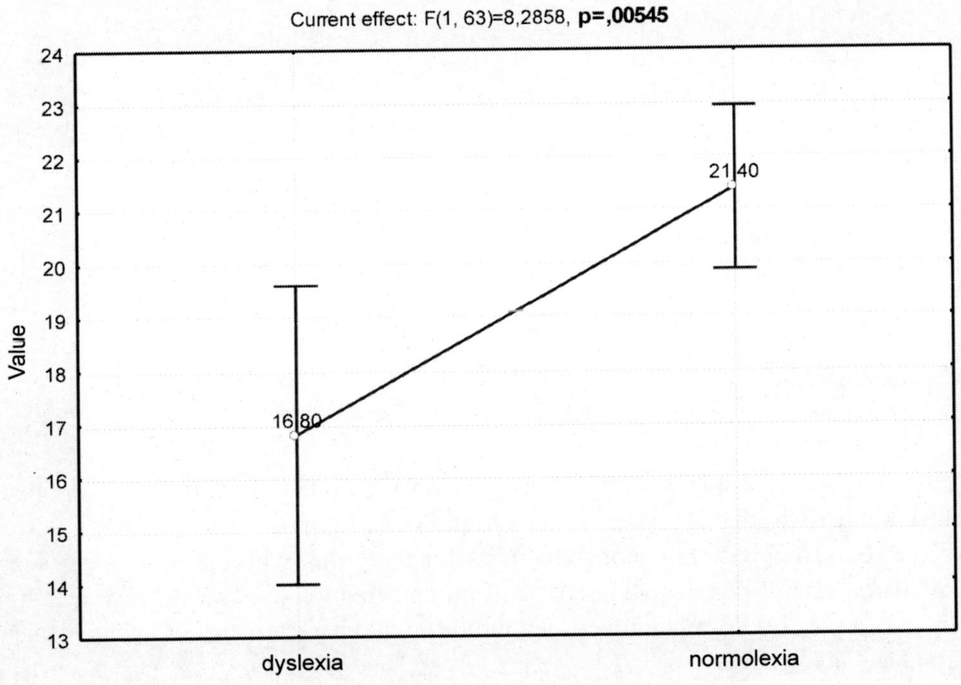

Figure 16. Family.

Figure 16 clearly shows that the attitude of the participants with dyslexia and that of the normal participants differs significantly. Gathering and analyzing the data from the four scales using the methodology of Renee Jill it can be concluded that the attitude of dyslexics towards their family is more detached. It is noticeable that the highest score of the children with dyslexia is lower than the lowest score of children without dyslexia. The significant difference between the two groups is confirmed by the comparison of the two average scores for the groups, for dyslexics it is 16,80, and for normolexics – 21,40. The analysis of the results for this variable showed a statistically significant difference between the two groups, $p = 0{,}005$.

This empirical research gives evidence to suggest the presence of differences regarding the characteristics of attention and psychosocial functioning in pupils with and without dyslexia. The established differences refer to:

1. Characteristics of attention
   - Attention range
   - Attention switching
   - Concentration of attention
   - Attention stability

2. Psychosocial functioning
   - Attitude to family
   - Attitude to friends
   - Sociability
   - Detachment
   - Social adequacy
   - Aggression

No difference between the two groups of participants was found for the following variables:

1. Attention distribution
2. Attention quality when processing linguistic and nonlinguistic stimuli
3. Attitude to sibling
4. Attitude to teacher
5. Curiosity
6. Dominance

The study has a within group design to which a correlation analysis was applied with variables - the five characteristics of attention which purpose was to find a correlation between three verbal and three nonverbal tests for the group with dyslexia. After analyzing the data it was established that all coefficients on the attention tests are positive which means that there is a positive correlation between the different characteristics of attention measured by verbal and nonverbal tests.

This means that children who have demonstrated low levels of attention on the verbal tests, have also demonstrated low levels of attention on the nonverbal tests. This finding gives evidence to reject the hypothesis that for participants with dyslexia there would be a difference in attention when processing linguistic versus nonlinguistic stimuli.

The latter part was designed as an experiment aiming at finding out whether the presence of dyslexia has an effect on the psychosocial functioning. A between group design was used with an independent and dependent variable. For testing that hypothesis the semi-projective test by Renee Jill was used to investigate the family and social relationships of the participants.

A multivariate analysis was conducted to establish the effect of the factor status for the participants on all variables simultaneously – attitude to family; attitude to sibling; attitude to friends; attitude to teacher; curiosity; dominance; sociability; detachment; social adequacy; and aggression. Significant difference was found in six of the ten scales – attitude to family, attitude to friends, sociability, detachment, social adequacy and aggression. After analyzing the results on scale "family" a statistically significant difference was found between the two groups. For both ends (lower, upper) the obtained scores for participants with dyslexia are significantly lower than the ones for normal controls. This means that participants with dyslexia exhibit a more detached attitude toward the family system. This result can be a due to the fact that parents of children with such a problem consider their children lazy, stupid and naughty. This in turn influences the formation of the level of expectations which facilitates the formation of self-esteem, social adequacy and adaptation abilities to cope with the changing environment. The adequate coping with everyday responsibilities, interactions with peers and adults, and perception and processing of emotions are strongly influenced by a number of family factors like family structure, models of interactions between the members of the family, type and way of dividing the roles in the family, family norms and values and family coalitions.

Family as a foundation for childhood development plays a leading role in the process of socialization of the child. However, gradually during the process of his development other factors start influencing this process – school, peers, and friends. It is interesting that the results on the two variables – "detachment" and "sociability" are very similar, i.e., the same tendency is observed on the two scales for children with and without dyslexia. The main source of anxiety at school is the fear of failure which leads to lowered self-esteem. It is very likely for children with low achievements to feel more anxious at school. This has an effect on the characteristics of attention which in turn influences task performance. The emotional tension has a strong negative effect on the adaptation of children to school life and leads to disturbances in communication with peers, detachment and behavior of poor social adequacy. There are different objective factors which might prevent the child from showing his real abilities at the beginning and gradually obtaining the status of being unsuccessful. The results give evidence to believe that participants with dyslexia show low scores on the scale "social adequacy" and high scores on the scale "aggression." Since these scales measure basic personality aspects of psychosocial functioning, it follows the hypothesis that there is a positive correlation between those two variables – "social adequacy" and "aggression" and they can be used to outline the type of interpersonal relationships of the child the way he or she perceives and experiences them.

Emotional reactions can be manifested in many different forms – conscious refusal to study, overt hostility, negative attitude to school, disobedience, extreme distractability and closing in one's own inner world. These emotional and social problems can lead to detachment from peers. After analyzing the scores on the scale "attitude to friends" a similar tendency is discovered – lower scores for the participants with dyslexia compared to the ones without dyslexia. The reason for that result can be explained by the fact that a person with dyslexia perceives the world around him as rejecting and charged with tension. The interaction with peers is an important factor which complements the everyday life of the child and helps the formation of knowledge about the self, the world and others, of the sense of belongingness and maintenance of self-respect. Dissatisfaction from the contact with people around has an impact on the self-esteem of the person with dyslexia and often he closes in himself realizing that he is unable to win approval and support and to prove himself in a new environment.

For the variables – "attitude to sibling", "attitude to teacher," "curiosity", and "dominance" there is no statistically significant difference between children with and without dyslexia.

For the scale "curiosity" there is no significant difference between the average scores for the two groups. It is interesting that the results of the participants with dyslexia are higher than the ones for the control group. For the last two scales "attitude to teacher" and "dominance" no significant difference between the two groups is observed. From a theoretical point of view it is believed that the personality characteristics of a person with dyslexia are due to secondary symptoms. In each stage of psychosocial development of the individual there are specific tasks that need to be addressed in such a way so as to enter a higher developmental stage. Otherwise, there is a higher risk that a number of external and internal factors will exert a negative influence on the personality of the individual including dysfunctional beliefs, lack of motivation for change and inability to account for reality.

References

Ainsworth, M. (1985). Patterns of attachment. *Clinical Psychologist, 38,* 27-29.

Ainsworth, M. (1993). Attachment as related to mother-infant interaction. *Advances in Infancy Research*, 8.

Bowlby, J. (1958). The nature of the child's tie to his mother. *The International Journal of Psychoanalysis*, 39.

Bowlby, J. (1978). Attachment theory and its therapeutic implications. *Adolescent Psychiatry,* 6.

Bowlby, J. (1983). Attachment and loss: Retrospect and prospect. *American Journal of Orthopsychiatry,* 52.

Brodie, R. (2008). Mary Ainsworth and Attachment Theory. *Child Development Media*. Retrieved from: http://www.childdevelopmentmedia.com/mary-ainsworth-and attachment-theory.html

DeWall, C. N., Lambert, N. M., Slotter, E. B., Pond, R. S., Deckman, T., Finkel, E. J., Luchies, L. B., & Finchman, F. D. (2011). So far away from one's partner, yet so close to romantic alternatives: Avoidant attachment, interest in alternatives, and infidelity. *Journal of Personality and Social Psychology,* 101.

Harms, P. D. (2011). Adult attachment styles in the workplace. *Human Resource Management Review, 21.*Main, M., & Goldwyn, R. (1994). Adult Attachment Rating and Classification System, Manual in Draft, Version 6.0. Unpublished manuscript: University of California at Berkeley.

Main, M., Kaplan, N., & Cassidy, J. (1985). Security in infancy, childhood and adulthood: A move to the level of representation. In I. Bretherton & E. Waters (Eds.), Growing Points of Attachment Theory and Research. Monographs of the Society for Research in Child Development (Vol. 50). Chicago: Chicago University Press.

Mcleod, S. (2007). Bowlby Attachment Theory. *Simply Psychology*. Retrieved from:http:// www.simplypsychology.org/bowlby.html

Mcleod, S. (2008). Mary Ainsworth-Strange Situation. *Simply Psychology*. Retrieved from: http://www.simplypsychology.org/mary-ainsworth.html

Mcleod, S. (2009). Attachment. *Simply Psychology*. Retrieved from: http://www. simplypsychology.org/bowlby.html

Natarajan, G., Somasundaram, C. P., & Sundaram, K. R. (2011). Relationship between attachment security and rejection sensitivity in early adolescence. *Psychological Studies,* 56.

Schultheis, E. (2009). Attachment Security: Born or Made?. *Psychology Today.* Retrieved from: http://www.psychologytoday.com/blog/family-affair/200901/ attachment security-born-or-made

Slough, N. M., & Greenberg, M. T. (1990). 5-year-olds' representations of separations from parents: Responses from the perspective of self and other. *New Directions for Child Development*, 48.

Solomon, J., George, C., & Dejong, A. (1995). Children classified as controlling at age six: Evidence of disorganized representational strategies and aggression at home and at school. *Development and Psychopathology*, 7.

Sroufe, L. A., Fox, N., & Pancake, V. (1983). Attachment and dependency in developmental perspective. *Child Development*, 54.

Wright, J. C., Binney, V., & Smith, P. K. (1995). Security of attachment in 8-22 year olds: A revised version of the Separation Anxiety Test, its psychometric properties and clinical interpretation. *Journal of Child Psychology and Psychiatry*, 36.

Zlatka, C. (2011). Relation between children's attachment to kindergarten teachers, personality characteristics and play activities. *Early Child Development and Care*, 18.

II. Diagnostic Issues in Clinical Psychology

In: New Developments in Clinical Psychology Research ISBN: 978-1-63483-223-6
Editors: D. St. Stoyanov and R.-D. Stieglitz

Chapter 4

ATTENTIONAL LAPSES AS A TRANSDIAGNOSTIC FACTOR TO TARGET TREATMENT IN MENTAL HEALTH DISORDERS: THE ROLE OF MINDFULNESS TRAINING

Sørensen Lin[1,2*], Osnes Berge[1,3], Binder Per Einar[4] and Schanche Elisabeth[4]

[1]Department of Biological and Medical Psychology, University of Bergen, Bergen, Norway
[2]K. G. Jebsen Center for Research on Neuropsychiatric Disorders, Bergen, Bergen, Norway
[3]Bjørgvin District Psychiatric Centre, Haukeland University Hospital, Bergen, Norway
[4]Department of Clinical Psychology, University of Bergen, Bergen, Norway

ABSTRACT

In contemporary clinical practice, treatment for individuals with mental health disorders is predominantly based on diagnostic categories. This practice, however, does not always ensure the best treatment for each individual patient.

A number of patients do not respond to or benefit fully from current treatments.

In response to this challenge, it has been suggested that treatments should address factors involved in distress and dysfunction across disorders (Barlow, Allen, & Choate 2004; Farchione et al. 2012; Clark 2009; Harvey 2008).

One such transdiagnostic factor is cognitive functioning. Across mental health disorders, psychopathology associates with attentional lapses. Compared to healthy controls, self-generated thought processes in mental health disorders seem to interfere with goal-orienting task-processing (i.e., cognitive control).

* Address all correspondance to: Dr. Lin Sørensen, Department of Biological and Medical Psychology, University of Bergen, Norway, lin.sorensen@psybp.uib.no.

This is supported by hyperactivation of the default mode brain network (DMN) interrupting target processing (Hanna-Andrews, Smallwood, & Spreng 2014; Whitfield-Gabrieli & Ford 2012) and with high behavioral variability on cognitive tests (Kaiser et al. 2008; Tamm et al. 2012).

Treatment targeting enhancement of the ability to sustain attention by reducing the level of attentional lapses, may therefore mediate better cognitive control functions, which may further lead the way to improved emotion regulation abilities. We will exemplify how mindfulness training can enhance the ability to sustain attention and act as a mediator in improving cognitive control functions and thereby normalize brain activation in patients with recurrent depression.

First, we will provide a background for why a focus on transdiagnostic factors in targeting treatment is needed, followed by a discussion of how commonalities in cognitive functioning can comprise one such transdiagnostic factor. Second, we will provide an overview of research showing that a high level of attentional lapses is a common trait across mental health disorder samples.

Third, we will suggest mindfulness training as one treatment that can enhance the ability to sustain attention, with emphasis on how such training may affect brain functions in patients with a depressive disorder. Fourth and finally, we will propose future directions for conducting research targeting sustained attention as an outcome measure,, and we will present data from a group of healthy adults on the relationship between mindfulness training and behavioral attention lapses.

Transdiagnostic Perspectives in Treatment of Mental Health Disorders: Attentional Lapses a Common Cognitive Problem

Transdiagnostic Perspectives

For approximately five decades, the predominant trend in clinical psychotherapy practice has been to target treatment to specific categories of mental health disorders (Barlow et al. 2004). Basing treatment on specific diagnostic categories can be challenging for practitioners in clinical psychological practice to implement. To become competent in the implementation of a given treatment protocol that targets a specific diagnostic disorder requires a substantial amount of training. Therefore, each clinician can only competently master a limited number of protocols (Barlow et al. 2004). Moreover, a large number of patients within the mental health field enter psychotherapy with symptoms qualifying for more than a single disorder. There is considerable overlap between the different diagnoses of mental health disorders in that individuals with one mental health disorder often have other comorbid mental health disorders or a high co-occurring symptom load from another mental health problem (Jacobi et al. 2004). One response to these challenges, which is the focus of this chapter, is a shift of focus from the unique nosology of each mental health disorder to common nosological factors across disorders (Barlow et al. 2004; Fairchione et al. 2012; Clark 2009; Harvey 2008).

Cognitive Dysfunctions Comprising Transdiagnostic Factors: Attentional Lapses

Cognitive dysfunctions may be promising transdiagnostic factors as targets of treatment across mental health disorders. Mental health disorders associates with cognitive dysfunctions. In particular, attention functions are often poorer in such disorder samples compared to healthy controls. A growing body of research shows consistently higher occurrence of attentional lapses as measured with brain activation patterns as well as behaviorally with cognitive tasks in individuals with mental health disorders (Hanna-Andrews et al. 2014; Whitfield-Gabrieli & Ford 2012). Attentional lapses lead to a poorer ability in sustaining attention accompanied by a tendency to be distracted from goal-oriented behavior (i.e., cognitive control processing; Miller & Cohen 2001). Attention allocation and the ability to sustain attention thus facilitate cognitive control in supplying the needed attentional resources for effortful processing (Fan, McCandliss, Fosella, Flombaum, & Posner 2005).

Cognitive control functions play an important role in regulating emotional processes (Ochsner & Gross 2005). One such function, cognitive reappraisal, makes an individual reinterpret the meaning of a stimulus or situation that elicits emotions. Such a stimulus can comprise self-generated maladaptive thoughts, such as the typical tendency to ruminate in patients with recurrent depression (Paul, Stanton, Greeson, Smoski, & Wang 2013). Cognitive control dysfunctions, such as limited abilities to flexibly adjust to changing context (i.e., cognitive flexibility), to inhibit maladaptive thought patterns (i.e., rumination; inhibitory control), and/or to allocate attentional resources to actively maintain information needed to achieve desired behavior (i.e., working memory) (Miyake et al. 2000), hinders the use of cognitive reappraisal in the process of emotional regulation. In depressive patients, this creates a vicious circle where the rumination tends to cause lack of cognitive control, otherwise needed to suppress the tendency to ruminate (Wagner et al. 2008). Multiple brain networks and trajectories between different areas of the brain are involved in the interplay between cognitive control and emotional processing (Etkin, Egner, & Kalisch 2011). For instance, in disorders of anxiety and depression, research shows an abnormal activation compared to healthy controls in the brain areas of the medial prefrontal cortex (mPFC; i.e., ventro mPFC and anterior cingulate cortex, ACC) and limbic structures (i.e., amygdala) (Drevets 2000; Ressler & Mayberg 2007). These activation patterns in the brain represent the dynamic interaction between regulation functions of cognitive control and emotional processing (Bush, Luu, & Posner 2000; Etkin et al. 2011). Thus, the cognitive control dysfunctions may manifest differently in behavioral expression and may also interplay differently with emotional processing across the disorders. Heterogeneous cognitive control profiles between and within mental health disorders (Bora, Harrison, Yücel, & Pantelis 2013; Joyce, Hutton, Mutsata, & Barnes 2005; Willcutt et al. 2005) make it challenging to target treatment to one specific cognitive control dysfunction. For instance, working memory training is an example of a treatment that targets cognitive control dysfunctions. Research shows this to be a successful approach only in small subgroups of patient groups (see Jacoby & Ahissor 2013; Melby-Lervåg & Hulme 2013; Onraedt & Koster 2014; Sonuga-Barke, Brandeis, Holtmann, & Cortese 2014). The common problem with frequent attentional lapses across disorders may thus constitute a more promising cognitive transdiagnostic factor as a target of treatment, or at least represent an alternative target of treatment to cognitive control dysfunctions. Enhancing the ability to sustain attention may mediate better cognitive control functioning and emotion regulation abilities.

Advancing a New Model

The overlap between mental health disorders and common nosological factors across mental health disorders points to the possibility of targeting treatment in a transdiagnostic perspective. In light of the importance of cognitive functions for mental well-being, common nosological cognitive traits may be one promising criteria as a target of treatment. We suggest attentional lapses to be such a transdiagnostic cognitive factor. In the next section, we will describe literature supporting this view.

Attentional Lapses in Mental Health Disorders: An Emphasis on Attentional Lapses Due to Rumination in Recurrent Depression

The Intrinsic Default Mode (DMN) Brain Network and Self-Generated Thought Processes

In our daily life, we need to focus on external tasks/stimuli intermittently with making internal reconstructions and evaluations of our experiences and memories. On a brain level, this intermittent alternation between an external and an internal focus in thought processes is reflected in the description of the reciprocal relationship between task-positive activation of brain networks related to cognitive control functions (i.e., fronto-parietal and cingulo-opercular networks: Dosenbach, Faire, Cohen, Schlaggar, & Petersen 2007; executive control network: Raichle 2011), and spontaneous activation of the intrinsic default mode brain network (Raichle et al. 2001; Shulman et al. 1997). The DMN is described as engaging in intrinsic modes of cognition in relation to memory retrieval, in visualizing future events, and in perceiving the perspectives of others (Buckner, Andrews-Hanna, & Schacter 2008; Sheline et al. 2009). This intrinsic network consists of the brain areas of dorsal and ventral mPFC, posterior cingulate cortex, precuneus, and medial and lateral parietal cortex, and parts of the medial and lateral temporal cortices (Raichle et al. 2001; Fox & Raichle 2007). The DMN is often referred to as a resting-state network as it is activated when individuals are not exposed to external stimuli or focusing on external cognitive tasks (Dosenbach et al. 2006; Mazoyer et al. 2001; Raichle et al. 2001; Shannon, Snyder, Vincent & Buckner 2006; Shulman et al., 1997). In such resting-states the DMN areas connect with each other (Greicius, Krasnow, Reiss, & Menon 2003; Greicius & Menon 2004). However, when an external stimulus is presented or when external focus is required, such as when performing cognitive tasks, the DMN is deactivated. DMN is thus said to be spontaneous and anti-correlated with active task processing (Kelly, Uddin, Biswal, Castellanos, & Milham 2008). The level of deactivation of the DMN seems to depend on the cognitive load of a task. For instance, the DMN appears to deactivate more when performing tasks with higher cognitive control load (see Broyd et al. 2009 and Whitfield-Gabrieli & Ford 2012. The reciprocal relationship between DMN activation and task-positive activation is suggested to have an adaptive role in that the activation of the DMN may ensure a mental state of alertness, preparing the brain for a quick shift in attention focus from internal thought processes to external goal-oriented processes (i.e., cognitive control processing) (Baird, Smallwood, & Schooler 2011; Sonuga-Barke & Castellanos 2007). It also seems that the DMN may be activated in goal-oriented processing when performing tasks that require internal self-generated processing (Andrews-Hanna 2012; Buckner et al. 2008). Such self-generated thought-processes include retrieving episodic autobiographical memories, mentalizing future events or the states of other peoples, or solving dilemmas or reevaluating emotional information. The activation of the DMN in relation to self-generated thought-processes may also have an adaptive role in reconstructing experiences relevant for future plans, in regulating social interactions, and in utilizing moments when there is no need of an external focus (Andrews-Hanna, Smallwood, & Spreng 2014; Buckner et al. 2008; Sheline et al. 2009).

Self-Generated Thought Processes and Attentional Lapses in Mental Health Disorders

The pattern and frequency of self-generated thoughts vary between individuals in functional outcome. However, maladaptive self-generated thought processes seem to characterize the psychopathology in mental health disorders (see review of Philippi & Koenigs 2014 and of Hanna-Andrews et al. 2014). This maladaptive pattern in internal thought processes can relate both to the content of the thought processes and to the frequency with which these thought processes occur. Across mental health disorders, it is the frequency of self-generated thought processes that seems to be the common problem (Hanna-Andrews et al. 2014). The tendency of falling into internal modes of thinking distracts the individual from task performance and goal-oriented behavior. This creates attentional lapses that encompass variable cognitive control and attention functioning over a sustained time period. However, in patients with depressive disorders, especially in patients with recurrent depression, the content of the self-generated thought processes also seems to be disrupted. The tendency to ruminate over past experiences, or over a perceived lack of future positive events may dominate the cognitive processing to such an extent, that it hinders the ability to flexibly shift between an external and internal mode of thought processing.

Attentional Lapses in Mental Health Disorders: DMN Activation Interrupts Cognitive Control Processes

In healthy adults, the DMN is interrupted when active task processing is required. Increased DMN activation associates in healthy samples with increased error responses (Eichele et al. 2008) and increased reaction time variability on cognitive control task processing (Weismann, Roberts, Visscher, & Woldorff 2006). This activation of the DMN while performing cognitive control tasks may represent a shift from an external mode of focus to an internal mode (Mason et al. 2007). Such a shift of focus will then act as a distraction from the attention focus on the external task at hand. Attentional lapses will likely occur with increased error rates and slower responses, which contribute to high intra-individual variability in reaction time in task performance (Broyd et al. 2009; Buckner et al. 2008; Sonuga-Barke & Castellanos 2007). Hyperactivation and hyperconnectivity of the DMN are typically found in mental health disorders compared to healthy controls (see Hanna-Andrews et al. 2014). Increased DMN activiation is shown to interrupt task processing in ADHD (Fassbender et al. 2009), depression (Berman et al. 2011: Sheline et al. 2009; see also Whitfield-Gabrieli & Ford 2012), and schizophrenia (Fryer et al. 2013; Landin-Romero et al. 2014; see also Whitfield-Gabrieli & Ford 2012). Furthermore, higher intra-variability in reaction times is observed foremost in relation to ADHD (see Tamm et al. 2012), but also in schizophrenia (Kaiser et al. 2008; Shin et al. 2013), depression, and borderline personality disorder (Kaiser et al. 2008). Self-reported self-generated thought processes associate with higher DMN activation, dominating task-positive activation levels (see Hanna-Andrews et al. 2014), also shown in patients with a major depressive disorder in relation to self-reported rumination (Hamilton et al. 2011). See Figure 1 illustrating the relationship between self-generated thought-processes and cognitive control functions, and how these self-generated thought processes disturb the cognitive control functioning in regulating ruminative thought processes in depressive patients.

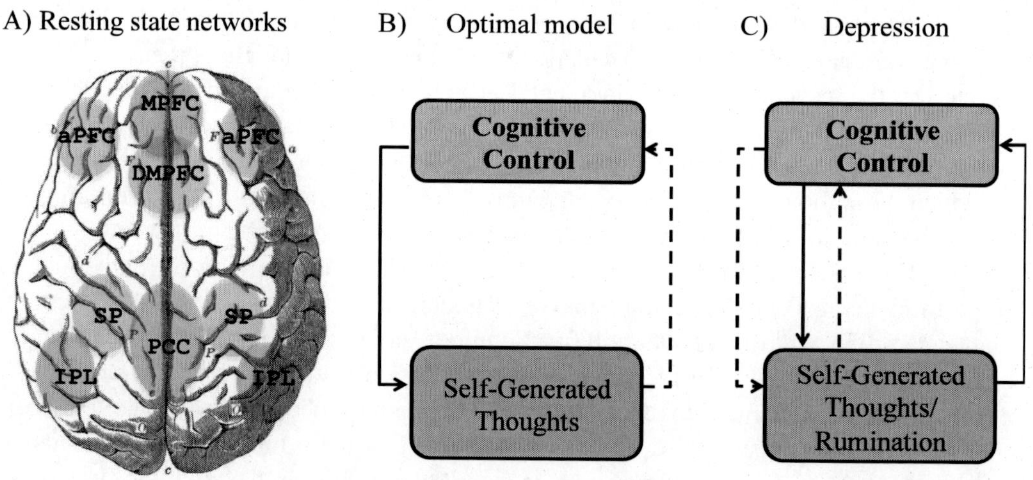

Figure 1. A) A substratal representation of the two brain networks; The Default Mode Network, represented by blue, and the Executive Control Network (i.e., cognitive control), represented by brown. aPFC = anterior prefrontal cortex, DMPFC = dorsal medial prefrontal cortex, IPL = inferior parietal lobule, MPFC = medial prefrontal cortex, PCC = posterior cingulate cortex, SP = superior parietal. B) A schematic representation of the optimal relationship between self-generative thought processes and cognitive control functioning, characterized by cognitive control regulation of intrinsic thought processes and C) A model showing the same relationship in patients with depression, where the self-generative thought processes interrupts cognitive control processing. The dotted line indicates that the interruption of cognitive control processes leads to a decreased regulation of the frequency and content of the self-generative thought processes. The blue line denote our suggestion of mindfulness training to improve the ability to sustain attention, which then lead to a decrease in self-generative thought processes interrupting cognitive control processing.

Mindfulness Training Targeting High Levels of Attentional Lapses

In summary, the intermittent shifts between activation and deactivation of the DMN, probably reflecting the dynamic shifts in modes of external and internal attention focus, seem to be dysfunctional in samples of mental health disorders compared to healthy control samples. For instance, the tendency in depressive patients to ruminate over negative thoughts and feelings seems to activate the DMN to interfere with goal-orienting control processing (Sheline et al. 2009). The occurrence of these attentional lapses may hinder cognitive control functions from suppressing these negative ruminative thought processes. Mindfulness training is suggested to be one treatment that may alter maladaptive thought processes, such as the ruminative tendencies of depressive patients, and thereby reduce the occurrence of DMN activation to interrupt with control processing (Hanna-Andrews et al. 2014). The UK National Institute of Health and Clinical Excellence (NICE) recommends one form of a manualized clinical oritented mindfulness training program, the Mindfulness Based Cognitive Therapy (MBCT) for treatment of recurrent depression (National Institute for Health and Clinical Excellence 2009).

A Goal in Mindfulness-Training to Increase Awareness and Regulation of Self-Generated Thought Processes: Reducing Ruminative Thought Processes in Recurrent Depression

Mindfulness-Training (MBCT)

Mindfulness can be defined as “the awareness that emerges through paying attention on purpose, in the present moment, and non-judgmentally to the unfolding experience moment-by-moment” (Kabat-Zinn 2003). Varying focus of attention is used in meditation practices with the goal to strengthen the capacity for mindful awareness. One such focus of meditation is the awareness of bodily sensations, such as the sensation of one’s breath. Extended focus on the breath is used as an anchor to develop both the ability to maintain a focused attention over time, and the ability to become aware when one’s attention wanders to other stimuli, such as thought processes. Training in maintaining a specific focus of attention (i.e., breath, physical sensations, sound) and gently returning awareness to this concrete focus each time one’s attention wanders is assumed to increase the awareness and regulation of internal thought processes (Bishop et al. 2004). The training in sustaining attention is thus suggested to improve the allocation of attentional resources (Malinowski 2013), which facilitates effortful cognitive processing (see Figure 1).

MBCT is a manualized eight-week group program aimed at raising awareness of negative ruminative thought processes in patients with recurrent depression. The theoretical foundation is that depressive lapses occur due to automatic negative self-generative thought processes hindering flexible cognitive and emotional functioning.

In MBCT, mindfulness practices (i.e., meditation techniques), in combination with psychoeducation, are used to break the vicious circle of ruminative thought processes fueling depressive moods. A central goal is to learn to become aware of and experience negative thoughts and feelings with an attitude of acceptance so that negative thoughts and feelings can be cognitively reappraised and thereby not be followed by an emotional stress reaction. By experiencing difficult thoughts and feelings with a non-judgmental attitude is thought to increase the individual's ability to tolerate these without automatically starting a ruminative cycle. Staying in touch with difficult emotions without judging this experience contains an element of exposure that may possibly also contribute to increased emotional tolerance. Through such mindfulness training, patients with recurrent depression can learn to take control over their self-generative thought processes.

Mindfulness-Training, Attention Functions and DMN Activation

MBCT is shown to have a positive effect in decreasing symptoms of depression and rumination (Kuyken et al. 2010) and in preventing relapses of depression (Kuyken et al. 2015). However, few studies have studied the effect of mindfulness training in depressive patients with psychophysiological measures. As far as we know, the scarcity of studies also encompasses a lack of studies using the level of attentional lapses as measured with DMN activation patterns and variable reaction times on cognitive tests as effect measures. One study, however, reports positive effects of MBCT in bipolar patients with increases in brain activation level in the mPFC and posterior parietal lobe during a mindfulness task (Ives-Deliperi, Howells, Stein, Meintjes, & Horn 2013). These brain areas are part of the DMN. Also, the same study found that the MBCT enhanced the working memory capacity in the bipolar patients. In another study of MBCT in adult ADHD, event-related potentials (ERP) were recorded during performance on a continuous performance test (Schoenberg et al. 2014). Increased amplitude in the components of Pe and NoGo-P3 following MBCT indicated effects in the ADHD sample of a less "restless" brain. The ERP P3 component is associated with attention allocation and the ability to sustain attention (Stevens, Pearlson, & Kiehl 2007). A pilot study of mindfulness training in adult ADHD found positive effects on both self-reported and performance-based measure of cognitive control functions (Mitchell et al. in press). Furthermore, several studies indicate a positive effect of meditation practice on brain activation level (Brefzzynski-Lewis, Lutz, Schaefer, Levinson, & Davidson 2007), including in DMN areas of the brain (Hansenkamp, Wilson-Mendenhall, Duncan, & Barsalou 2012; Taylor et al. 2011).

The research on nosological factors endorse that attentional lapses as measured by the interaction between the DMN activation and task-positive activation are a common trait across mental health disorders. However, as far as we know, research on the effects of mindfulness training in mental health disorder samples seems not to have incorporated the same measures of attentional lapses as effect measures.

In light of our suggested new model, we advise a focus in future research on the relationship between DMN activation pattern and task-positive activation in the brain as an effect of mindfulness training. Attentional lapses can be measured behaviorally at the same time by including cognitive test that allows for calculating intra-individual reaction time variability. In this way, the ability to sustain attention can be assessed at two levels of brain function.

FUTURE DIRECTIONS FOR STUDYING LEVEL OF ATTENTIONAL LAPSES AS AN OUTCOME EFFECT OF MINDFULNESS TRAINING: THE RELATIONSHIP BETWEEN MINDFULNESS TRAINING AND ATTENTIONAL LAPSES IN A SAMPLE OF HEALTHY ADULTS

Future Directions

We argue in favor of applying experimental cognitive methods and advanced statistics in calculating attentional lapses. Traditional neuropsychological test measures are often included in studies using cognitive measures as an effect of treatment (i.e., effect of mindfulness in ADHD; Mitchell et al., in press). In such test measures, the error rates are typically used as a measure of attentional lapses (omission errors) which seldom follow normal distribution. Using test measures including a high number of trials where the reaction time is recorded on each trial, provides the opportunity to study a more statistically sound measure of attentional lapses than through error rates. Thus, moving the field of cognitive testing in effect studies of treatment towards more challenging methods and statistics will require cooperation between clinical psychologists and cognitive experimental psychologists. This also incorporates the possibility of including psychophysiology in combination with cognitive testing, such as neuroimaging techniques, which permit the study of the relationship between DMN activation levels and task-processing as an outcome effect of treatment. There may be effects of treatments that can be detected only through combining the expertise of clinical psychologists in diagnostic assessment and treatment with experimental psychologists' keen competence in cognitive and neurophysiological methods.

In the next section, we will illustrate how the level of attentional lapses can be used as an effect measure by calculating intra-individual variability in reaction time (IIV RT) on a cognitive test that contains a higher number of trials.

THE RELATIONSHIP BETWEEN 4 WEEKS MINDFULNESS TRAINING IN HEALTHY ADULTS AND LEVEL OF ATTENTIONAL LAPSES

We have run a pilot study on the effect of mindfulness training on attention functions in a group of 25 university students. The participants were 19 to 28 years old (mean age = 23.12, standard deviation = 2.03), and 15 of them were females. These students performed the revised attention network test (R-ANT) (Fan et al. 2009) before (pre-testing) and after (post-testing) they participated in a four-week course in mindfulness training. The r-ANT was run on a desktop PC. The participants were presented with a target stimulus (an arrow) in the center of a horizontal row of 5 distractor stimuli (identical arrows).

The instruction was to decide the direction of the center arrow by pressing a key with the index finger for the left direction and with the ring finger for the right direction on a mouse. The row of arrows appeared either on the left hand side of the screen or on the right hand side. A cue could be presented before the target appeared, indicated by flashing boxes (see Fan et al. 2009 for more details).

We will currently focus on the level of attentional lapses as measured with the intra-individual reaction time (IIV RT; standard deviation of the reaction time intra-participants) on the r-ANT. A high IIV RT indicates that a participant has a high frequency of occasional slow reaction times, which results in a variable reaction time pattern throughout the test. The r-ANT includes 288 trials. We included only accurate trials with a reaction time of 200 milliseconds and above. A total mean of the IIV RT for each participant was calculated from the pre- and post test sessions, respectively. In addition, we collapsed the four runs (each containing 72 trials) of the r-ANT into two test blocks, and IIV-RT was calculated for each of these two test blocks.

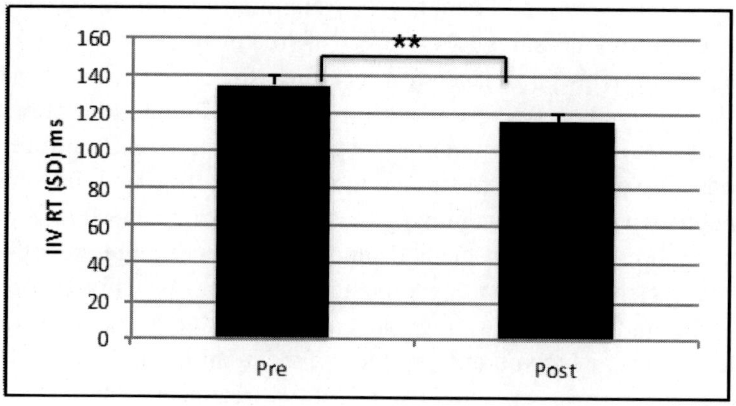

a

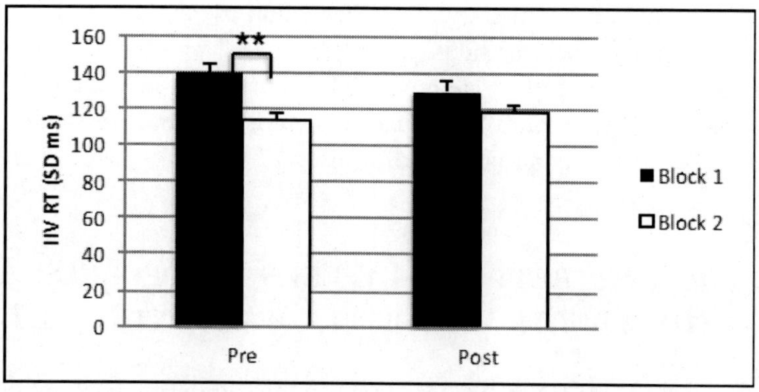

b

Note. ** $p < .01$. IIV RT = intra-individual variability in reaction time. The IIV RT was calculated with standard deviations (SD) for each participants in two blocks of the r-ANT.

Figure 2. The means of IIV RT from the r-ANT in pre- and post test sessions in a), and of the blocks 1 and 2 in the pre- and post test session in b).

Linear regression analyses were run, and the results showed that the level of IIV RT was explained neither by age nor by the sex of the participants. Furthermore, the pre-testing of IIV RT explained 38 percent of the variance of the post-testing IIV RT in relation to test blocks 1 of the r-ANT, and 34.6 percent of the post-testing IIV RT in the test blocks 2. Repeated univariate analysis (rANOVA) was conducted including the test blocks and the two test sessions as repeated variables (2 x 2 factorial design). The results showed a significant within main effect of test session ($F(1,24) = 26.26$; $p < .001$) and a significant within interaction effect between test session and test block ($F(1,24) = 8.41$; $p < .01$). Figure 2 a) shows the level of IIV RT decreasing from the pre test session to the post test session across all blocks. Figure 2 b) shows the mean scores of the IIV RT in each block in the pre- and the post test sessions, where there is a higher level of IIV RT in test block 1 in both test sessions. In addition, there is a larger decrease in IIV RT from test block 1 to test block 2 in the pre test session compared to in the post test session. Post-hoc paired t-tests revealed only a significant difference between test block 1 and 2 in the pre test session ($t(1,24) = 3.07$; $p < .01$) and not in the post session.

The results thus indicate that the mindfulness training had an effect in reducing the level of attentional lapses from the pre- to post test sessions in this pilot study. The level of attentional lapses as measured with IIV RT was highest in test block 1 in both test sessions, and the decrease in level of IIV RT from the pre- to the post testing appeared in test block 1 (see Figure 2 b). The r-ANT takes around 30 minutes to complete, and it seems like the effect of mindfulness training on reducing the level of attentional lapses appeared in the first 15 minutes of performing the r-ANT. However, it is important to note that the reduced level of IIV RT from the pre- to the post test session may be a result of a test practicing effect for which we cannot control in the absence of a control group.

This pilot study contained a small sample with no control group. The results still seemed to support the use of IIV RT as a measure of behaviorally attentional lapses in effect studies of treatment.

Considerations of the Mind-Brain Relationship in Advancing a New Model of Attentional Lapses as Target of Treatment

The use of common cognitive dysfunctions such as attentional lapses as target of treatment in mental health disorders imply that measures of brain activation and brain behavior can be transferred to real-life events. This has proven to be challenging, and the lack of relationship between clinical factors and brain measures of either neural or behavioral phenomena is therefore referred to as the "mind-brain problem" (Stoyanov, Stanghellini, & Broome 2012). This relates especially to the search for unique neural signatures of diagnostic categories, which has proven to produce inconsistent findings (e.g., Gillihan & Parens 2011; Fahrah & Gillihan 2012). Applying multifaceted constructs such as diagnostic categories in research has been shown to limit implications for the scientific study of psychopathology, e.g., understanding etiological factors in psychopathology (Olbert et al. 2014). Nosographical (diagnostic) categories are specified in a medical, normative and cultural context with limited overlap with concepts in cognitive neuroscience (Stoyanov et al. 2012). As such, the diagnostic criteria used in mental health disorders comprise common behavioral characteristics for each disorder and do not specifically relate to common cognitive/brain dysfunctions (Goldberg 2011; Buckley et al. 2009). This follows from samples of patients with specific mental health disorders, such as depression, to comprise a heterogeneous functioning group of individuals. Despite the fact that some specific cognitive dysfunctions, such as cognitive control differentiate groups of depressive patients from healthy control groups, only subgroups of patients demonstrate these cognitive control dysfunctions on performance-based measures (Bora et al. 2013). This is demonstrated, for instance, in relation to ADHD, in which the common trait of an inhibitory problem is only apparent in about 40 to

50 percent of patients when using a 90 percentile as cut-off scores on performance-based measures (Nigg, Willcutt, Doyle, & Sonuga-Barke 2005).

Thus, these challenges are why we suggest a shift from targeting treatment after diagnostic categories to use brain dysfunctions as a transdiagnostic target for treatment. Brain dysfunctions can be operationalized and tested, either with performance-based measures and/or with brain imaging. Cognitive neuroscience is characterized by the use of operationally defined tasks and/or procedures. Hence, the validity, reliability, theoretical soundness and sharp operational definition are of the greatest importance in cognitive neuroscience (Uttal 2001). The investigation of a more demarcated and singular aspect of psychopathology, e.g., transdiagnostic factors such as attentional lapses, may be promising to use in clinical psychology for several reasons. Firstly, such a construct is part of existing theories across diverse research fields such as neuropsychology, psychopathology and cognitive neuroscience, hence, it constitutes an inter-correlative construct as defined by Stoyanov et al. (2012). Secondly, the construct can be operationally defined and tested both within and across these fields. Thirdly, and more specific related to cognitive neuroscience, the phenomenon of attentional lapses is a dimensional phenomenon that can more easily be parametrically varied, and this is superior to categorical contrasts in cognitive neuroscience when making inquiries into the specificity (Uttal 2001).

It is noteworthy that all methodologies applied in research are associated with shortcomings. This is also the case in the use of neuroimaging in research of mental health disorders. Researchers use different procedures and operationalize differently when measuring DMN activation. This comprises measuring DMN in a resting state mode (i.e., no active task), with contrasting task-positive activation from task-negative activation, and with interpreting increased activation in brain areas part of DMN during task-positive activation to indicate interference by the DMN. The different approaches in measuring DMN activation may result in the fact that the different studies do not measure the same phenomenon. Furthermore, the use of performance-based measures in laboratory settings is a reductionist method of measuring phenomena, and this is associated with poorer ecological validity. The lack of sensitivity and specificity for diagnostic categories in use of performance-based measures has triggered a search for instruments with higher ecological validity.

Questionnaire measures, such as the “Behavior Rating Inventory of Executive Functions” (BRIEF), are one such instrument, where informants (self- and comparing reports) are asked about their cognitive control functions in the everyday life (Roth, Isquith, & Gioia 2005). However, the use of questionnaire measures seems to capture other aspects of brain functions than measures of performance-based measures (Toplak et al. 2013). So in the end, the use of measurement methods of either imaging and performance-based tests place limitations on the assessment of a specific phenomenon, and it is therefore important that studies applying these methods identify and discuss such possible limitations in the interpretation of findings. Having said this, attentional lapses as measured with IIV RT in individuals with ADHD have been shown to relate to real-world ADHD behaviors (Antonini, Narad, Langberg, & Epstein 2013), to have a genetic origin (Kuntsi & Klein 2012; Bellgrove, Hawi, Kirley, Gill, & Robertson 2005), and to decrease with the use of stimulant medications (Spencer et al. 2009). This supports the hypothesis that in ADHD attentional lapses may be a strong candidate for a disorder endophenotype (Castellanos & Tannock 2002). Attentional lapses are most broadly studied in relation to ADHD (Kuntsi & Klein 2012), but the literature that is referred to in this chapter strongly points to attentional lapses having a putative role in mental health disorders in general (Broyd et al. 2009).

Conclusion

We suggest a new model involving the use of attentional lapses as a target of treatment in patients with mental health disorders. Attentional lapses, as measured by DMN hyperactivation and high behavioral variability on cognitive tests, are shown to be a cognitive dysfunction across mental health disorders. These attentional lapses may have different causality across disorders, with both lack of cognitive control and level of arousal affecting the activation of the DMN. Thus, the interference of DMN in task-positive activation suggests that a reduced level of attentional lapses will mediate improved cognitive control functions by an increased ability to sustain attention. The research showing attentional lapses to be a consistent problem across mental health disorders does not seem to have been utilized in target of treatment, which should be the next step so that patients with mental health disorders can achieve improved quality of their life. Traditionally, research on treatment effects has tended to focus on the level of reduced disorder symptoms. This requires informants, and for adults this often consists of self-reports on questionnaires. Patients who have invested time and resources on treatment may report a falsely perceived positive effect. This phenomenon is observed in children with ADHD. Their parents, who have invested in the children's treatment, seem to report greater effects of treatments compared to the children's teachers, who have not invested in the treatment of the children. In fact, inclusion of teacher reports has shown some treatments of ADHD to have no effect, compared to higher reported effects when only including parent reports (Sonuga-Barke et al. 2013). Neuroscientific methods and measures can expand the possibilities for measuring different aspects of effects of treatments that may not be captured with the use of questionnaires. We suggest mindfulness training as one intervention that can enhance the ability to sustain attention and to regulate self-generative thought processes. Including imaging and performance-based measures as effect measures in research studies can pave the way for using the same measures as targets for treatment in conjunction with mindfulness training in future clinical psychotherapy practice.

Acknowledgments

The present chapter was sponsored by Kenneth Hugdahl, who also read and commented on the manuscript. We thank Steinunn Adolfsdottir for commenting on the manuscript and helping with data analysis.

References

Andrews-Hanna, J.R. 2012. The brain's default network and its adaptive role in internal mentation. *Neuroscientist*, *18*, 251–270.

Andrews-Hanna, J.R., Smallwood, J., & Spreng, R.N. (2014). The default network and self-generated thought: component processes, dynamic control, and clinical relevance. *Annal New York Academy Science*, 1316, 29-52.

Antoni, T.N., Narad, M.E., Langberg, J.M., & Epstein, J.N. (2013). Behavioral correlates of reaction time variability in children with and without ADHD. *Neuropsychology*, *27*(2), 201-209.

Baird, B., Smallwood, J., & Schooler, J.W. (2011). Back to the future: autobiographical planning and the functionality of mind-wandering. *Consciousness and Cognition*, *20*, 1604–1611.

Barlow, D.H., Allen, L.B., & Choate, M.L. (2004). Toward a unified treatment for emotional disorders. *Behavior Therapy*, *35*, 205-230.

Bellgrove, M.A., Hawi, Z., Kirley, A., Gill, M., & Robertson, I.H. (2005). Dissecting the attention deficit hyperactivity disorder (ADHD) phenotype: sustained attention, response variability and spatial attentional asymmetries in relation to dopamine transporter (DAT1) genotype. *Neuropsychologia, 43*(13), 1847-1857.

Berman, M.G., Peltier, S., Nee, D.E., Kross, E., Deldin, P.J., & Jonides, J. (2011). Depression, rumination and the default mode network. *Social Cognitive and Affective Neuroscience*, *6*, 548-555.

Bishop, S.R., Lau, M., Shapiro, S., Carlson, L., Anderson, N.D., Carmody, J., … Devins, G. (2004). Mindfulness: A proposed operational definition. *Clinical Psychology: Science and Practice*, 230-241.

Bora, E., Harrison, B.J., Yücel, M., & Pantelis, C. (2013). Cognitive impairment in euthymic major depressive disorder: a meta-analysis. *Psychological Medicine*, *43*(10), 2017-2026.

Brefzynski-Lewis, J.A., Lutz, A., Schaefer, H.S., Levinson, D.B., & Davidson, R.J. (2007). Neural correlates of attentional expertise in long-term meditation practitioners. *Proceedings of the National Academy of Sciences of the United States of America*, *104*, 11483-11488.

Broyd, S.J., Demanuele, C, Debener, S., Helps, S.K., James, C.J., & Sonuga-Barke, E.J.S. (2009). Default-mode brain dysfunction in mental disorders: A systematic review. *Neuroscience Biobehavioral Review*, *33*, 279-296.

Buckley, P.F., Miller, B.J., Lehrer, D.S., & Castler, D.J. (2009). Psychiatric comorbidities and schizophrenia. *Schizophrenia Bulletin*, *35*(2), 383-402.

Buckner, R.L., Andrews-Hanna, J.R., & Schacter, D.L. (2008). The brain's default network: anatomy, function, and relevance to disease. *Annual New York Academy Sciences*, *1124*, 1–38.

Bush, G., Luu, P., & Posner, M.I. (2000). Cognitive and emotional influences in anterior cingulate cortex. *Trends in Cognitive Sciences, 4*(6), 215-222.

Castellanos, F.X., & Tannock, R. (2002). Neuroscience of attention-deficit/hyperactivity disorder: the search for endophenotypes. *Nature Review Neuroscience, 3*(8), 617-628.

Clark, D.A. (2009). Cognitive behavioral therapy for anxiety and depression: possibilities and limitations of a transdiagnostic perspective. *Cognitive Behaviour Therapy*, *38*(S1), 29-34. doi:10.1080/16506070902980745

Dosenbach, N.U., Fair, D.A., Cohen, A.L., Schlaggar, B.L., & Petersen, S.E. (2007). A dual-network architecture of top-down control. *Trends in Cognitive Sciences*, *12*(3), 99-105.

Dosenbach, N.U., Visscher, K.M., Palmer, E.D., Miezin, F.M., Wenger, K.K., et al. (2006). A core system for the implementation of task sets. *Neuron*, *50*, 799–812.

Drevets, W.C. (2000). Functional anatomical abnormalities in limbic and prefrontal cortical structures in major depression. *Progress in Brain Research, 126*, 413-431.

Eichele, T., Debener, S., Calhoun, V.D., Specht, K., Engel, A.K., Hugdahl, K., ... Ullsperger, M. (2008). Prediction of human errors by maladaptive changes in event-related brain networks. *Proceedings of the National Academy of Sciences of the United States of America, 105*(16), 6173-6178.

Etkin, A., Egner, T., & Kalisch, R. (2011). Emotional processing in anterior cingulate and medial prefrontal cortex. *Trends in Cognitive Sciences, 15*(2), 85-93.

Fan, J., McCandliss, B.D., Fossella, J., Flombaum, J.I., & Posner, M.I (2005). The activation of attentional networks. *Neuroimage, 26*, 471-479.

Fan, J., Gu, X., Guise, K.G., Liu, X., Fossella, J., Wang, H., & Posner, M.I. (2009). Testing the behavioral interaction and integration of attentional networks. *Brain and Cognition, 7*(2), 209-220.

Farah, M.J. & Gilihan, S.J. (2012). The puzzle of neuroimaging and psychiatric diagnosis: echnology and nosology in an evolving discipline. *American Journal of Bioethics Neuroscience, 3*(4), 31-41.

Farchione, T.J., Fairhome, C.P., Ellard, K.K., Boisseau, C.L., Thompson-Hollands, J., Carl, Barlow, D.H. (2012). Unified protocol for transdiagnostic treatment of emotional disorders: a randomized controlled trial. *Behavior Therapy, 43*, 666-678.

Fassbender, C., Zhang, H., Buzy, W.M., Cortes, C.R., Mizuiri, D., Beckett, L., & Shweitzer, J.B. (2009). A lack of default network suppression is linked to increased distractibility in ADHD. *Brain Research, 1273*, 114-128.

Fox, M.D. & Raichle, M.E. (2007). Spontaneous fluctuations in brain activity observed with functional magnetic resonance imaging. *Nature Reviews Neuroscience, 8*(9), 700-711.

Fryer, S.L., Woods, S.W., Kiehl, K.A., Calhoun, V.D., Pearlson, G.D., Roach, B.J. Mathalon, D.H. (2013). Deficient Suppression of Default Mode Regions during Working Memory in Individuals with Early Psychosis and at Clinical High-Risk for Psychosis. *Frontiers in Psychiatry, 10*(4), 92.

Gilihan, S. & Parens, E. (2011). Should we expect "neural signatures" for DSM diagnoses? *Journal of Clinical Psychiatry, 72*(10), 1383-1389.

Goldberg, D. (2011). The heterogeneity of "major depression." *World Psychiatry, 10*(3), 226-228.

Greicius, M.D., Krasnow, B., Reiss, A.L., & Menon, V. (2003). Functional connectivity in the resting brain: a network analysis of the default mode hypothesis. *Proceedings of the National Academy of Sciences of the United States of America, 100*, 253–8.

Greicius, M. D., &Menon, V. (2004). Default-mode activity during a passive sensory task: uncoupled from deactivation but impacting activation. *Journal of Cognitive Neuroscience, 16*, 1484–92.

Hamilton J.P., Furman, D.J., Chang, C.C., Thomason, M.E., Dennis, E., & Gotlib, I.H. (2011). Default-Mode and Task-Positive Network Activity in Major Depressive Disorder: mplications for Adaptive and Maladaptive Rumination. *Biological Psychiatry, 70*, 327-333.

Hanna-Andrews, J.R., Smallwood, J., & Spreng, R.N. (2014. The default network and self-generated thought: component processes, dynamic control, and clinical relevance. *Annal New York Sciences, 1316*, 29-52.

Harvey, A.G. (2008). Insomnia, psychiatric disorders, and the transdiagnostic perspective. *Current Directions in Psychological Science*, *17*(5), 299-303.

Hasenkamp, W., Wilson-Mendenhall, C.D., Duncan, E., & Barsalou, L.W. (2012). Mind-wandering and attention during focused attention: a fine-grained temporal analysis of fluctuating cognitive states. *Neuroimage*, *59*, 750-760.

Ives-Deliperi, V.L., Howells, F., Stein, D.J., Meintjes, E.M., & Horn, N. (2013). The effects of mindfulness-based cognitive theray on patients with bipolar disorder: A controlled functional MRI investigation. *Journal of Affective Disorders*, *150*(3), 1152-1157.

Jacobi, F, Wittchen, H.U., Hôlting, C., Pfister, M., Mûller, N., & Lieb, R. (2004). Prevalence, co-morbidity and correlates of mental disorders in the general population: results from the German Health Interview and Examination Survey (GHS). *Psychological Medicine, 34,* 597–611.

Jacoby, N. & Ahissor, N. (2013). What does it take to show that cognitive training procedure is useful? A critical evaluation. *Progress in Brain Research*, *207*, 121-140.

Joyce, E.M., Hutton, S.B., Mutsaba, S.H., & Barnes, R.E. (2005). Cognitive heterogeneity in first episode schizophrenia. *British Journal of Psychiatry*, *187*, 516-522.

Kabat-Zinn, J. (2003). Mindfulness-based interventions in context: Past, present, and future. *Clinical Psychology: Research and Practice*, *10*, 144-156.

Kaiser, S., Roth, A., Rentrop, M., Friederich, H.C., Bender, S., & Weisbrod, M. (2008). Intra-individual reaction time variability in schizophrenia, depression and borderline personality disorder. *Brain and Cognition*, *66*(1), 73-82.

Kelly, A.M., Uddin, L.Q., Biswal, B.B., Castellanos, F.X., & Milham, M.P. (2008). Competition between functional brain networks mediates behavioral variability. *Neuroimage*, *39*, 527–537.

Kuntsi, J. & Klein, C. (2012). Intraindividual variability in ADHD and its implications for research of causal links. In Stanford, C. and Tannock, R. (eds). Behavioral neuroscience of attention deficit hyperactivity disorder and its treatment. Current topics in behavioral neurosciences. Springer-Verlag Berlin-Heidelberg.

Kuyken, W., Hayes, R., Barrett, B., Byng, R., Dalgleish, T., Kessler, D., ... Byford, S. (2015). Effectiveness and cost-effectiveness of mindfulness-based cognitive therapy compared with maintenance antidepressant treatment in the prevention of depressive relapse or recurrence (PREVENT): a randomised controlled trial. *Lancet*.

Kuyken, W., Watkins, E., Holden, E., White, K., Taylor, R.S., Byford, S., … Dalgleish, T. (2010). How does mindfulness-based cognitive therapy work? *Behaviour Research and Therapy*, *48*(11), 1105-1112.

Landin-Romero, R., McKenna, P.J., Salgado-Pineda, P., Sarró, S., Aguirre, C., Sarri, C., … Pomarol-Clotet, E. (2014). Failure of deactivation in the default mode network: a trait marker for schizophrenia? *Psychological Medicine*, *21*, 1-11.

Malinowski, P. (2013). Neural mechanisms of attentional control in mindfulness meditation. *Frontiers in Neuroscience*, *7*(8).

Mason, M.F. et al. (2007). Wandering minds: the default network and stimulus-independent thought. *Science*, *315*, 393-395.

Mazoyer, B., Zago, L., Mellet, E., Bricogne, S., Etard, O., Houdé, O., … Tzourio-Mazoyer, N. (2001). Cortical networks for working memory and executive functions sustain the conscious resting state in man. *Brain Research Bulletin*, *54*, 287–98.

Melby-Lervåg, M. & Hulme, C. (2013). Is working memory training effective? A meta-analytic review. *Developmental Psychology*, *49*(2), 270-291.

Miller, E. K., & Cohen, J. D. (2001). An integrative theory of prefrontal cortex function. *Annual Review of Neuroscience*, *24*, 167–202.

Miyake, A., Friedman, N. P., Emerson, M. J., Witzki, A. H., Howerter, A., & Wager, T. D. (2000). The unity and diversity of executive functions and their contributions to complex “frontal lobes” tasks: A latent variable analysis. *Cognitive Psychology*, *41*, 49–100.

Mitchell, J.T., McIntyre, E.M., English, J.S., Dennis, M.F., Beckham, J.C., & Kollins, S.H. (in press). A Pilot Trial of Mindfulness Meditation Training for ADHD in Adulthood: Impact on Core Symptoms, Executive Functioning, and Emotion Dysregulation. *Journal of Attention Disorders*. doi:10.1177/1087054713513328.

National institute for health and clinical excellence (2009). *Depression: Treatment and management of depression in adults, including adults with a chronic physical health problem.* Retrieved 26.12.2013, from http://www.nice.org.uk/nicemedia/live/12329/45890/45890.pdf

Nigg, J.T., Willcutt, E.G., Doyle, A.E., & Sonuga-Barke, E.J.S. (2005). Causal heterogeneity in attention-deficit/hyperactivity disorder: do we need neuropsychologically impaired subtypes?. *Biological Psychiatry*, *57*, 1224-1230.

Ochsner, K.N. & Gross, J.J. (2005). The cognitive control of emotion. *Trends in Cognitive Sciences*, *9*(5), 242-249.

Olbert, C.M. & Tupler, L.A. (2014). Quantifying heterogeneity attributable to polythetic diagnostic criteria: theoretical framework and empirical framework. *Journal of Abnormal Psychology*, *123*(2), 452-462.

Onraedt, T., & Koster, E. H. W. (2014). Training working memory to reduce rumination. *PLOS one, 9*(3).

Paul, N.A., Stanton, S.J., Greeson, J.M., Smoski, M.J., & Wang, L. (2013). Psychological and neural mechanisms of trait mindfulness in reducing depression vulnerability. *Social Cognitive and Affective Neuroscience*, *8*(1), 56-64.

Philippi, C. & Koenigs, M. (2014). The neuropsychology of self-reflection in psychiatric illness. *Journal of Psychiatric Research*, *54*, 55-63.

Raichle, M. (2011). The restless brain. *Brain Connectivity*, *1*(1), 3-12.

Raichle M.E., Macleod, A.M., Snyder, A.Z., Powers, W.J., Gusnard, D.A., & Shulman, G.L. (2001) A default mode of brain function. *Proceedings of the National Academy of Sciences of the United States of America, 98*:676–682.

Ressler, K.J. & Mayberg, H.S. (2007). Targeting abnormal neural circuits in mood and anxiety disorders: from the laboratory to the clinic. *Nature Neuroscience*, *10*(9), 1116-1124.

Roth, R.M., Isquith, P.K., & Gioia, G.A. (2005). BRIEF-A: Behavior rating inventory of executive function – adult version. Professional manual. *Psychological Assessment Resources*.

Schoenberg, P.L., Hepark, S., Kan, C.C., Barendregt, H.P., Buitelaar, J.K., & Speckens, A.E. (2014). Effects of mindfulness-based cognitive therapy on neurophysiological correlates of performance monitoring in adults attention-deficit/hyperactivity disorder. *Clinical Neurophysiology*, *125*(7), 1407-1416.

Shannon, B. J., Snyder, A. Z., Vincent, J. L., & Buckner, R. L. (2006). Spontaneous correlations and the default network: effects of task performance. *Social NeuroscienceAbstrac*t, 119.5.

Sheline, Y.I., Barch, D.M., Price, J.L., Rundle, M.M., Vaishnavi, N., Snyder, A.Z., Raichle, M.E. (2009). The default mode network and self-referential processes in depression. *Proceedings of the National Academy of Sciences of the United States of America, 106*(6), 1942-1947.

Shin, Y.S., Kim, S.N., Shin, N.Y. Jung, W.H., Hur, J.W., Byun, M.S., … Kwon, J.S. (2013). Increased intra-individual variability of cognitive processing in subjects at risk mental state and schizophrenia. *PLoS One*, *8*(11).

Shulman, G.L., Fiez, J.A., et al., 1997. Common blood flow changes across visual tasks: II. Decreases in cerebral cortex. *Journal of Cognitive Neuroscience*, *9*(5), 648–663.

Sonuga-Barke, E.J.S., Brandeis, D., Cortese, S., Daley, D., Ferrin, M., Holtmann, M., Sergeant, J. (2013). Nonpharmacological interventions for ADHD: systematic review and meta-analysis of randomized controlled trials of dietary and psychological treatment. *American Journal of Psychiatry*, *170*, 275-289.

Sonuga-Barke, E., Brandeis, D., Holtmann, M., & Cortese, S. (2014). Computer-based cognitive training for ADHD: a review of current evidence. *Child and Adolescent Psychiatric Clinics of North America*, *23*(4), 807-824.

Sonuga-Barke, E.J., & Castellanos, F.X. (2007). Spontaneous attentional fluctuations in impaired states and pathological conditions: a neurobiological hypothesis. *Neuroscience Biobehavioral Review, 31*(7), 977-986.

Spencer, S. V., Hawk, L.W., Richards, J.B., Shiels, K., Pelham, W.E., & Waxmonsky, J.G. (2009). Stimulant treatment reduces lapses in attention among children with ADHD: the effects of methylphenidate on intra-individual response time distributions. *Journal of Abnormal Child Psychology, 37*(6), 805-816.

Stevens, M.C., Pearlson, G.D., & Kiehl, K.A. (2007). An FMRI auditory oddball study of combined-subtype attention deficit hyperactivity disorder. *Am J Psychiatry, 164*(11), 1737-1749.

Stoyanov, D., Stanghellini, G., & Broome, M. (2012). Conceptual issues in psychiatric neuroimaging: An update. *Current Topics in Medicinal Chemistry*, *12*, 2348-2356.

Tamm, L., Narad, M.E., Antonini, T.N., O`Brien, K.M., Hawk Jr., L.W., & Epstein, J.N. (2012). Reaction time variability in ADHD: A review. *Neurothreapeutics*, *9*, 500-508.

Taylor, V.A., Grant, J., Daneault, V., Scavone, G., Breton, E., Roffe-Vidal, S., Beauregard, M. (2011). Impact of mindfulness on neural responses to emotional pictures in experienced and beginner meditators. *NeuroImage*, *57*, 1524-1533.

Toplak, M. E., West, R. F., & Stanovich, K. E. (2013). Practioner review: Do performance-based measures and ratings of executive function assess the same construct? *Journal of Child Psychology and Psychiatry*, *54*(2), 131-143.

Uttal, W.R. (2001). The new phrenology: the limits of localizing cognitive functions in the brain. *Cambridge*. MIT Press.

Wagner, G., Koch, K., Schachtzabel, C., Reichenbach, J.R., Sauer, H., & Schlösser, R.G.M. (2008). Enhanced rostral anterior cingulate cortex activation during cognitive control is related to orbitofrontal volume reduction in unipolar depression. *Journal of Psychiatry Neuroscience*, *33*(3),199-208.

Weissman, D. H., Roberts, K. C., Visscher, K. M., & Woldorff, M. G. (2006). The neural bases of momentary lapses in attention. *Nature Neuroscience, 9*(7), 971-978.

Whitfield-Gabrieli, S. & Ford, J.M. (2012). Default mode network activity and connectivity in psycholpathology. *Annalual Review of Clinical Psychology*, *8*, 49-76.

Willcutt, E. G., Doyle, A. E., Nigg, J., Faraone, S. V., & Pennington, B. F. (2005). Validity of the executive function theory of attention-deficit/hyperactivity disorder: A meta-analytic review. *Biological Psychiatry*, *57*, 1336–1346.

In: New Developments in Clinical Psychology Research
Editors: D. St. Stoyanov and R.-D. Stieglitz
ISBN: 978-1-63483-223-6

Chapter 5

DIFFERENTIAL DIAGNOSIS OF AUTISTIC SPECTRUM DISORDERS

Vanya Matanova*[*], *PhD, DSc, CertCBT
Sofia University "St. Clement of Ohrid", Bulgaria

ABSTRACT

Diagnosis and differential diagnosis of developmental disorders are rapidly developing areas, although many questions remain under discussion. From a historical point of view, for a long time there has been an unfounded transfer of knowledge about the mature person to children's mental functioning. The wide continuum of the autistic spectrum – from relatively mild to extremely severe disorders hinders substantially the diagnostic process, furthermore the separate nosological entities in this spectrum have similar manifestations, even if they belong to different nosologies. This requires great attention to detail during the diagnostic procedures by a team of specialists for a sufficient amount of time in order to determine the diagnosis, therapy and prognosis.

INTRODUCTION

Diagnosis is the process of determining whether the observed problems meet the criteria for a disorder, defined by the international manuals and the speciliazed literature. The diagnostic process is a dynamic stereotypy of the syndromes – their emergence, development, enrichment or extinction.

The differential diagnosis is an unseparable part of the diagnostic process. According to Bleicher, V. M. (1979) the differential diagnostic process can be divided into several phases:

- Defining the leading symptom,
- Comparison of the differential diagnostic importance of the present pathological symptoms,

[*] Email: v_matanova@yahoo.com.

- Description of the disorder considering its similarities and differences with other disorders.

For an adequate differential diagnosis it is necessary to follow a number of basic principles:

- Diagnosis cannot be based solely on a monosymptomic picture.
- The process needs to continue for a sufficient amount of time to analyze the necessary information and to consider the dynamics of the symptoms.

Diagnosis and Differential Diagnosis of Developmental Disorders

Diagnosis and differential diagnosis of developmental disorders are rapidly developing areas, although many questions remain under discussion. From a historical point of view, for a long time there has been an unfounded transfer of knowledge about the mature person to children's mental functioning. Just in ICD – 10 new themes about specific disorders in children and adolescents have been identified. An adequate diagnosis requires a distinct consideration of the stage of childhood development and the conditions in which it takes place. This means that in case of a mental disorder in childhood, elements of disontogenesis are always present. What is extremely important is that the symptoms and syndormes in that period are age-specific. Often the age-specificity obscures the nosological specificity. Taking into account the systemic approach, a child is dependent upon the functions of the system he belongs to. In childhood the age specificity reflects the reactivity of the child, and not so much the nosological essence of the disorder.

The need for differentiating between autistic spectrum disorders and other similar conditions as well as within their own structural levels emerges with the first clinical observations and descriptions of such individuals. The wider and more in-depth psychiatric and psychological research of autism evolves in the 1940's /Bleuler 1911; Kanner 1938-1943; H. Asperger 1944/. In the beginning of the 20-th century specialists describe autistic manifestations under different names. Some refer its main characteristics to the familiar forms of schizophrenia and some psychotic disorders. Others view the condition as a manifestation of an organic failure of the central nervous system and thus assign it to mental retardation variations.

In psychiatry there are childhood psychoses resembling the symptomatology of autism. However, the observed clinical profile there is different, specifically regarding the primary and secondary symptoms compared to the classical definition by Leo Kanner. It is widely accepted that the autistic manifestations emerge during the first years of the life of a child and the full clinical picture usually develops by the age of 3.

Many of the difficulties in diagnosing and differentiating autism are related to the variability of manifestations of the syndrome and to methodological problems. A number of authours accept that the psychological development of the child with autism is pathological from the first months of his life. Indications for that can be found in the peculiarities of the reactions and behavior of children with autism like impairment of the muscle tone, weak affective reactions, pathological sensitivity to weak sensory signals etc. During the first years of life of the child the possibility to make a differential diagnosis is hindered by the fact that this type of disontogenesis manifests some common symptoms and reactions with other types of abnormal childhood development, for instance neuropathy, mental retardation, attachment disorders, deafness, complex forms of speech pathology etc.

In case of autistic spectrum disorders, the onset of abnormal functioning serves as a criterion for the differential diagnosis. Due to the lack of precise age criteria regarding the development of the different areas of functioning, it is necessary to look for qualitative impairments and the absence of progress in the acquisition of skills and knowledge.

The importance of differential diagnosis in children with autistic spectrum disorders is strengthened by the fact that usually these children manifest a number of problems and symptoms, characterizing other nosologies as well. The high variability of the manifestations of the autistic spectrum as well as the controversial validity and specificity of some of the symptoms, make the differential diagnosis extremely complex. For its adequate implementation an assessment procedure according to a multiple axis system is required. The first step is to determine the intellectual level of the child. For practical purposes it is necessary to evaluate it by the non-verbal skills of the child. The second step is related to establishing a discrepancy between speech development and mental age. Mental and speech development do not proceed entirely in parallel, as in early childhood they evolve independently, and later on speech becomes meaningful and thinking takes the form of speech. In order to diagnose autistic spectrum disorders after establishing the typical clinical symptoms it is necessary to put them in a hierarchical order and to distinguish them from other conditions with similar symptomatology. This requires a thourough analysis not only of autistic spectrum disorders but also of some developmental disorders since part of their symptoms resemble that of the autistic spectrum.

In 1943 Leo Kanner introduces the term autism in childhood psychiatric practice, however, it is still one of the biggest misteries in childhood abnormal development. Today it is certainly known that autism is not psychosis nor is it a form of emotional disorder or childhood schizophrenia. Autism is a developmental disorder involving a cognitive deficit, having common characteristics with other developmental disorders but still preserving its own specific symptomatology.

Autism is a generalized developmental disorder defined by the presence of abnormal development prior to the age of three. The main symptoms are autistic isolation and a strive for permanence. These children have a cogenital inability to communicate and to react adequately in a situation. Still in infancy there is an absence of a shoulder twisting and head raising when the child is picked up as well as no adaptation to the body of the adult. The lack of eye contact is considered a typical sign although many empirical studies disprove this statement. Such children handle different objects in a stereotypical manner, perceive different body parts without being able to consider them as a whole, do not initiate and maintain relationships with other people their own age, as if they do not notice their presence and actively avoid them. Many authors stress the lukewarm interactions of intellectual parents and their children and see a psychogenic reaction caused by an impaired mother-child relationship. The play of autistic children is marked by the lack of imagination and symbolism. The traditional social elements are missing from their plays. The play as an activity is stereotypical and the use of toys is not according to their intended function.

Almost all children with autism have some speech and language impairments which could vary greatly. It is possible a complete absence of verbal production as well as a relatively good speech development. The common thing to all people with autism is that the speech does not serve as a means of communication and information exchange. The early speech activity in those children is expressed in a random usage of names of different objects, names or idiosynchratic phrases. What stands out are the pronounced pragmatic speech disturbances defined by a lack of congruence between their own verbal production and the requirements of others and the situation. This speech activity, in fact, reflects a world incomprehensible to others – it is chaotic, senseless, not designed for communication, demonstrating good mechanical, fragmentary memory. Verbal production is usually variegated by multiple phonological, morphological and syntax mistakes.

Difficulties in communication are manifested not only in the verbal but also in the non-verbal aspect. Most authors accept that speech of people with autism does not serve its communicative function. There are many studies that refute this statement. Scientists claim that children with autism still communicate through speech however its form and functions are limited compared to that of children with other developmental disorders. Children with autism name objects, make comments and ask questions but these communication acts are not conscious and do not have social significance.

They use declarative statements that are situation-based and are not coded as an address to other people. Usually they are able to formulate statements about confirmation/agreement or refutal/disagreement. It is difficult for them to keep the conversation and their answers seem irrelevant and persevering. They find it difficult to understand the context of the statement, they show literality in their understanding and production of verbal and non-verbal signals. They are incapable of using expressive gestures to comprehend or convey emotional states. In place of such non-verbal signals they use idiosynchratic ones. Even in people with high-funcitoning autism facial, vocal and gesture expressions seem strange. There are instrumental gestures that children master correctly and use them for social interactions. According to Happe (1994) speech development of children with autism can be predicted not by standard tests but by the results from the measured non-verbal gestures and shared attention.

Behavior of children with autism is characterized by a variety of rituals and obsessions that usually accompany their actions related to eating, dressing, washing etc.They make the impression of being confined in another world while nothing from this one attracts them or awakes any desires or activity.

Their face is frozen, emotionally passive, irritated after change in the envirnement, negative and rejecting any attempt by others to make contact.

In early age in children with autism the domineering disorders are those of neuro-autonomic and instinctive systems which are manifested as sleep distrubances, lack of sucking reflex etc. At an older age the dominant impairments pertain to the behavioral sphere and are related primarily to social adaptation. In some cases the symbiotic relationship with the mother is preserved for a long time, expressed in a painful attachment to her and a prominent fear of losing her. Still the opposite tendency is possible – emotional alienation, disregard, rejection and indifference to other people including the primary caregivers. Isolation and confinement to one's own inner world is caused by fears and hyperreactivity to extrinsic stimuli.

AUSTISM: CLINICAL MANIFESTATIONS

The clinical manifestation of autism can be summarized by the characteristics of abnormal functioning in three areas – social interactions, communication and behavioral impairments. Autism is a complex compilation of emotional and behavioral features, of which the most prominent are emotional coldness, indifference toward others and the world, active avoidance of contact, displayed permanent shutting in from the outside world etc. Intellect, speech and sociability operate in a strict individual disharmony.

Many authors believe that the intellectual quotient in people with autism is lower than the norm but higher than the one in individuals with mental retardation. The thing that remains unfamiliar to people with autism is the perception of themselves as similar to others which is a consequence of the absence of a need for social interaction and joint activities with family and friends and the lack of eye contact. There is evidence that children with autism show better results in manipulative and visual spatial skills and in tests requiring the instant recall of information. These findings pose the question about the definition of autism and classification of its symptoms. It remains unresolved whether we can talk about autism and mental retardation when it is clear that in cases of mental retardation there is secondary symptomatology demonstrated as autistic manifestations and social isolation. In that sense the validity of the diagnosis atypical autism brings huge doubts. Today the term autism is used in two aspects: theoretical – reflecting non-pathological phenomena, the tendency to be absorbed by personal fantasies and dreams, in which one seeks pleasure, and clinical – for classification of a generalized developmental disorder.

Autism has a great variety of forms and a wide range of individual reactions. Here is why the investigation of its etiology is difficult from a clinical point of view. The wide range of disorders categorized as autism include congenital attention regulation disorders, high basic levels of natural opiates, endocrine disorders, developmental disorders of the left hemisphere etc.

According to Baron-Cohen (1988, 1992) the main difficulty of a child with autism is his inability to comprehend mental states of other people. The researcher believes that a mental state cannot be observed directly but could only be inferred for which purpose the child needs a complex cognitive mechanism. To understand what someone thinks is more complicated than to grasp how he feels because hope and desires are always directed at something.

Frith (1989) believes that children with autism lack the ability to accept and explore other people's thinking. She suggests that this is a deficit developed during the first weeks of the life of a child, it is a deficit in the ability and desire to accept a different way of thinking which can provide the child with the pleasure of perceiving a new object. This is probably related to the indifference of such children to the so called "joint attention". They find their own ways to elicit engagement and attention, for instance, by performing repetitive behaviors. It is possible that these manifestations are related to the lack of symbolism and their inability to recreate their sensations due to an impairment of the "central cohesive force."

Autism is associated with an impairment of the mechanisms for emotional adaptation as a result of an uncompleted structure of emotional organization of behavior. Although that primary structure of defect is not known throughout the entire hierarchy of distribution of impaired and preserved components, there is evidence which suggests that the basic nature of autism is a pathology of affect.

During the period following the clinical discovery of Leo Kanner, the studies and theories about autism develop around the biological and social-affective reasons. Soon after the syndrome is accepted as valid most researchers accept autism not as an endogenic disorder but as a negative affective reaction to an inadequate environment. Suggestions in that direction, however, do not support the presence of a psychogenic or environmental factor.

The next direction researchers take is searching for common symptoms and etiological factors between autism and other cognitive, perceptual and speech disorders. In the period 1978-1982 the concept that the main impairments in autism are a result of neuro-biological deficits is resuscitated. For that period of time the study of the social and emotional development of people with autism remain in the background. Because of that the main hypothesis of that time is that social deficits are secondary to a common cognitive deficit. Cognitive deficits are manifested in situations which require the processing of emotionally and socially conditioned phenomena and sings. Children with autism respond to situations in which other children or adults actively engage them in social interactions. In those cases an active social behavior is observed based on engagement and cooperation.

There is contradictory evidence regarding social engagement in children with autism. One of the research methods of social engagement is using the attachment paradigm. It is known that children can initiate more prominent social behavior toward their caregivers compared to strangers and demonstrate clearly differentiated reactions of separation/reunion/ with the caregiver. It has been found that during spontaneous play children with autism look for closeness with their caregiver more than with a stranger. These results compared to those of children with mental retardation show that the former address vocalizations, look for visual and tactile contact with their caregiver for a longer period of time compared to that with a stranger. Attachmen behavior of children with autism does not differ from that of children with other developmental disorders or mental retardation. This does not refute the existence of attachment disorders in children with autism, a statement primarily based on the observation that they do not use positive emotionality so often when demonstrating their attachment although it is not entirely absent.

Social behavior in children with autism is determined by their mental age. The ones with higher mental age demonstrate a higher frequency of active social behavior especially when adults actively seek social interaction with them. This data puts into question the validity of the diagnostic criteria in DSM regarding social deficits in children with autism. In a survey among parents of children with autism, 40% claim that until the age of 6 their children have manifested elements of social behavior as a response to the behavior of the mother and have been aware of her presence.

These findings suggest more quantitative results than qualitative characteristics of the social behavior of children with autism. Apparently they are capable of manifesting act of social conduct but simultaneously they show significant impairments in social judgment which determines to a larger degree the deficits in their social functioning. How then to distinguish between children with autism and those with developmental disorders? Due to the fact that most children with autism demonstrate non-verbal behavior specialists are forced to investigate precisely that. Affect or emotion can be demonstrated through vocalization, facial expression, body posture, gestures. In an experiment from 1979 4 groups of children – with mental retardation, with a developmental disorder, with autism and a control group are put in a situation stimulating the expression of four basic states – surprise, pleasure, frustration and desire. Vocalization of children with autism are strictly specific and this is the reason why it is hard to be adequately interpreted by people different from their caregivers. In 1986 a similar experiment is conducted but considering the facial expression of the children. The results show that children with autism manifest a significantly larger number of combinations of emotions compared to the other groups.

It is known that the main feature of autism is the undifferentiated perception of oneself as well as the inability to distinguish between one's self and non self. This widely accepted statement is refuted by the results of an experiment about visual self-recognition based on discerning a change in the reflected image. Self-recognition is reported when there is touching of a real part (not reflected), when the child smiles or uses vocalization etc.

Children with autism between 5 and 11 years recognize themselves but do not show the same kind of affect as the one manifested by normal children. There is some data that children with autism smile to their own image as often as normal children, although another study shows that 79% of children with autism manifest full indifference to self recognition. Apparently the response of children with autism to self-recognition varies. Reactions of children with autism resemble those of children with mental retardation. However, there are differences in the frequency of smiling addressed at reflected images. This definitively proves that people with autism have impairments of vocal, gesture and facial expression of affect.

Impairments of social conduct in children with autism are expressed in the deficit of skills for indicating rather than for sharing or demanding. There is no answer to the question whether the deficit in the skills for sharing is specific for autism or common for developmental disorders. The impaired nonverbal behavior of children with autism is related to deficits in symbolic representational thinking i.e., in the capacity of the child to use an object to present or create another object. It can be assumed that the impairments of the nonverbal behavior in regard to joint attention are relatively independent from the impairments for symbolic representation.This is important regarding the question whether nonverbal behavior requires a certain developmental level of symbolic thinking or not. Direct convey of affective signals precedes development of nonverbal gesture communication. This allows the child to enhance his comprehension about similarities between his emotional experience and that of other people. Shared experience refers to the ability of the child to express different emotional states as well as to respond to emotions of others.

Impairments of children with autism regarding nonverbal skills for indication can be considered as secondary resulting from a deficit in the ability to share emotional experience with the parents.

In the middle of the 20-th century emerges the idea that children with autism have a disability of the arousal-regualting systems which influences the way these children treat and behave in the environment. In the 1960's it becomes popular to believe that children with autism have chronically high arousal and in fact stereotypical and repetitive behavior aims at reducing that high arousal. This idea is later modified by accepting the existence of fluctuations between high and low arousal activity. These variations are considered a result of the unsuccessful processing of sensory information. Sensitivity and attention to external stimuli vary depending on whether the child with autism is in a state of high or low arousal activity. This theory explain the functional meaning of repetitive behavior but leaves unanswered questions about the asynchronous development of children with autism.

It is known that as a response to unfamiliar aspects of a situation children with autism can increase their self-stimulating behavior as the frequency of stereotypical acts depends on the developmental level of the child.

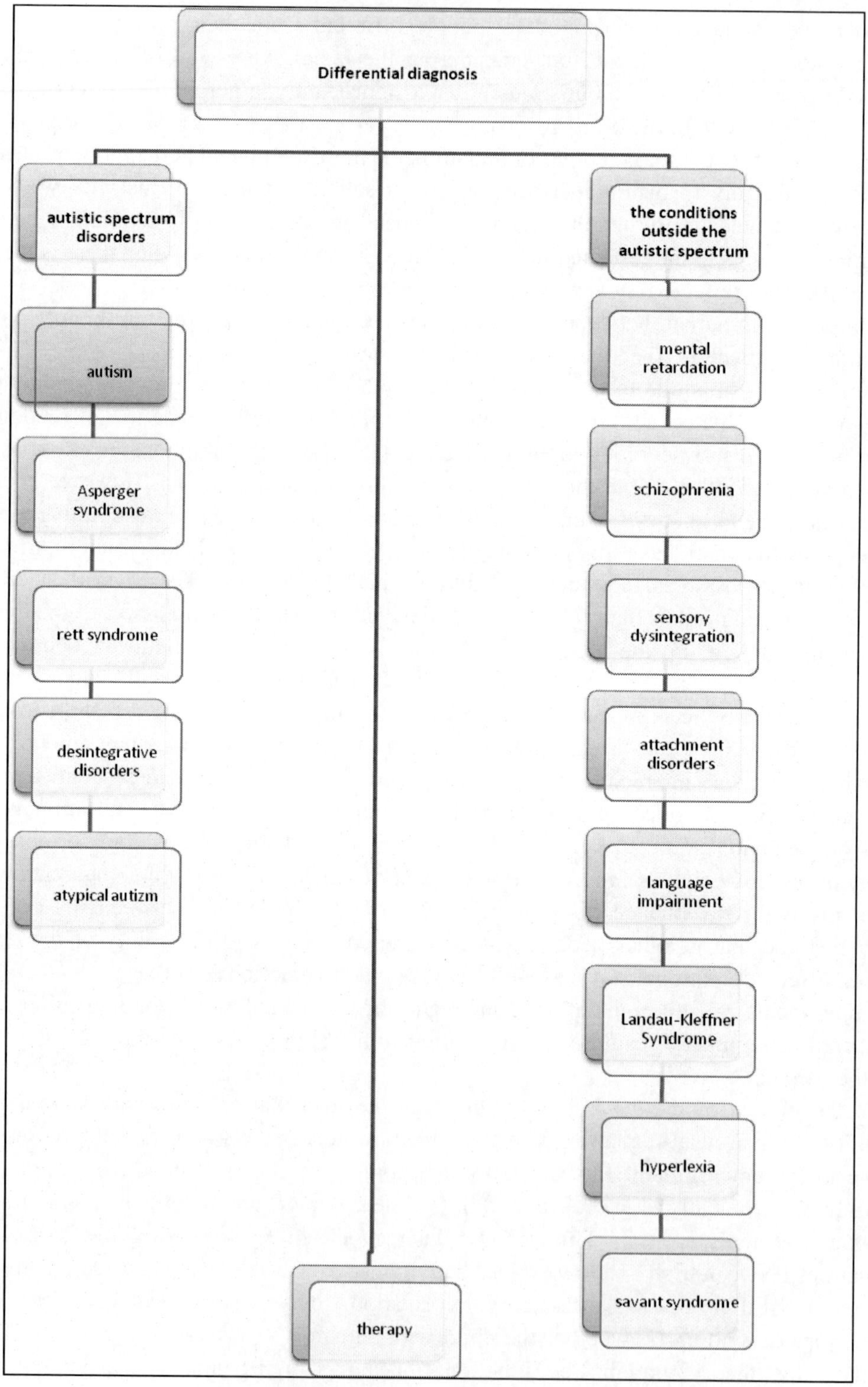

Figure 1. Differential diagnosis of autistic spectrum disorders.

Often children with autism cope with excessively powerful stimuli through different means – gaze aversion, ear plugging, avoidance, constant questions asking, ritualistic behavior, stereotypical movements etc. Motor stereotypes can serve different functions including seeking social attention. The question how arousal deficits in children with autism selectively influence the processing of social and language information and at the same time do not have the same impact on the processing of nonverbal information is of great importance. In that regard it is interesting that in children with autism the range of optimal stimulation is narrower than that in normal children. It is possible that this fact influences the processing of social information. Unlike objects that have permanent qualities people are unpredictable to a great extent. This makes it difficult for children with autism to process that type of information due to a low threshold of saturation or rejection of the stimulus.

Apart from these specific characteristics children with autism often suffer from other non-specific problems like fears, phobias, sleep and eating disturbances, momentary outbursts of anger and aggression. There is often self-harming like hand biting etc. The specific manifestation of the deficits of autism changes with time and growth of the child but continue in adulthood as they continue to pose problems in socialization, communication and choice of interests.

Differential Diagnosis Inside the Autistic Spectrum

Asperger Syndrome

In 1944 Hans Asperger independently of Leo Kanner uses the term autism to describe a syndrome with an onset in early childhood. H. Asperger provides a description for that condition similar to the one given by Leo Kanner in 1943. The reported features again are related to behavior. He describes 4 children (boys) with the so called by him "autistic psychopathy." H. Asperger believes that the syndrome described by him is different from the one of Leo Kanner. There are two main differences between the two descriptions: the children described by Leo Kanner have organic speech while the ones from the group of Asperger express themselves well, however, they show some general motor clumsiness. H. Asperger believes that the main disability affects social functioning. Many authors validate Asperger syndrome as autism without mental retardation (Klin 2003).

It seems like a strange and unexpected coincidence two scientists independent of each other to choose the same term to characterize the nature of the disorder they try to describe. In fact, the term has been previously introduced by Bleuler and was meant to describe schizophrenia. In those first descriptions H. Asperger avoids short formulations. He gives detailed, lively and empathic descriptions. H. Asperger attempts to relate autistic behavior to the normal variations of personality development which constitutes a unique approach in understanding autistic disorders.

He believes that such children have a "fundamental disability that is manifested in all behavioral and expressive phenomena." As a result of this disability difficulties in social interaction arise. He underlines the variability of manifestations of those difficulties – from inability to integrate in a social group to compensation by peculiar originality of thinking and experience. He and Leo Kanner assert that there is "an impairment of the emotional contact" on some deeper level of affect and/or instinct. H. Asperger underlines the peculiarities in communication, specificities of facial expression, lack of "eye contact," presence of stereotypical movements and a perplexing uneven pattern of intellectual achievements.

According to H. Asperger these children have personality disorders expressed in social isolation (Klin 2003). Some authors believe that "autistic personality disorder" is a term which better matches the original despricption by H. Asperger (Volkmark, Klin, Schultz, Rubin, Bronen 2000). The children observed by H. Asperger show problems with social interactions and nonverbal communication, have idiosyncratic production and express egocentric preoccupation with unusual interests. He notes that these individuals have difficulties in regard to empathy and intuition as well as a tendency for climsiness.

The term "Asperger syndrome" is used for the first time by Lorna Wing (Wing 1981) to designate those capable individuals with autism who do not meet Kanner criteria of being silent and detached individuals. For L. Wing the difference between the two syndromes is in their severity. In the late 1980's most authors begin to use the term in that sense. In that way, however, the original idea by H. Asperger that the disorder can exist at different intellectual levels is lost. L. Wing recommends this diagnosis to be used in cases that are hard to be referred to any other category. There is some ground to believe that Asperger syndrome is not well defined yet. L. Wing believes that a child can be Kanner type but in his teenage years to develop Asperger syndrome. This idea contradicts the classification by Szatmari (1989) according to which criteria for Asperger syndrome are not met by those for an autistic disorder. This author does not take into account the possibility for a developmentally conditioned change of the clinical picture.

L. Wing includes many additional difficulties that children demonstrate during the first 2 years of their life. Some of them are lack of normal interests and satisfaction from the presence of others, diminished quality and quantity of speech, noticeable decrease in joint interests and desire for communication, delay in impressive speech development, lack of imaginery representations and role play. In the original paper by Lorna Wing on problems with Asperger syndrome from 1981 high levels of anxiety and depression are reported as well as other affective disorders.

Clinical studies confirm the presence of depression episodes and suicidal risk. During the early periods of development children with Asperger syndrome do not notice or care that they are different from others. Their life is constrained to their family and their social contacts are limited. During adolescence they begin to realize the existing differences between them and people around them. When a child with Asperger syndrome tries to find friends, to tell a joke or to attract attention, he is usually excluded from the group, victimized or insulted.

H. Asperger describes symptomatology close to that described by Leo Kanner. He concludes that the disabilities in these children are related to the emotional and behavioral areas. Speech appears much earlier, then, a period of low verbal activity follows due to the experience that other people cause problems and one should avoid contact with them. This leads to introspection and isolation. Speech production emerges prior to walking habits. The child lives in his own social environment in his own idiosyncratic manner.

Leo Kanner not only is the first to describe and analyze the behavior of children with autism but he also sets the beginning of discussions about diagnosis of autism. In the 1940's in psychiatric literature descriptions by Leo Kanner and H. Asperger appear about disorders with similar behavioral deviations, united under the common term "autism." If the provided descriptions are closely inspected it will be found the the cases are very similar. H. Asperger completes the evolution of the disorder following its dynamics in later age and believes that autistic psychopathy is different from early childhood autism in which there is an organic disability or dementia. Good prognosis gives reasons to Asperger to classify the syndrome as part of psychopathies.

Social criteria for Kanner and Asperger syndromes are identical. Children with Asperger syndrome are isolated but make attempts to present themselves to others although using inappropriate means. Their speech is pedantic often unnecessary, without direction and limited in topics. They are often described as loners who show some interest into making friends and contacts. They are chronically frustrated by their unsuccessful attempts to engage others and to establish relations with them. They usually misinterpret the context of the affective interactions based on their lack of sensitivity to the emotions of other people.

Unlike Kanner syndrome, in Asperger syndrome the qualitative impairments of communication are not present as a symptom in his definition. Problems with speech prosody have been reported as opposed to speech in Kanner syndrome which is rigid and monotonous. A second feature constitutes in an egocentric communication style. The chosen topics are related to favourite objects and events without taking into consideration the interests of the listener. The object of interest changes every year or every two years. Motor clumsiness in Asperger syndrome is manifested in delayed acquisition of general and fine motor skills like riding a bike, throwing and catching a ball, climbing as well as particularly pronounced difficulties in visual-motor coordination.

Going through the original articles by L. Kanner and H. Asperger one is left with the impression for the lack of grounds to consider that the latter has described entirely different type of children. The definition of H. Asperger about autism is much more detailed than that of L. Kanner but his article remains unheeded compared to that of L. Kanner which is widely discussed and cited.

Today Asperger syndrome is defined as a generalized developmental disorder which is a term-umbrella, comprising of a spectrum of disorders that differ in the quantity and quality of their symptoms or age when they appear (Szatmari 2000). Nowadays there is a tendency to relate Asperger syndrome to an exceptionally intelligent with high verbal abilities close to the norm autistic child. This definitely is not the disorder H. Asperger had in mind but the existence of such special category is actually clinically convinient. In fact, there is not a unified accepted definition of Asperger syndrome. Lack of agreement between different authors brings lots of confusion since clinical professionals feel free to use the label depending on their own interpretations of what Asperger had on mind.

In ICD – 10 Asperger syndrome is classified as similar to autism but lacking language or intellectual disabilities. Such individuals manifest pronounced ineptness in communication as they are either too silent or too verbose and do not take into consideration the situation or the interests of their communication partner. Nonverbal communication skills and movement coordination is impaired to a great extent. There is inadequate intonation, wrong pronoun usage, verbal stereotypes. However, high achievements are observed in narrow fields of interest.

The theoretical ties between Kanner and Asperger syndromes determine a vicious circle in scientific studies looking for differences between autism and Asperger syndrome. Until this day research has not been able to discover apparent differences between the two syndromes. Even if it is accepted that Asperger syndrome is in fact autism combined with high intellectual levels there emerges a question whether that is a form of autism or the only existing type of autism. In cases of low intellectual functioning is it not advisable to talk about intellectual deficit which inevitably causes the development of autistic features and affective inability? L. Wing believes that Asperger syndrome is the only form of autism. Other authors, however, claim that Asperger syndrome comprises a distinguishable group defined as a group at the upper end of the autistic spectrum (Gillberg 1992).

According to the paradigm of the theory of mind Asperger syndrome could be related to those individuals who acquire metarepresentations and theory of mind after a substantial and harmful delay. Like other individuals with autism they do not possess such skills in their early years and because of that they do not develop normal social interactions, normal perception and expression of internal states.

Eventually they develop a theory of mind but not like in normal children since they miss the "critical period" and they adapt themselves to the different perceptual and cognitive schemas too late. The latter usually develop in parallel with the theory of mind and metarepresentations. Therefore, in Asperger syndrome this theory is not going to be useful in the usual sense – people with that syndrome will succeed on tasks which elements are obvious but will not be able to handle simple real life situations that include imperceptible signs. This theory can explain the high frequency of psychiatric disorders among these individuals (Tantam 1991). Depression can be due to the insight they have about their difficulties and emotions.

Psychotic symptoms could be caused by inadequate and untimely development of a theory of mind. According to Frith (1991) people with Asperger syndrome who acquire a theory of mind late and therefore in an abnormal way, are exposed to a high risk of developing an abnormal theory of mind. This assumption leads to the conclusion that in Kanner syndrome there cannot be such symptomatology. In that sense Asperger syndrome can be viewed as intermediate – between classical autism in which a theory of mind is absent and schizophrenia in which case the theory of mind is hyperactive (Ozonoff, Bowler 1996). This hypothesis suggests redirection of attention from superficial behavioral manifestations to basic cognitive disabilities. A criterion often used for differential diagnosis is the distinction of the use of speech in children with Kanner and Asperger syndromes. It is widely accepted that speech in people with autism do not serve a communicative function. Speech activity is related to the accidental use of names of different objects, names of people or mechanically memorized expressions showing good procedural and fragmentary memory. Unlike them in people with Asperger syndrome speech does serve a communicative, however, interactions are avoided because others are perceived as intruders. Behavioral reactions toward others also differ for the two syndromes. The child with autism does not notice people around him, while children with Asperger syndrome know others exist they just need to be avoided.

All features characterizing Asperger syndrome can be observed to some degree in the normal population. People differ from one another in terms of their skills in social interactions and in considering the nonverbal behavior of the people they communicate with. Many individuals who are independent and capable as adults have specific interests but that fact does not mean that they belong to the group of people with Asperger syndrome. H. Asperger himself notes that isolation in one's own world and presence of specific interests is common among the normal population. The difference between people suffering from Asperger syndrome and people with normal development is that the latter do not find it difficult to lead a two-way conversation while the former experience difficulties in their interactions. All individuals from the normal population have their own inner world which often is influenced by social experiences while people with Asperger are isolated, detached from others.

Rett Syndrome

Unlike other developmental disorders Rett syndrome is encountered predominantly among girls. It is first described in Germany in 1966 but becomes popular in 1983 when observations are published in English books and magazines. Concordance in identical twins is close to 100% and in siblings around 0% allows for the assumption about the genetic neuro-degenerative nature of the disorder by a spontaneous mutation of a specific gene.

Rett syndrome is accompanied by progressive motor disabilities, spinal atrophies and severe motor defects. Gradually with age the child begins losing muscle volume, changes are observed in the joints and the spinal column. Many children lose their ability to move independently.

For diagnosing someone with Rett syndrome the first manifestations observed between 7-24 months are especially important. The most distinctive symptom is the loss of purposeful hand movements, distinctive stereotypical movements resembling twisting or washing the hands. Stereotypical wetting of palms with saliva, defective chewing, excessive salivation and tongue thrusting as well as loss of social engagement against a relatively preserved social smile.

Such children look towards or through people without making contact with them. Characteristic of the disorder are the posture and the walk against muscle hypertonus. In later childhood there is a tendency for developing ataxy and somatopraxy related to scoliosis or kyphoscoliosis and sometimes with choreoathetosis. Often in early or late childhood seizures appear which are usually small seizures with onset prior to the age of 8. These disabilities result in a pronounced delay in mental functioning. Progressive motor disability confirm the diagnosis.

In order to make a Rett syndrome diagnosis the condition needs to meet the following criteria:

- Clear normal psychomotor development during the first five months and normal head circumference at the time of birth.
- Retention of the head enlargement retention in the period 6 months – 4 years and loss of acquired manual habits until the age of 2 years and 6 months.
- Severe impairment of the impressive and expressive speech.
- Stereotypical hand movements demonstrated in parallel with loss of manual skills.

Unlike autism in Rett syndrome there is motor discoordination, characterized by a walk with widely placed legs, "washing" of the hands with saliva, hyperventilation and the most characteristic of the syndrome – the presence of a period of normal psychomotor development.

In case of Rett syndrome, normal early development is followed by a partial or full loss of acquired manual skills and speech as well as by a delay of head growth. Especially typical is the loss of purposeful hand movements, the emergence of stereotypes like hand twisting and hyperventilation.

Rett syndrome is a neurological disorder characterized by severe cognitive and physical impairments. The classical form is encountered only among girls. In the last couple of decades there is an increase in the agreement among specialists regarding developmental disorders namely that different genetic disorders have a specific effect on behavior. Behavior in those disorders has general and specific features that comprise the behavioral phenotype. Rett syndrome is a homogenic disorder with different variability of symptoms which gives grounds to describe different types of the syndrome. There is no consensus regarding the biological markers and this is further exacerbated by the fact that the different disorders demonstrate similar symptomatology. Development of girls with the syndrome is normal for the first 6 months of their life which does not refute the notion that the disorder is present at birth.

Language development on the level of single words in a way develops prematurely. General and fine motor movements develop according to the age norm. Development between 6 and 18 months slows down or stops. This period of stagnation is followed by a period of regress which continues between 1 and 4 years. During the regression phase it can be observed loss of social and communication skills, of manipulative actions, of speech and words. The regression is specific for the skills in those three spheres and is not observed in others. In the period between 2 and 10 years development is in a state of plateau. Neuromotor functions may continue to digress but this is not always observed. Individuals with Rett syndrome can acquire some new skills in that late phase. In the progressive phase severe cognitive impairments are observed. In that period some individuals can demonstrate mental age corresponding to the age of 8 months.

Repetitive hand movements are one of the required diagnostic criteria for the classical Rett syndrome. There is a wide variability of stereotypical hand movements including: repetitions, very simple or primarily clumsy movements of touching, rubbing, squeezing or pinching, washing, twisting, hand licking, finger twisting and clapping; also putting the hands in the mouth and finger licking as hands are associated with dyskinetic movements of the mouth and tongue. For some individuals with Rett syndrome – hand movements are executed around the center of the body with both hands. Manual stereotypes are defined by the age of the individual.

Abnormal breathing is encountered when the child is awake and is absent when she is asleep. Irregular breathing is observed during periods of extremely fast and shallow breathing. Periods of apnea are situated 60 to 120 seconds apart. This model of periodic hyperventilation and breathing retention happens more often to younger girls. Among girls with the syndrome there are difficulties with inspiration as well.

Results from studies about sleep patterns are contradictory probably due to the use of different methodologies. Some authors report that individuals with Rett syndrome have problems falling asleep at night, wake up early in the morning and fall asleep often during the day. This means that individuals with Rett syndrome sleep less at night but more for 24 hours compared to healthy controls. Sleep hours do not correlate with age. Day sleep is positively correlated to age as opposed to night sleep which is respectively negatively correlated to age.

Autistic-like behavior gives grounds to many authors to accept Rett syndrome as a subtype of autism. In contemporary classification manuals – ICD, DSM, Rett syndrome is part of the pervasive developmental disorders. More than two decades researchers have been focusing on the possibility to differentiate the syndrome from autism. There is a consensus that a large number of behavior reactions are common for both conditions:

- Lack of eye contact
- Lack of appropriate interests and facial expression
- Speech and language disabilities

These symptoms are usually present during the first stages of Rett syndrome, during the stagnation and regression periods. The absence of facial expression is observed in 71% of cases during the first year, lack of motor adaptation – in 69%, lack of eye contact – in 63%, isolation and indifference – in 63%. The percentage of children who never point with a finger is 68%, there is lack of verbal expression, difficulty in understanding movements executed by others is encountered in 87%, self-stimulating behavior – in 73%, sudden laughter and screams – in 73% (Nomura, Y.; Segawa, M. 1990).

Diagnosis and differential diagnosis of Rett syndrome is hindered by the presence of symptoms observed in other autistic spectrum disorders. Still the presence of normal psycho-motor development during the first months of life and gender of carriers of that syndrome can serve as differential diagnostic criteria.

Rett syndrome is one of the relatively rare genetic disorders in childhood. With development of genetic research it has become possible to differentiate distinct subtypes. This refutes the understanding that Rett syndrome follows a single course of regress of already acquired skills.

Diagnosis in those cases is based on the clinical assessment and the use of diagnostic criteria for atypical Rett syndrome which should include at least three of the six main criteria and at least five of the eleven additional criteria for classical Rett syndrome. Differential diagnosis includes Angelman syndrome, autism, congenital metabolic disorders and intellectual deficit. Childhood degenerative disorder is another type of generalized developmental disorder that defines the presence of a period of clearly normal development until the onset of the disorder and of clearly defined phase of loss of already acquired skills which comprises at least several developmental areas and coincides with the onset of some typical abnormal features in social, cognitive and behavioral functioning.

This condition is observed in 3-4-year-old children and is characterized by a substantial drop in intellectual, emotional and language functioning during a period of several months. This rarely encountered condition had been described long before autism but it has been recognized only in recent years.

Children with that syndrome develop all autistic spectrum features but after a long period of completely normal development. The condition differs from autism in its onset, development and result. Due to the fact that it is rare it is often misdiagnosed as autism. The following several criteria are mandatory for the correct diagnosis of the syndrome:

- loss of social skills
- loss of bladder and sphincter control
- loss of expressive and receptive speech
- loss of motor skills
- loss of play

- inability to develop personal relationships with children own age
- impairments of nonverbal behavior
- inability to initiate and maintain conversation

Prognosis is ususally not good – most individuals are left with severe mental retardation. There is uncertainty to what degree this condition differs from autism. In some cases the disorder is due to an accompanying encephalopathy, but the diagnosis should be based on behavioral symptoms.

The onset is usually around the age of 3 or 4. Before that the child becomes anxious, tense, increases his physical activity, demonstrates stereotypical movements and compulsive behavior. Differential diagnosis should be made with the syndromes in the group of autistic spectrum disorders, with Landau Klephner syndrome and receptive speech disorders.

Often there is a period of unclear illness: the child becomes dopy, aroused, anxious and hyperactive.

A decline follows and then a loss of speech and language accompanied by behavioral disintegration. In some cases the loss of skills is persistently progressive – usually when the disorder is accompanied by a progressive neurological disorder, but usually the decline lasts several months and then it is followed by a plateau and after that - by a slight improvement.

Diagnosis is based on the presence of clear normal development at least until the age of 3, followed by a loss of acquired skills accompanied by abnormal quality of social functioning. Usually there is a substantial regress or loss of speech, regress in skills for play, in social skills and adaptive behavior. These symptoms are accompanied by a general loss of interest to the environment, by stereotypical, repetitive motor mannierisms.

The described characteristics of Rett syndrome and "Other disintegrative disorder" are not observed in Asperger syndrome and therefore differentiation is facilitated. However, difficulties can be encountered when distinguishing between different conditions even outside the group of pervasive disorders.

Many objections and discussions are raised by the formulation of the nosological unit "atypical autism".

Atypical autism differs from childhood autism by the onset of the disorder. Abnormal development can manifest itself for the first time at the age of 3 and there might not be enough abnormalities in social interaction, communication and stereotypical behavior.

Typical for atypical autism is that it emerges most often in individuals with mental retardation in whom the low intellectual level does not give an opportunity to express specific behavioral deviations necessary for diagnosing someone with autism.

Moreover, atypical autism can emerge as a result of a severe impairment of the receptive speech which hinders the formation of proper verbal production and deprives the child from communication means.

The disorder is represented by at least two of the following categories – joint social interaction, communication problems, stereotypical, limited behavior. The observed abnormalities bear autistic-like character and are a consequence of other deficits like mental retardation or severe receptive speech disorder. The autistic behavior is based not on mental isolation but on the lack of means for communication and as a result others become uninteresting and useless.

The use of this nosological unit puts into question the necessity for a hierarchy of symptoms, their unification in symptom-complex as a necessary requirement for making a nosological diagnosis.

Another reason for objection is the fact that as a nosological unit is used a term characterizing the consequences of the presence of an established primary deficit. This creates too many misunderstandings among specialists and results in a substantial number of diagnostic mistakes.

DIFFERENTIAL DIAGNOSIS OF CONDITIONS OUTSIDE THE AUTISTIC SPECTRUM

Language Developmental Disorders

In most part of the cases communication disorders accompany the abnormal childhood development. They can be both the reason and the consequence of disabled childhood functioning.

In case of impaired language development all subsystems of the language system are affected not necessarily to the same degree. These children show deficits in cognitive development as a confirmation of the fact that language development is indicative of cognitive functioning. The realization/awareness of one's own language incompetence in some cases results in a change of psychological conditions and manifestations of neuroticism, anxiety, depressivity as well as a change in social interactions with children own age and adults. Such children are often labeled as different, even mentally retarded.

The first indication for the presence of a problem is the lack of active speech. Undeniable indicaitons in early childhood for the presence of a developmental disorder are:

- Lack of latent speech until 12 months of age;
- Lack of joint interest with other people towards objects;
- Lack of single words until the age of 16 monts as well as two-word sentences until 24 monts;
- Loss of language and social skills at every age.

The etiology of motor language disorders has not been entirely clarified yet. It is assumed the presence of developmental problems of the cerebral mechanisms, however, this has not been expressly confirmed. Such children usually make eye contact, take part in nonverbal play and activities, use toys and objects for their designated purpose.

The development of language subsystems is impaired. This poses a serious difficulty in education and adaptation for these children. Gradually a secondary mental retardation can be observed as a result of the impossibility for thinking to become processed through speech and in turn speech to become meaningful.

Expressive speech disabilities need to match the following criteria:

- Expressive speech skills, defined by tests, should not be less than two standard deviations below the level corresponding to the chronological age of the child;

- Data from expressive speech development correlates with level of nonverbal intellect within one standard devidation;
- Test results for impressive language skills are normal or are within two standard deviations corresponding to the age of the child;
- Understanding and use of nonverbal signs corresponds to age norm;
- There are no neurological, sensory or somatic disorders which might directly affect expressive speech;
- Intellectual quotient is higher than 70.

Widely discussed is the communication disorder, diagnosed through the years as alalia, general underdevelopment of speech, dysphasia of development, specific language disorder etc. The existence of multitude of terms for one nosological entity is a clear sign for ambiguity and uncertainty regarding the definition and identification of that disorder as well as regarding its etiology. Regardless of how the disorder is named, it should be kept in mind that it can be diagnosed only when visual and auditory senses and intellect are intact. In spite of the absence of intellectual, sensory or somatic impairments the child does not acquire the necessary for the age and sociocultural environment language skills. In that regard there should be distinguished two conditions – delayed language development and impaired language development.

In case of delayed language development there is a preserved speed of progression and succession of development but the onset of language development is shifted in time with minimum of 6 months from the presumable age norm. Children with delayed language development do not manifest deficits in impressive speech, the delay usually affects only expressive speech. Communication in most cases is implemented through paralinguistic means which do not complement but substitute specific verbal information. Such children do not show deviations in cognitive functioning but depending on the period of delay they become gradually isolated from the group of children their own age which changes their future personal and social development. Moreover those children are often given negative labels, which influences their functioning as a whole.

In case of expressive language disorders, assessment with standard developmental tests for expressive speech is significantly under the level of nonverbal intellect and impressive speech. This incongruence is manifested clinically through symptoms including limited dictionary, grammar mistakes in speech formation, difficulties in sentence production in terms of their complexity and completeness. These difficulties influence school skills and social interacitons.

In case of mixed type impressive-expressive impairments development of the impressive as well as the expressive speech is significantly below the level of nonverbal intellect. The clinical picture comprises of inadequate comprehension of words, sentences, entire text as well as difficulties in speech production.

Impairments of impressive speech are always manifested also as impairments of speech production. The etiology is unspecified but usually many signs of brain cortex failure are observed. Those children show impaired speech understanding against relatively well preserved nonverbal intellect. They have autistic-like behavior and often perceive themselves as such but respond in an adequate way to nonverbal stimuli. There is a heightened threshold of auditory sensitivity, absence of ear for music and inability to localize the source of the sound.

Specific developmental disorder of receptive speech is characterized by the fact that the ability of the child to understand speech is below the level of his mental age. In almost all cases the expressive speech is also impaired and there are abnormalities in word and sound pronunciation. Diagnosis is justified only when symptoms are outside the norm. Placing a diagnosis can be hard due to the inability to understand grammatical structures (negation, questions, comparisons, etc.) and incomprehension of the fine aspects of language. Receptive speech disorder can be considered only when the criteria for generalized developmental disorder are not met. Moreover, from all variations of specific disorders in this case the accompanying emotional, behavioral and social impairments are with the highest frequency.

Such disorders do not take any special form but are usually manifested as hyperactivity, attention deficit, low social adaptability, isolation, anxiety, sensitivity or excessive timidity. In children with a severe form of the disorder social development can be delayed, they can show echolalia without understanding what they have heard and to have limited interests. They differ from children with autism because usually show normal emotional bonding, normal mock play, normal parent seeking for comfort, normal use of gestures and only mild impairments in nonverbal communication.

Receptive language disorders include:

- Verbal auditory agnosia
- Comprehension deficit
- Delayed speech

Early symptoms are:

- Echolalia, repetitive speech – spontaneous or delayed.
- Inability to follow instructions.
- Inapproprite answers to asked questions.
- Repetition of asked questions before giving an answer.
- Difficulties in answering yes/no questions and questions about when, where and how.
- Lack of attention to oral speech in cases of high level of activity.
- Jargon phasias etc.

All children with autistic spectrum disorders have to some degree a receptive language disorder. It is possible, however such type of language disorder to be specific without its presence to be defined by sensory, neurological or psychological illnesses and disorders. Pragmatic language disorders often remain undiagnosed because of the possibility the behavioral and emotional peculiarities of the child to be explained with isolation and shyness. Pragmatic language disorders are manifested in an inability to use the appropriate language code corresponding to the situation and the communication partner. These disorders include: constant question asking, loss of eye contact, excessive talk about specific objects in detail, indifference to others, talking only about oneself, dialogue disengagement, literal comprehension of speech, inability to answer open questions, difficulties in understanding abstract speech – understanding multiple meaning of jokes, inability to put oneself in the position of the listener, inability to understand and interpret body language and facial expression, inability to express feelings, disregard for the situation and the collocutor. Differential diagnosis between autistic spectrum disorders and language developmental disorders is especially difficult due to the fact that language disabilities are diagnostic criteria for autistic spectrum disorders. In case of children with language disorders social isolation can be observed but as secondary symptomatology, as a result of the lack of or limited number of verbal means for communication with others. Unlike children with autistic spectrum disorders, they look for contact with others, do not live in their own world, for them others exist although communication is difficult.

Landau-Kleffner Syndrome – Acquired Aphasia with Epilepsy

Landau-Kleffner syndrome is a disorder in which after an initial normal language development the child loses his receptive as well as expressive speech skills but preserves his general intellect. The difference is that the onset of this type of pathology is accompanied by paroxysmal records in the EEG, almost always in the temporal lobes usually bilateral. The onset is usually between 3 and 7 years but its onset can happen earlier or later in childhood. In ¼ of cases the loss of speech occurs gradually for a period of several months, but sometimes this loss can be sudden – for a couple of days or weeks. In some cases the quality of voice is affected as the normal intonations are lost. In the months following the initial loss of speech behavioral and emotional problems are often observed but they gradually die down and children acquire some other means for communication. The etiology of this disorder is unknown but the clinical picture presupposes the presence of an inflammatory process. It is necessary to make a differential diagnosis with pervasive developmental disorders characterized by early normal development followed by regress – like Rett and Heller syndromes. A mandatory part of the instruments for differential diagnosis is an EEG test. The difficulties are caused by the possibility for the existence of comorbidity between epilepsy and an autistic spectrum disorder. Landau-Kleffner syndrome (acquired aphasia with epilepsy) can be diagnosed in accordance with the following criteria:

- The loss of impressive and expressive speech skills should be of a duration not less than 6 months.
- There is normal language development until the moment of speech loss.
- The presence of mono or bilateral paroxysmal changes in EEG results in temporal lobe areas in between up to two years before or after the onset of the speech impairments.
- Normal nonverbal intellect.
- Apart from paroxysms there are no other neurological disorders.
- The condition does not match the symptoms of a general developmental disorder.

It is necessary to make a differential diagnosis with Rett and Heller syndromes in which case there is early normal development followed by a loss of impressive and expressive speech abilities. The differential diagnostic criterion is the presence of EEG abnormalities in the temporal lobes.

SENSORY INTEGRATION AND DISINTERGRATION

Sensory integration signifies reception, processing, integration and order of sensory perceptions so that thay are used in a purposeful and meaningful way. These sensations give information about our physical condition, our presence in the world, the relations of the self with others and the world etc.

Mental activity is accomplished through the simultaneous participation of the three functional brain units. According to A. Luria the energetic unit or the unit for regulating cortical tone and waking receives signals from internal organs and from sensory analyzing systems by catching events from the outside world. This unit processes the signals that energize the brain cortex. In case of impairment in cortical tone and waking there are three types of phases – equalizing, paradoxical and ultraparadoxical, varying in the relationship stimul-recation. The second functional unit of the brain according to Luria is for reception, analysis and storage of information. It consists of three sections – visual (occipital), auditory (temporal) and general sensory (parietal).

Primary zones break down the incoming information into a large quantity of comprising elements, secondary zones synthesize these characteristics and the tertiary ones integrate the information in different sensory channels. The third functional unit is responsible for programming, regulating and verifying conscious activity. It implements planning and organization of behavior, transition from one operation to the next, manages the implementation of the program, checks the final product against the initial plan, corrects mistakes etc. As a result of the joint action of these three functional units, implementing the analysis and synthesis of incoming information, a plan for action is designed. If the program cannot solve a task, a new program is designed until there is an adequate reaction of the organism to the incoming signals.

In case of sensory disintegration the brain cortex is not able to systemize the constant flow of incoming sensory impulses carrying sensory information i.e., sensory disintegration is related to brain dysfunction. Lack of an adequate sensory perception processing leads to an inability to form socially adaptive patterns of behavior. In case of an absence of an adequate sensory integration the processes that suffer the most are the ones related to learning, there is inability to cope with constant every day increasing demands from the environment and the accompanying stress situations. The most affected ability is the one for processing past experience which lowers to a great extent the adaptation ability.

The term "sensory disintegration" is introduced for the first time by A. Iris to signify an inability to process particular information received through senses. Sensory disintegration is an impairment of the process of acceptance, organization and integration of sensory information. It hinders the ability of the individual to plan and organize actions necessary for adequate behavior required by the changes in the environment. According to Carol Kranowitz neurological brain disintegration can be manifested in three ways:

- Brain incapacity to receive signals due to severed ties in nervous cells

- Inconsistency of received sensory signals and
- Consistent reception against inadequate coordination with other sensory messages.

In case of impaired processing of sensory information the individual is not able to provide a motor response and to manifest adequate beahavior. Each person in his life has moments of sensory disintegration due to the inability to sustain constant optimal regulation of his body. For instance, when an individual is deprived of sleep for a long period of time reflexes and concentration suffer.

Contemporary understanding of sensory disintegration is related to impairments of sensory modulation. It is discussed that the individual cannot regulate the entry of sensory information in an adequate way which negatively affects his ability to maintain adequate behavior. The main aspects of sensory disintegration can be systemized in two categories:

- Receiving an excessive amount of sensory information which results in "overload." The individual is overly sensitive and responds inadequately to ordinary sounds.
- Receiving an insufficient amount of sensory information which leads to a craving for intense sensory stimulation.

This means that the individual can react intensely to an insignificant sensory stimulus or to ignore intense stimulation from the environment. Many authors believe that the autistic isolation is a result of a similar sensory instability. Perceived objects through different sensory modalities do not make sense because they do not stay constant in time. Such children cannot develop correct and accurate perceptions. This leads to increased levels of anxiety. It is possible that the individual blocks sensory information in order to protect himself from an "overload" by "closing" some of the sensory modalities especially when it is related to information that he experiences as threatening.

In case of sensory disintegration of the auditory modality there are difficulties in ignoring unnecessary information. For instance, at a loud place all sounds are heard with the same intensity. This results in behavioral problems caused by the frustration and inability to neglect insignificant sensory stimuli. Such children often plug their ears or have an exaggerated response to loud and unexpected sounds. Those suffering from a lack of sufficient sensory information feel anxious and tense in quiet situations and aim at causing some kind of noise that would provide them with a kind of protection.

Individuals who are hypersensitive to visual stimuli often experience fear in public places with many people or in very bright rooms. Their behavioral reactions are extreme – they either become hyperactive or seek isolation. They prefer to stand in the dark, avoid vivid colors and eye contact, they feel insecure when they climb up or down stairs. Those who suffer from insufficient visual stimulation peer intently into objects and faces or put them too close to their own face. Sensory disintegration of the visual mode can lead to ineffective communication face to face due to the lack of understanding of the expression of the other person.

In case of disintegration of the gustatory modality children experience severe tension and frustration when they are presented with strong smells or tastes regardless of whether they are pleasant or not. They avoid certain foods either because of how they taste or because of what they are comprised of. Those who are not sensitive enough often aim for strong and specific smells and food, bring to their nose or mouth all kinds of objects in order to feel them better and because of that often seem to have weird food preferences. Such children are easily distractible and find it difficult to perform any purposeful actions.

In tactile modality disintegration children show extreme reactions to insignificant or gentle touch, avoid touching as a whole or certain materials and surfaces. They do not like walking barefoot, playing with sand, glue, plasticize, soiling their hands or touching unfamiliar objects. The low threshold to tactile stimulation makes children insensitive to pain, they do not act adequately by retracting their hand from hot surfaces, they do not "remember" they have to wear certain clothes when it is hot or cold. In case of such low sensitivity children may experience serious injuries. In situations of frustration they often bite their fingers or nails, play with their hair, they are constantly moving and looking for tactile stimulation.

Sensory disintegration of the vestibular system leads to high or low sensitivity to movement. These children are afraid of heights and have "gravitational insecurity". In order to avoid such discomfort they keep their head straight up and they look stiff. On the other hand, low sensitivity to movement leads to behavior of stimulation seeking. Such children are constantly moving, hanging or turning for long periods of time which does not make them unstable. They often experience severe problems keeping their balance – they bump into walls and objects and lack an instinct to protect themselves from blows. Due to these characteristics children are often diagnosed as hyperkinetic.

Impairments of the proprioceptive system processing result in problems with planning motor actions or with the ability to use one's own body. This may have an impact on the implementation of every day life activities like writing, drawing, dressing, eating. Since the child does not realize the extent of his body he often bumps into objects or falls down. These children are clumsy and awkward and have difficulty solving relatively simple problems.

Sensory disintegration results in four main groups of problems:

- Related to attention and activity regulation. The ability to take part in an assignment transforms into an ability to identify and maintain sensory information or background noise.
- Protection from sensory stimulation – a behavioral reaction of fear and flight reaction. Such children are easily aroused, they prepare their body for survival without recognizing that a particular stimulus is not threatening. The answer to this fear is usually aggression, flight or isolation from ordinary every day activities which the child experiences as frustrating or threatening.
- Impairments of activity levels. These children are disorganized, they lack purpose or interest, they do not calm down easily after physical activity.
- Adaptation and behavior: These children are either explosive or aggressive, it is hard for them to adapt to new conditions of the environment, they often cry and are very irritable. Very often such actions are a result of the lack of tolerance to loud noises, visual or tactile stimuli.

The enormous amount of problems that children with sensory disintegration can develop explains the lack of emotional stability and adequate social skills. Behavioral models and interactions of the child with others define to a great extent the attitude of others towards him.

Sensory disintegration diagnosis is made difficult by the fact that many psychological, neurological or psychiatric problems resemble sensory disintegration. Often sensory disintegration symptoms are misidentified as "psychological" problems. It is known that sensory information deprivation results in serious changes in brain functioning which are manifested as memory impairments, mental difficulties, personality changes, hallucinations etc.

Sensory disintegration is manifested in different ways in children. Symptoms can be systemized in several main groups:

- Hypersensitivity to touch. There is withdrawal from touch, avoidance of certain foods and clothes solely based on their texture, fear reaction to everyday activities for example bathing, washing etc.
- Low sensitivity to sensory stimulation. Such children usually seek intense sensory experiences.
- Unusually high or low level of activity.
- Coordination problems.
- Speech and language retardation.
- Problems with mastering school material. These problems are observed against normal intellectual functioning.
- Behavioral disorganization. There is inability to plan or to adapt.
- Low self-esteem. This is related to the negative reactions of others toward the behavior and reactions of the child.

Children with sensory disintegration demonstrate more than one symptom and can manifest social and emotional disabilities, loss of self-control, inability to stay calm and alone as well as difficulties in transition from one situation to the next.

Sensory disintegration is not included as a separate nosological unit in diagnostic manuals. Elements of sensory disintegration are present in many developmental disorders. Disintegration symptoms impact other areas of functioning. Information processing in different sensory modalities as well as the the ability to transfer that information from one sensory modality to another can be based on cognitive, emotional and behavioral deviations. Sensory disintegration diagnosis in autistic spectrum disorders will make the therapeutic strategies and social measures for children more precise.

ATTACHMENT DISORDERS

Attachment disorder is characterized by permanent abnormalities in the structure of social interactions of the child which are associated with emotional dysregulation and reactivity to environmental change. Phobias and anxiety are common. It is difficult to calm the child. There are impaired relationships with children own age accompanied by manifestations of aggression and self-aggression.

It is considered that the syndrome develops as a consequence of gross neglect by parents, maltreatment, unmet needs or bad upbringing. A sensitive parent satisfies the basic needs of the child which soothes the discomfort and arousal of the child. Children with secure attachment trust others and believe their needs are valid. Those who do not develop a secure attachment have a high risk of developing low self-esteem, needy or clinging behavior, pseudoindependence, decompensation in times of stress, loss of self-control, inability for initiating and maintaining friendships, separation and oppositional attitude towards parents, antisocial behavior, aggression and violence, inability to trust and show intimacy, pessimistic attitude toward oneself, family and society, lack of empathy, compassion and guilt, behavioral and learning problems etc.

Attachment disorders do not result solely in emotional and social problems but also in biochemical specificities in the developing brain. Children growing up without love and security have extremely high levels of stress hormones which may be harmful for brain and body growth and development. Neurolobiological consequences of emotional neglect can lead to change of behavioral patterns, psychological states and achievements.

One of the most harmful consequences of an insecure attachment of the child is his chronic inability to modulate his emotions, behavioral patterns and impulses. Attachment plays an important role in mastering self-control by the child. It is known that more than 80% of maltreated children develop disorientational and disorganizational attachment styles resulting in a wide range of symptoms.

Emotion and behavior regulation is an important part of psychological health which is viewed in the process of parent-child interaction. Signals by the child (gazes, screams, cooing etc.) enhance emotional reactions in the parent. Depressive, maltreating or neglecting parents cannot discern the signals the child sends them and because of that do not respond to the emotions and needs of the child and he grows up without the necessary internal regulating support which results in three main reactions:

- Feelings of alienation and loneliness, impaired representation for own body.
- Inability to control impulses – physical and sexual aggression, self-disfiguration.
- Lack of trust and intimacy – perceiving others as threatening (Cole & Putnam 1992).

Reasons for the disorder should be sought in the development of a parent-child relationship and the attachment between them. There are a number of factors that refer both to the parent and the child as well as to the environment the child grows in and develops. 40-70% of mothers experience postpartum depression as a result of the radical change in hormone levels. And about 30% have a prolonged and severe postpartum depression. Such mothers find it difficult to take good care of their children which is a result of the depressive symptomatology as well as of their insensitivity towards the signals of the child. If the depression continues during the first six months after birth a delay in child development will affect locomotion, body growth and lower social responsiveness. When depression of the mother continues throughout the first year of life, the child shows a profile of behavioral and physiological dysregulation. Those characteristics can result in behavioral problems and aggression in preschool age.

Reactions of children to separation and encounter have an impact on the history of parent-child interactions as well as on the parental style and the psychosocial functioning of the child (Brettherton 1985).

Children with a disorganized attachment are labeled as indecisive, fearful and traumatized. They do not complain of losses, they are afraid to admit past traumas (Main

1994). They actively and condescendingly devalue attachment etc. Mothers of such children often have a history of family violence and abuse. Such mothers are not responsive to their children needs and give inaccurate, inappropriate or contradicting cues to their children (Lyons-Ruth 1994). They show high levels of negative affect toward their children and low levels of tenderness. Often parents who grew up in abusive families, transfer their fears and insecurity to their own children, behave as insensitive, abusive, depressive people without showing love or attachment. Children of such parents are put in a paradoxical situation: closeness to parents increases the fears of the child, however, at the same time the child needs soothing contact and support.

In 1969 Bowlby defines the term "attachment" as the "presence of a continous psychological connection between two human beings". In the first months after birth there are some specific behavioral activities on the part of the baby that provoke certain actions on the side of the mother. These relations are the basis for child ego and identity development. The specific behavioral activity on the part of the child and the mother are a prerequisite for attachment formation. When a caregiver responds adequately to the needs of the child, the latter begins to develop trust toward the world. This process is known as "cycle of trust." Children who develop an ability to internalize security and safety and can "use" their emotions are able to accept and learn from their failures.

Children who develop a reactive attachment disorder for some reasons do not succeed in establishing a strong psychological attachment to the caregiver and do not learn to trust others. There are different studies which show that mothers are "tuned" to perceive and respond to the emotional expression of their child even when emotions as such have not appeared yet. In the beginning the emotional patterns of the child are primitive but gradually they become more complicated and differentiated. This expression stimulates the empathic resources of the mother by which she is able to feel the internal condition of the child. Children are also "tuned" to perceive the emotions of their mother. In the second half of the first year children demonstrate an ability to use perception of emotion of the mother to receive support and also to use her facial expression to adapt to an unknown situation i.e., there is already social reference.

There are certain specificities of child development in regard to the development of the mother-child relationship which directly influence the future emotional and social functioning of the child. Due to his immaturity the child needs a symbiotic relationship with the mother which gradually weakens through the process of maturation of sensorymotor functions and the acquisition of independence. Insufficient or inconsistent satisfaction of emotional needs and "signals" of the child can lead to emotional and/or cognitive impairments. In the period between two and four years the child begins to separate from his mother experiencing a sufficient amount of frustrating experience. In relation to that he formulates a passion toward discoveries and learns to say "no." This period is of the so called "ambivalence conflict" when the symbiotic relationship with the mother exists simultaneously with the striving of the child to separate from her.

Reactive attachment disorder is characterized by an inability to establish normal relations with others. Such children react strongly to changes in the environment, they are restless and are difficult to soothe. The symptoms of the reactive attachment disorder tentatively can be divided into 4 groups: social, emotional, behavioral and developmental symptoms.

Social symptoms are manifested in the fact that a child with such a disorder do not make "eye contact," often asks infinitely long and sensless questions or babbles without ceasing, tries to control everything around him which aggravates his relations with children his own age. Reacitons to strangers are emotionally indiscriminative. Those children often seem inadequate, threatening or clinging, with low self-esteem who do not show love towards their parents.

Behavioral symptoms are expressed in destructive behavior toward oneself, others and things.

They often are violent toward animals and siblings, have an impaired emotional control, they find appealing activities related to fire, blood, and viscera. In some cases they might steal, lie and have abnormal eating habits. Together with these symptoms there are other developmental peculiarities manifested as general retardation, absence of causal thinking, lack of awarenss as well as abnormal speech patterns.

Typical for reactive attachment disorder is the presence of a "negative attachment cycle" in the family.

The child has a markedly negative behavior which cannot be ignored and which in turn brings strong emotional reaction on the part of the parents thus creating intense but unsatisfactory relationship. As a result of that parent and child distance from one another and their relationship is destroyed.

The main symptoms are inability to establish contact and inadequate reactions in almost all social interactions as well as clinging to ill-known people.

The first signs of "hospitalism" or "anaclytical depression" (R. Spitz) are an absence of tracing, social smile, simple plays and nonverbal pleas to be picked up (after the age of 5 months), absence of clear behavioral signs of attachment toward the parents (after the age of 8 months). Such children do not aim for contact and do not show reciprocity although their ability for social interaction is preserved. They are not interested in the environment and the toys around them.

In that type of disorder the diagnostic criteria are:

- Onset prior to the age of 5.
- Contradicting or ambivalent social reactions in different social situations.
- Emotional impairments – loss of reciprocity, isolation, aggressive reactions and increased anxiety.
- At large preserved abilities for social interaction.

The large range of symptoms in reactive attachment disorder sometimes makes it difficult to diagnose it. It is obligatory to make a differential diagnosis with generalized developmental disorders. It always needs to be considered the fact that children with reactive attachment disorder have normal abilities for social bonding unlike the ones with generalized developmental disorder.

When raised in normal conditions the abnormal style of social reactions decreases to a large degree, an observation that cannot be made in the case of generalized developmental disorders.

Although there are abnormal speech and language patterns in the reactive attachment disorder, they cannot be referred to the qualitatively abnormal characteristics of language development encountered in generalized developmental disorders. In children with reactive attachment disorder there are not any steady or gross cognitive deficits, nor are there stereotypical patterns of behavior, activity and interests.

Zeanah, Mammen, and Lieberman (1993) propose that attachment disorders constitute deep pervasive disorders of emotions of children about security and safety. They propose criteria for 5 types of attachment disorders that differentiate this condition from generalized developmental disorders:

- Children with an attachment disorder reactive type have normal abilities for social bonding and reciprocity unlike the ones with generalized developmental disorder.
- Regardless of the abnormal style of specific reactions in case of reactive attachment disorder the main feature of the behavior of the child in variety of situations is manifested by the fact that this abnormal style can be reduced and mitigated to a great extent if the child is put in normal raising conditions which provide constant care adjusted to the needs of the child. While such possible reduction is not observed in cases of generalized developmental disorder.
- Although children with reactive attachment disorder can have an impaired language development they do not show qualitatively abnormal characteristics of interaction typical for autism.
- Unlike autism eactive attachment disorder is not accompanied by steady and gross cognitive deficits which do not improve substantially after a change in the environment.
- Steadily limited, repetitive and stereotypical patterns of behavior, interests and activities are not typical of the reactive attachment disorder.

Reactive attachment disorder unlike autism and other autistic spectrum conditions almost always emerges as a result of grossly inadequate child care.

MENTAL RETARDATION

Many authors express doubts about the statement by Leo Kanner that the children he described have normal intelligence. Those doubts are based on the hypothesis that considering the gross impairment of emotions and social bonding, intellectual development cannot remain unaffected. This suggests age and not nosological specificity that can be observed in different disorders of the central nervous system. In support of that is the fact that most children diagnosed with autism later develop epileptic seizures and precisely because of that some authors believe that the diagnosis is encephalopathy with unknown origin.

Many authors claim that a large portion of children with autism are also mentally retarded. Around 80% of them have a proven IQ below 70. The connection between autism and low levels of intelligence represent a diagnostic challenge because the overall picture of mental retardation suggests an autistic type of behavior. Diagnostic procedures need to recognize the retardation of the intellectual development which to a great extent is related to impairments in communication, social skills and imagination. Some authors believe that classical autism described by Leo Kanner is the typicial version of a combination of autistic type of behavior and low IQ, while Asperger syndrome is the typical version of autistic behavior and high IQ.

For a diagnosis of mental retardation to be made there should be a lowered level of intellectual functioning leading to reduced possibilities for adaptation to every day requirements of the normal social environment. In order to diagnose correctly this condition it should be taken into account the global assessment of abilities and not only the specific impairments or skills in specific areas.

Goldberg, Benjamin and Creed (1992) underline the age as a diagnostic criterion for establishing mental retardation. In relation to term unification a group of experts from UNESCO propose a definition that differentiates two main features of mental retardation – delayed general development and limited learning abilities. The formation of cognitive functions is delayed and particular difficulties are observed in attention and verbal memory development. In some cases emotional reactivity is preserved but it is often inadequate and disproportionate to the stimulus. Emotions are extreme and unstable and they define the frequent mood change accompanied by motor arousal and stereotypical behaviors. Language system development is delayed but we cannot describe it as delayed language development, rather as impaired. There are impairments of the impressive as well as the expressive speech. Changes in language functioning have a more qualitative than quantitative nature. All those characteristics are manifested to a different degree depending on the type and degree of mental retardation.

According to most researchers the delay in psychosocial development in individuals with mental retardation is considered a result of the combination of genetic, organic, biochemical, social and other factors. There is a consensus about the fact that in most cases mental retardation is not caused by a single factor. In spite of that there is a tendency to seek for an isolated case of brain injury leading to brain dysfunction. In case of brain injury – in adults it causes loss of funcitons while in children it leads to a disorder of the psychosocial functioning.

In that sense still Vygotsky differentiates two types of disorders – primary defect and secondary impairments. Depending on the time of onset of the disorder there is either development or disintegration of the respective psychological function. Primary impairment is related to the so called matrices or systems of early stages of development, and secondary defects are connected to relatively stable structures, for instance, the brain cortex. From a developmental point of view slow pace of motor skills acquisition in a mentally retarded child shows that there is immaturity of all cortex zones. There are instances, however, of normal motor development in mentally retarded children. This is explained by the fact that possibly there is a dissonance in brain zones maturation. According to Luria (1973) retarded development and maturation of tertiary zones is a shared feature among children with mental retardation. This hinders the systematization and generalization of new experience in cognitive and emotional schemas.

Against all diversity in mental retardation symptoms there are some common features that are related to underdevelopment of psychological activity particularly cognitive processes and personality as a whole. Another common feature is based on the fact that impairments high-level cognitive processes have a leading role in the structure of the psychological defect, particularly abstract thinking against relatively good phylogenetic development of the older components.

In early childhood impairments of the cognitive activity are manifested in delayed development of psychomotor abilities, impairment of visual and auditory reflexes, change in emotional reactions, delayed speech and language development, weak cognitive interest etc. In school age the main characteristics of the clinical picture are – situational nature of thinking, inability to summarize/generalize, inability for differentiation and classification. In adolescence the most prominent is personality immaturity – increased suggestibility, lack of critical thinking, inability to make independent decisions, impulsivity, situational dependence of behavior etc. Mental retardation is related to an alteration of all psychological processes which is manifested in impairments of perception, attention, memory, and emotions. There is also inadequacy of affect considering the situation, insufficient initiative and motivation. The specificity of the clinical picture is determined by whether it is a hereditary or exogenously determined type of mental retardation.

Personality development suggests a simultaneous development of cognitive, emotional and social structures. The level of cognitive development is a keystone for the respective emotional and social growth. In every day practice, however, it is possible for the level of social functioning to outgrow the cognitive level, but this is usually a consequence of a specialized training in a protected environment. Low social skills are determined also by the isolation of those individuals and by their neglect of social interactions with others and by the non-compliance with the fact that childhood development to a great extent is influenced by the interaction with coevals which is a way to overcome segregation and to achieve a better level of development for those individuals.

Problems with assessment of intellectual development usually and traditionally are an important part of psychological assessment of childhood development. This is essential for childhood disorders since intellectual underdevelopment or deficits determine to a great extent the diagnosis and as a result the social status and the prognosis. The characteristics of the cognitive functioning when used for differential criteria should be considered carefully since secondary and tertiary impairments have a negative impact on the potential developmental possibilities of the child. Historically tests for intellectual assessment have been designed to record intellectual failure. Results of such tests are always descriptive in nature and because of that there is very low probability through them to provide an explanation for the way a task is executed. In relation to that there are many cases in which a low intelligence quotient does not necessarily mean intellectual deficit.

An important task of differential diagnosis is the differentiation of mental retardation from other similar conditions. This task is complicated by the fact that in the area of pathological development there is no symptom that is strictly specific and by whose presence or absence a differential diagnosis can be made.

Other disorders that require a differential diagnosis from mental retardation are speech and language disorders. Speech and especially language pathology is one of the main characteristics of children with mental retardation. In order to establish a preserved intellectual ability in children with speech and language pathology it is necessary above all to establish their ability to successfully execute tasks that do not require the use of speech. Difficulties in differential diagnosis are due mainly to the lack of clear and concrete objective criteria for mental retardation, even less an objective instrument for intellectual measurement and assessment. All techniques are to some extent subjective and depend on the professional and personal experience of the investigator. A large number of diagnostic methodologies consist of material that is abstract and cognitive in nature and the resolution of the different problems on the test is determined by training and environment. The group of children with mental retardation is very heterogenous and manifestations are diverse which puts into questions results from the same instruments for all children with mental retardation. In many studies it has been convincingly proven that the level of cognitive activity, of social adaptability and volition regulation as well as emotional reactions to success-failure to a great extent are defined by situational factors and influence the execution of intellectual tasks.

The thorough understanding of the symptomatology and the clinical picture of the different levels of mental retardation, the precise differentiation of primary impairments from secondary and tertiary ones again present the question about the validity of the diagnosis of atypical autism as well as the validity of the intelligence quotient as a differential diagnostic criterion in distinguishing between disorders within the group of pervasive developmental disorders.

For the correct diagnosis of autism it is necessary to look into its internal structure tentatively divided into four substages. According to developmental disorders of the different levels of basal affective organization, some authors define four groups of children with autism. The nature of disadaptation depends on the contacts of the child and the predominant role of one of the levels the functions of which always suffer from some deficit.

The first group of autism is related to a predominant influence by the deficits in the first affective level mechanisms. It is associated to the primitive and passive forms of mental adaptation. These forms take part in providing the individual with safety and control in his own psychological domain. Children from this group cannot develop their potential due to the pathological isolation in their own domain. There is an absence of motor and speech contact with the environment as well as an underdeveloped sense of pleasure, pain and hunger. The child strives for a primitive affective adaptation that would ensure comfort and safe position in the environment. There are no attempts for emotional contact and active interaction with other people.

In the second group of autism a dominant place in affective regulation is taken by the differentiated second level which designs adaptive reactions securing psychosomatic needs by developing stereotypical reactions in active sensory contact with the environment. Although he establishes a selective emotional contact with the environment, the child with autism from this group is satisfied by using a limited number of speech and motor patterns, adequate only in a number of situations. Typical for his behavior is a sense of fear and manifestations of aggression in response to any change. As a reaction to the violated internal emotional stability the child manifests self-stimulation in terms of tracing moving objects, playing with squeaky objects, arranging long lines of small objects, jumping continuously, freezing in strange body positions, designing own rituals to get rid of fear etc.

Disadaptation of the child with autism from the third group depends on the deficits in the mechanisms from the third level of affective behavioral organization which is connected to the general structure of the psychological domain. It is related to an active overcoming of obstacles and managing changes in the environment. This type of behavior aims at overcoming inner fear from the environment by transforming negative influences into positive. The child cannot develop an adequate stereotypical reaction to the negative external factors and attempts to compensate for that weakness by recreating the situation of fear and horror many times. Although he is afraid he becomes attracted to the real source of his fear. For many years the child looks for the same source of experiences and fantasies which determines their pathological nature and the aggressive behavior of the child. On that basis the child does not use the dialogue as means for communication and in his behavior the dominant patterns are those of an active monologue.

As a special type of autism are defined the cases from the fourth group in which there is a deficit in the predominating fourth level. In the basis of this level there is a design and mastering of rules of emotional contacts as well as of adequate perception of needs and experiences of other people. In this case there is a pathological dependence on caregivers, especially the mother. This dependence is observed mainly in case of a need to contact other people. Children show motor awkwardness, limited, agrammatical, delayed speech. There is a specific delay in the general intellectual development. Children often perceive situations literally and it is hard for them to master new models of behavior. Disorders from this level hinder in a specific way the independent adaptation of the child and influence in a negative way the development of the other lower emotional levels.

The described four groups of disordered affective adaptation are not practically encountered in a clear form due to the various and complex combinations of hypo and hyper functions of the different structural levels. Of main importance is the early differentiation of autism from some cases of mental retardation. Often in cases of unfavorable social conditions as well as in cases of complicated forms predominately with cerebral-organic etiology, it is possible for mental retardation to occur. The differential diagnosis is particularly legitimate in those cases in which the observed mental retardation is defined not by a real intellectual underdevelopment but by the specific behaviors and acitivities of the child. Therefore, the most frequent reason for diagnostic error is the autistic syndrome itself, related to an impaired contact with other people. Children from the first group are often considered as mentally retarded due to the absence of the so called complex animation, interest toward the mother and other close people, and to human facial expression. The reactions to discomforting influences from the environment like hunger and pain are weak. In early childhood the diagnosis is complicated by the absence of speech reactions, grooming habits and underdeveloped play activity. The main symptoms are often related to some visual and motor manifestations. In children with mental retardation there is a desire for eye contact with others and there is no negative attitude to environmental change. However, the development of spatial orientation is delayed. Motor development of children with mental retardation is characterized by adynamia and frequent aimless clumsy gestures. The typical expressive hand plasticity of children with autism is not encountered. Diagnostic errors in children from the second group are due to difficulties similar to the ones manifested by children with mental retardation like inadequate contact with the environment - in drawing attention to certain objects, developing simple household habits, delayed speech and motor development. As differential criteria can be considered also the absence of extrinsic fears characteristic of children with mental retardation, lack of peculiarities in speech intonation, of neologisms and echolalia. There are no typical for autism manifestations like self-stimulation and interest in signs and symbols. Children from the fourth group come closer to the ones with mental retardation mainly because of their passivity, unexpressed interests, poor speech and delayed development of fine motor movements. Of great importance for the correct differentiation of mental retardation is the analysis of developmental mechanisms during the first two years of life. In children with autism there is an apparent lack of synchrony in the hierarchy of mental functions as the ones with more complicated structure and later manifestation in normal ontogenesis demonstrate faster development.

SCHIZOPHRENIA

Leo Kanner believes that a distinguishing characteristic of childhood schizophrenia is its procedural character. It occurs after a period of normal psychophysical development and outlines processes of decomposition, loss of already developed characteristics and abilities by the child. Schizophrenia causes gradual deviation from the standards of normal thinking and interactions with reality and others.

In the aspects of age manifestation of the two conditions there are substantial differences as well. While schizophrenia suggests aggravation of pathological processes, autism brings its specific periods of compensation and obliteration of difficulties in the social maturation of the person.

In order to make the right differential diagnosis the professional should be aware of the diagnostic criteria and the clinical picture of schizophrenia The onset of the condition can be acute or prodromal, manifested with strange ideas and behavior. Typical of schizophrenia is the presence of:

- Thought echo,
- Insertion or subtraction of thoughts,
- Delusions,
- Influence or passivity of the body and the limbs,
- Hallucinations in different modalities or the presence of persisting delusions,
- Catatonic behavior – arousal, postures or wax flexibility, negativism, mutism,
- Negative symptoms like pronounced apathy, poverty of speech and stubbed or inadequate emotional reactions.

Unlike schizophrenia that has at least a two-year period of normal development, in autism the child is as if born with a congenital disability to connect in a normal way with people and to respond adequately to situations. Everything that comes from outside in order to violate the invariability of the situation and to bring the child out of his isolation is averted.

Other authors like M. Sh. Vrono consider early childhood autism as a manifestation of schizophrenia in the earliest stages of the life of the child. L. Kanner himself in his first descriptions claims that the syndrome in many respects resembles schizophrenia. It is considered that these are the first disontogenic expressions of the illness. In very few cases, however, in catamnesic follow-ups an outbreak of schizophrenic attacks are observed in later years. The general tendency is that of compensation as the main symptoms of the syndrome remain but undergo age modification. People suffering from the syndrome and characterized by lack of empathy, strange communication, social isolation and hypersensitivity have the same traits that are included in the definition for a schizoid personality.

It has been established that the chances a child having an Asperger syndrome to develop schizophrenia is many times higher than that for normal children. In fact out of the 200 children observed by Hans Asperger only one has developed schizophrenia. Contemporary research proves that around 5% of Asperger syndrome carriers develop schizophrenia as adults. The difference is that people with schizophrenia have a much higher threshold for stressful factors and in hyperintensity of these factors they develop clear signs of schizophrenia including hallucinations and illusions. In Asperger syndrome it can be reported hearing of voices because of the literal understanding of speech and misidentification of the hidden meaning of the asked questions.

Another major difference is related to speech. In Asperger syndrome there is no blockage of thoughts as described by Bleuler. Speech in Asperger syndrome can be slow and irrelevant to the asked questions but that is a result of the tendency of the individual to creep into the conversation rather than to the creation of new ideas. Speech is always logical even when it is not connected to the asked questions although sometimes it may seem strange and peculiar. In spite of that there is a very clear difference between the unclear schizophrenic speech and the concrete, meticulously studied information part of the speech of people with Asperger syndrome. The latter do not have thought echo, replaced or inserted thoughts, voices commenting their actions and behavior, voices talking to one another, the feeling that external forces exert control over their desires, emotions and behavior.

The difficulty in making differential diagnosis emanates from the fact that both conditions affect language, social interactions and cognitive activities. The onset of expression and the nature of the disorders are different, but there are similarities in the possible chronic defects that are present in both conditions.

HYPERLEXIA

In both widely accepted manuals – DSM and ICD, there is no identification of the term hyperlexia although similar symptomatology is described in several nosological units.

A differential diagnosis should be made with Kanner syndrome, Asperger syndrome, specific learning disabilities, expressive-impressive language disability, Savant syndrome, schizoid personality.

For the first time the term hyperlexia is used in the 1960's. Then it was defined as a disorder in which word decoding is at a very high level of development compared to understanding. It is accompanied by improved learning abilities based on the premature specific brain development.

In the 1970's Silverberg excludes deficits in understanding from criteria for diagnosing hyperlexia. Then hyperlexia starts to be considered as a specific learning disability. A little later Huttenlocker (1976) discovers language impairments in children with hyperlexia. Cobrinik and Richman introduce them as diagnostic criteria. In the late 1980's Healy provides the following diagnostic criteria:

1. Spontaneous reading of words before the age of 5.
2. Impaired comprehension in reading and listening.
3. Word recognition is above the level of linguistic and cognitive abilities.

In 1990 Aaron defines hyperlexia as a type of reading disability in which the assessment of the dimensions of decoding and understanding are contrary to the assessment in dyslexia. That is in hyperlexia there is a good decoding but bad understanding. According to the author hyperlexia is a specific learning disability accompanied by language, cognitive and social deficits.

The last 10-15 years hyperlexia is associated with autistic spectrum disorders. There are too many discrepancies and contradictions regarding the nature, etiology and classification of hyperlexia. Pennington (1996) associates hyperlexia with autism and right hemispheric disabilities. Rourke (1996) relates it to nonverbal impairments of the learning ability and with Asperger syndrome.

According to L. Richman (1998) hyperlexia should be defined as a syndrome coexisting between autism and language learning disabilities or between Asperger syndrome and nonverbal learning disabilities. According to that definition children with hyperlexia should be categorized as part of the group suffering from a language disability. The thing that distinguishes them is the pronounced difficulty they experience in social skills and perception.

Nowadays hyperlexia is defined by the following features:

1. Premature unexpected agewise development of the ability to read words which might be accompanied by an intensive use of letters and digits.
2. Pronounced difficulties in understanding of oral speech.
3. Inadequate social skills, difficulties in socialization and interactions with others.

Additional criteria are:

4. Special way of acquiring expressive speech.
5. Procedural memorization of sentences without understanding their meaning.
6. Difficulties in initiating conversations.
7. Intensive need to maintain habits.
8. Elements of ritualistic behavior.
9. Increased visual, auditory and/or tactile sensitivity.
10. Self-stimulating behavior.
11. Specific, unusual for the respective age fears.
12. Very well-developed auditory and visual memory.
13. Thinking in conrete and literal terms and presence of difficulties in using abstract terms.

Thus described the diagnostic criteria in reality resemble autistic spectrum disorders. The wide range of listed behaviors makes it difficult to identify hyperlexia and to differentiate it from similar disorders. It is required to make a very precise differential diagnosis with autism, behavioral disorders, communication disorders, emotional disorders, attention deficit, auditory disability, mental retardation etc. Moreover it is necessary to distinguish between the primary, core symptoms and their organization in a symptom-complex from the secondary impairments – consequence of the impact of the primary ones. The question whether hyperlexia is a separate nosological unit in the group of specific learning disabilities or it can be categorized as a generalized developmental disorder remains open. According to Richman (1998) when we talk about hyperlexia we should talk about language difficulties. When we talk about both we should not forget the features autistic spectrum disorders.

Until recently hyperlexia was understood as a nonverbal learning disability. The characteristics of these disorders combined with hyperlexia, however, very much resemble Asperger syndrome. All these symptoms undoubtedly are accompanied by attention deficit.

Children with hyperlexia are usually diagnosed as having autism. The increased abilities to decode a text are accepted as premature development without taking into account deficits in other areas of functioning.

Considering the results from a one-year long observation we can positively report that the group is very diverse or heterogeneous. Because of the small number of participants at this stage the results are primarily descriptive aiming to make a qualitative interpretation of the observed specificities. In spite of that two groups are relatively clearly defined.

The first group consists of children with language disabilties regarding understanding and verbal production. They exhibit difficulties in text comprehension as well as in single words comprehension especially multiple meanings of one word. It is also difficult for them to understand complex logic-grammatical structures especially prepositions. It is obvious that in this group language disabilities stand out, particularly those of language content.

In the second group, the children have visual-spatial and motor disabilities. These impairments, however, are observed only in regard to non-linguistic stimuli, and because of that word and phrase decoding is preserved.

In children from the first group a low verbal IQ and a high nonverbal IQ is observed. Almost in all cases good visual memory is reported.

In the second group we observed the opposite results – low nonverbal IQ and high verbal IQ. These children show good auditory memory and pronounced deficit in cognitive functioning. Although both groups are able to decode words well, in the first group there are isolated phonetic errors.

The first group of children have autistic-like symptoms associated predominately with delayed language development, persevering behavior, echolalia and problems in comprehension. This, however, cannot be considered as a generalized developmental disorder but rather the observed autistic behavior is a consequence of a language disability. Language content disabilities undoubtedly lead to symptoms manifested as underdevelopment of the communicative function of speech. This condition is always manifested as remoteness, isolation, reclusion and inadequate communication.

In the second group the symptoms resemble more Asperger syndrome due to the presence mainly of pragmatic language deficits in expression and interpretation of what is experienced through speech.

In the first group, problems with understanding a text may not be manifested during the first stages of acquisition of reading skills because of the excellent memory of the children. What is striking is their general immaturity, their inability to take into account the reactions of other people and to consider the consequences of their own behavior. They are usually absent-minded and impulsive but these symptoms are related to the language deficit and it can be expected that they will decrease with the development of the language system.

In the second group the understanding of words is better. However, they have more severe disabilities in social perception as well as problems considering nonverbal behavioral signal which leads to lack of learning efficiency and perseveration of the same errors.

The observed children pose the question about the nosology of developmental disorders. The excessive expansion of the number of nosological units has a dual effect. On one hand, this is a result of a more precise assessment which is always a prerequisite for a successful therapy. On the other hand, however, the excessive fragmentation leads to "loss" of the general picture. In turn this leads to the design of inadequate therapeutic strategies. Some of the symptoms of childhood developmental disorders are nonspecific i.e., they can be encountered in several nosological units but may play a different role in the general picture of the specific disorder. Exactly that nonspecificity requires an assessment of the overall funcitoning of the child with precise consideration of reasons and consequences.

Apparently hyperlexia is one of the disorders which has not found a place in the system of childhood developmental disorders. In this case what defines the group with hyperlexia is that in it there are children with different manifestations of the disorder.

What unifies them are the unusual learning abilities that create a certain developmental disbalance – in certain areas they show premature development, in others development is delayed. Premature development is usually demonstrated regarding the early acquisition of reading skills without systematically targeted training. The delay can be observed in one or several areas but here the possibilities are much more. The observed symptomatology in children with hyperlexia disproves another myth that reading skills are formed on the basis of relatively well-developed language system and intentional training.

SAVANT SYNDROME

In 1887 Dawn presents a series of lectures in London in which he describes his 30-year long professional experience. He presents 10 cases including one about a boy with perfect memory about operas. Dawn makes a series of observations which are valid to this day, a century later, and the individuals described by him are called autistic savants. His observations determine that:

- Skills are always limited to a very narrow area of special skills - music, art, math, technical and spatial. This narrow area of abilities is usually intriguing considering the wide variety of human skills.
- These exceptional and special skills are always associated with a phenomenal and unique memory – very narrow but extremely deep. Often memory is accompanied by a limited understanding of what is being said. Dawn defines that as verbal adhesion, other authors call it "memory without estimation."
- These cases are observed more often in boys than in girls.

Savants are people who have serious mental and physical disorders but who possess significant sometimes phenomenal talants. This is a very rare phenomenon. In the literature there are a couple of very well documented cases (Sacks 1986, 1995, Treffet 1989).

Savant syndrome is probably one of the strangest and least understood phenomena in studying human differences and cognitive skills. Usually, it is called like this because of the unusual skills expressed by the carriers of this syndrome. It is going to be very difficult for us to understand human memory and knowledge until we have not understood people-savants.

Autistic savants is one of the most fascinating phenomena in psychology. Autistic savants are individuals who have unusual skills that are not observed in other people. From the autistic population 10% have savant abilities, and from the population of individuals with mental retardation – around 1%. There are many forms of savant abilities but in general they can be grouped in – mathematical calculation, exceptional memory, art and musical skills. From the mathematical abilities in individuals with autism there is the so called calendar memory. Exceptional memory is manifested in memorizing details about famous people – date of birth/death, details about family members, members of the government etc. The reasons for these abilities are not clarified yet. These abilities are often called fragmentary skills of amazing/astonishing savants. Savant abilities can be encountered in other developmental disorders as well as in mental retardation but not more often than 1:2000. 50% of people with savant syndrome have an autistic disorder and 50% have some of the other forms of developmental disorders including mental retardation. 10% of people with autism have a wide spectrum of savant abilities. These abilities are called " fragmentary skills" and are manifested in excessive engagement and memorization of details like sport events, dates, routes etc. Talented savants are people with special skills and abilities that are rare in the normal population. There exist the so called "phenomenal savants" whose skills are so extraordinary that they exceed the abilities of normal people. There are 50 cases of such savants described in the literature, half of which are autistic savants.

The condition early childhood autism is described as a separate nosological entity 56 years after the original description by Dawn. As is known, only in 1943 Leo Kanner describes a similar condition and calls it "early childhood autism". Autistic savants usually have impairments of the left hemisphere with right hemispheric functional compensation. These disabilities can be prenatal, perinatal or postnatal. Left hemispheric disabilities relate to impairments of the high cognitive levels and they are being compensated by the lower levels of the so called procedural memory.

In order to understand Savant syndrome it is useful to have knowledge about autism and pervasive developmental disorders in general. One of the most popular definitions is that Savant syndrome is extremely rare but distinguishable condition in which people with autism or other serious mental disabilities or severe mental illnesses have isolated islands of abilities which are in contrast to the other disabilities they have. The condition can be hereditary or acquired as a result of a disability of the central nervous system. It is useful to group those special skills in the following three categories:

- Fragmentary specific skills that are in contrast with the other levels of functioning.
- Talanted savants whose individual levels of skills are high but are in contrast to their disabilities.
- Phenomenal, exceptional savants whose skills are extraordinary and in contrast to their disabilities. Such skills are rarely observed in the normal population. The accidental assessment of savant syndrome can vary to a great extent. There are less than 100 registered cases of phenomenal savants in the world literature for the past 100 years.

Exceptional memory is a sign of savant syndrome but it can also be a special skill. There are cases of savants memorizing populational statistics, telephone books, bus timetables (Sacks 1986).

- Facilitated calculation – oral calculation of complex mathematical operations.
- Calendar calculation – the ability to identify day of the week or date in the nearest 40 000 years (Sacks 1986).

- Musical abilities – savant abilities close to musical genius. Such savants can play a complete musical piece after they have heard it once (Hermelin 2001).
- Art skills – exceptional drawing, sculptural and specific drawing skills (Hermelin 2001).
- Language skills – encountered very rarely, however, there is one well-documented case of a savant with a congenital central nervous system disability who can read, write and translate in 15-20 languages (Hermelin 2001).

The reasons why some people with autism or another disability have savant abilities are still unknown. There are many theories but none can be accepted as undeniable. The biological theories refer to genetic and neurochemical reasons, the theory of left hemispheric dysfunctions, temporal lobe disabilities etc.

All etiological theories can be unified in a couple of groups. Cognitive theories explain the presence of savant syndrome with a deficit in executive functions and abstract thinking while the theory of the impaired (unstable, weak) coherence - with a well developed memory and representations (Happe 1994, Schopler & Mesibov 1995). All theories search for a connection with the autistic spectrum and the so called islands of exceptional abilities.

Savant syndrome diagnosis is facilitated to a certain degree by the presence of pronounced abilities. A diagnostic error is to classify all individuals with savant syndrome as autists, Kanner type. In any case savant syndrome remains one of the unknown conditions of the human brain especially regarding the cognitive functioning of individuals with that syndrome.

The wide continuum of the autistic spectrum – from relatively mild to extremely severe disorders hinders substantially the diagnostic process, furthermore the separate nosological entities in this spectrum have similar manifestations, even if they belong to different nosologies. This requires great attention to detail during the diagnostic procedures by a team of specialists for a sufficient amount of time in order to determine the diagnosis, therapy and prognosis.

REFERENCES

Baron Cohen, S. (2008). The Facts: Autism & Asperger Syndrome. Oxford University Press.

Beaumont R.B., Sofronoff K., (2008). A New computerised advanced theory of mind measure for children with Asperger syndrome: The ATOMIC. 38(2).

Begeer, S., El Bouk, S., Boussaid, W., Terwogt, M. M., & Koot, H. M. (2009). Underdiagnosis and referral bias of autism in ethnic minorities. *Journal of Autism and Developmental Disorders,* 39.

Chawarska, K., Klin, A., Paul, R., Macari, S., & Volkmar, F. (2009). A prospective study of toddlers with ASD: Short-term diagnostic and cognitive outcomes. *Journal of Child Psychology and Psychiatry,* 50(10).

Dyches, T. T. (2011, January 18). Assessing diverse students with autism spectrum disorders. *The ASHA Leader.*

Ganz, J. B., Earles-Vollrath, T. L., Heath, A. K., Parker, R. I., Rispoli, M. J., & Duran, J. B. (2011). A meta-analysis of single case research studies on aided augmentative and alternative communication systems with individuals with autism spectrum disorders. *Journal of Autism and Developmental Disorders*, 42(1).

Gokcen, S., Bora, E., Erermis, S., Kesikci, H., Aydin, C. (2009). Theory of mind and verbal working memory deficits in parents of autistic children, *Psychiatry research.* 166(1).

Gutstein, S. E., & Gutstein, H. R. (2009). *The RDI book: Forging new pathways for autism, Asperger's and PDD with the relationship development intervention program.* Huston, TX: Connections Center Publications.

Huerta, M., Bishop, S. L., Duncan, A., Hus, V., & Lord, C. (2012). Application of DSM-5 criteria for autism spectrum disorder to three samples of children with DSM-IV diagnoses of pervasive developmental disorders. *American Journal of Psychiatry,* 169(10).

Iacoboni, M., (2009). Imitation, Empathy, and Mirror Neurons. *Annual Review of Psychology*, 60.

Itzchak, E.B., Lahat, E., Burgin, R. & Zachor, A.D. (2008). Cognitive, behavior and intervention outcome in young children with autism. *Research in Developmental Disabilities*, 29.

Kaland N., Callesen K., MollerNielsen A., Mortensen E.L., Smith, L. (2008). Performance of children and adolescents with Asperger syndrome or highfunctioning autism on advanced theory of mind tasks. *Journal of Autism and Developmental Disorders,* 38(6).

Kanner, Leo. (1943). Autistic Disturbances of Affective Contact. *Nervous Child*, 2(3).

Kasari, C., Paparella, T., Freeman, S., & Jahromi, L. B. (2008). Language outcome in autism: Randomized comparison of joint attention and play interventions. *Journal of Consulting and Clinical Psychology*, 76(1).

King, M., & Bearman, P. (2009). Diagnostic change and the increased prevalence of autism. *International Journal of Epidemiology*, 38 (5).

Landrigan, P. J., Lambertini, L., & Birnbaum, L. S. (2012). A research strategy to discover the environmental causes of autism and neurodevelopmental disabilities. *Environmental Health Perspectives*, 120(7).

Lanter, E., & Watson, L. R. (2008). Promoting literacy in students with ASD: The basics for the SLP. *Language, Speech, and Hearing Services in Schools*, 39(1).

Pickett, E., Pullara, O., O'Grady, J., & Gordon, B. (2009). Speech acquisition in older nonverbal individuals with autism: A review of features, methods, and prognosis. *Cognitive and Behavioral Neurology*, 22(1).

Prelock, P., Paul, R., & Allen, E. (2011). Evidence-Based Treatments in Communi-cation for Children with Autism Spectrum Disorders. In F. Volkmar & B. Reichow (Eds.) *Evidence-based treatments for children with ASD*. New York: Springer.

Seltzer, V. C. (2009). *Peer-impact diagnosis and therapy: A handbook for successful practice with adolescents.* New York, NY: New York University Press.

Shelton, J. F., Hertz-Picciotto, I., & Pessah, I. N. (2012). Tipping the balance of autism risk: Potential mechanisms linking pesticides and autism. *Environmental Health Perspectives,* 120(7).

Spector, J. E. (2011). Sight word instruction for students with autism: An evaluation of the evidence base. *Journal of Autism and Developmental Disorders*, 41(10).

van der Meer, L. A., & Rispoli, M. (2010). Communication interventions involving speech-generating devices for children with autism: A review of the literature. *Developmental Neurorehabilitation*, 13(4).

Volkmar FR, et al. (2009). Autism and autism spectrum disorders: Diagnostic issues for the coming decade. Journal of Child Psychology and Psychiatry, 50.

Volkmar FR, et al. (2009). Pervasive developmental disorders. In BJ Sadock, VA Sadock, eds., Kaplan and Sadock's Comprehensive Textbook of Psychiatry, 9th ed., vol. 2.

Watson, L. R., Crais, E. R., Baranek, G. T., Dykstra, J. R., Wilson, K. P., Hammer, C. S., & Woods, J. (2013). Communicative gesture use in infants with and without autism: A retrospective home video study. *American Journal of Speech-Language Pathology*, 22(1).

Williams, D. (2012, March). *Neurological basis for autism: Implications for speech-language pathologists.* Miniseminar presented at the Ohio Speech-Language-Hearing Association, Columbus, OH.

Woodbury Smith M.R. & Volkmar, F.R. (2008). Asperger syndrome. *European Child & Adolescent Psychiatry,* 18.

In: New Developments in Clinical Psychology Research
Editors: D. St. Stoyanov and R.-D. Stieglitz
ISBN: 978-1-63483-223-6

Chapter 6

Differential Diagnosis of Attention-Deficit/Hyperactivity Disorder (ADHD)

Rolf-Dieter Stieglitz*, Sandra Baumgartner, Salvatore Corbisiero, Beatrice Mörstedt and Berit Oetsch
The University of Basel, Switzerland

Abstract

The hallmarks of Attention-Deficit/Hyperactivity Disorder (ADHD) are reflected in the symptom areas of inattention, impulsivity and hyperactivity. ADHD was long regarded as a childhood disease, but various studies have since found that adults are equally affected by the disorder. Differential diagnostic considerations, therefore, as well as the need for regard to potential comorbidity are of great importance for the diagnostic process. As possible examples are mentioned autism spectrum disorder, substance use disorders, schizophrenia, affective disorders, anxiety disorders and personality disorders. These groups of disorder form the subject of discussion in this chapter.

1. Introduction

The hallmarks of Attention-Deficit/Hyperactivity Disorder (ADHD) are reflected in the symptom areas of inattention, impulsivity and hyperactivity. ICD-10 subdivides these symptom areas into those of simple impaired activity and attention deficit disorder (F90.0: disturbance of activity and attention), hyperkinetic disorder with impaired social interaction (F90.1: hyperkinetic conduct disorder), other hyperkinetic disorders (F90.8 or F90.9) and attention deficit disorder without hyperactivity (F98.8). Compared to DSM-IV, DSM-5 no longer lists explicit subtypes for ADHD but instead focuses on three so-called 'specifiers'

* E-mail: rolf-dieter.stieglitz@upkbs.ch.

based on predominant phenotypes, i.e., the combined presentation, the predominantly inattentive presentation and the predominantly hyperactive-impulsive presentation.

ADHD was long regarded as a childhood disease, but various studies have since found that adults are equally affected by the disorder. It is today believed that around 50% of those diagnosed with ADHD during childhood and adolescence continue to be affected by the disorder in adulthood. With a world-wide prevalence rate of 1-7%, ADHD represents one of the most common disorders in adulthood (de Zwaan et al. 2012; Fayyad et al. 2007; Kessler et al. 2006). Figures for prevalence rates vary considerably depending on the country and the samples researched. With a gender ratio of 1.6:1, more men than women are affected by the disorder in adulthood (Stieglitz et al. 2012).

In the context of phenomenology, the diagnostic criteria relate to symptoms which also feature as diagnostic criteria for other disorders or which can frequently appear as concurrent clinical phenomena. Thus, for example concentration difficulties represent a diagnostic criterion for manic and depressive episodes but can occur equally with many mental disorders (e.g., schizophrenia). This raises poignant questions in relation to the differential diagnostic process. In addition, ADHD shows a high frequency of comorbidity with a series of other disorders with estimated prevalence rates reaching a figure of as high as 80%. This is important because comorbid patients represent a substantial number of people in treatment and present greater disorder severity from both the clinical and social perspectives than those people diagnosed with only one type of disorder (Torrens et al. 2012: 1005).

Differential diagnostic considerations, therefore, as well as the need for regard to potential comorbidity are of great importance for the diagnostic process. DSM-5, for example, at criterion E carries a reference to the fact that ADHD symptoms are not exclusively particular to schizophrenia or other psychotic disorders but may be explained in the context of other mental disorders. As possible examples are mentioned autism spectrum disorder, substance use disorders, schizophrenia, affective disorders, anxiety disorders and personality disorders. These groups of disorder form the subject of discussion in this article.

2. Diagnostics of ADHD

Compared to other disorders, the diagnostic process of ADHD in adulthood presents itself as rather more complex. This is not so much for psychopathological reasons but rather as a result of the lifespan perspective which warrants particular consideration, as is similarly the case with personality disorders. The following factors can in some cases render establishing a diagnosis difficult:

- The root of the symptoms must be sought in childhood. This is particularly important on account of the fact that many adult ADHD patients were never diagnosed during childhood or adolescence.
- As a consequence, the patient's own reliable personal memories or those of third parties involved (e.g., parents) play a significant role in the diagnostic process.
- Additional sources of data such as school reports must form part of the assessment process. School reports are, however, often not available or limited to lists of grades only which are of little value. The availability of detailed accounts of displays of

irregular forms of behaviour (e.g., disruptive behaviour in class, absent-mindedness) or performance levels (eg. concentration problems) is rare.
- Testing for potential comorbidities is essential.

Weiss et al. (1999) recommend various practical steps to be included in the diagnostic process which do not mandatorily need to be followed in the order listed here: the clinical interview, testing for ADHD symptoms through the implementation of rating scales, testing for other psychiatric disorders, testing for symptoms in childhood, further tests, and the recording of impairments.

Step 1: The clinical interview. The purpose of the clinical interview is to document the patient and their life history as well as their present life experience and behaviour. It serves to diagnose ADHD symptoms and other disorders and to evaluate the patient's current level of functioning.

Step 2: Testing for ADHD symptoms through the implementation of rating scales. Rating scales in the form of self-evaluation and third party evaluation procedures can facilitate the quantification of present and past symptoms.

Step 3: Testing for other psychiatric disorders. As already mentioned, prevalence rates of comorbidity with other psychiatric disorders are high. Comprehensive screening for other psychiatric disorders is therefore of primary importance. Where indications of other psychiatric disorders exist, diagnostic criteria of potential comorbid disorder(s) require thorough examination (e.g., in the form of diagnostic interviews).

Step 4: Testing for symptoms in childhood. A diagnosis for ADHD in adulthood is based on information relating to the patient's childhood. Adults diagnosed with ADHD often relate extremely vivid childhood memories. Noteworthy examples are e.g., emotional reactions of teachers and parents.

In cases where patients find it difficult to recall childhood memories, the examining clinician is forced to rely on external sources of information. Consulting school reports can in some cases yield fruitful results. The implementation of diagnostic scales may further assist the diagnostic process.

Step 5: Further tests. Although there are no compulsory testing procedures to assess a patient's levels of performance in order to establish an ADHD diagnosis, such tests can nevertheless deliver useful supplementary information. These include e.g., (neuro-)psychological examinations in relation to performance levels in either pencil-and-paper or computerised forms. Such tests, however, are no replacement for the clinical interview and the rating and recording of the psychopathology by means of specific scales.

Step 6: Recording of impairments. As ADHD is accompanied by various impairments, differentiated investigation into possible affected areas such as quality of life, family situation or work, personal relationships, education and training as well as activities in everyday life is necessary. Here, too, the use of rating scales may prove helpful.

As with other mental disorders, the starting point of the diagnostic process for ADHD lies in the careful recording of a patient's medical history, whereby with ADHD special regard must be paid to certain particularities and additional aspects. Table 1 summarises the most important areas in relation to medical history-taking as well as supplementary diagnostic findings.

The core areas of a medical history in ADHD cases are similar to those of medical histories in cases of other disorders (e.g., family medical history, physical illnesses).

Table 1. Diagnostic components of adult ADHD

■ complete psychiatric anamnesis
■ ADHD-specific contents of the interview
■ differential diagnoses and comorbidities
■ exclusion of organic mental disorders
■ internistic and neurological examination
■ interview with parents and/or care givers
■ complete ADHD related psychometric assessment
■ neuropsychological assessment

The following aspects require special attention:

- *(early) Childhood development:* e.g., complications at birth, irregularities observed already before school age (such as delayed development)
- *School:* e.g., problems during class and with homework, problems with discipline, behavioural problems, comments in school reports, early diagnostic assessment
- *Work:* e.g., training and education, recurring difficulties, change of work place

Psychological testing procedures can, in view of the assessment targets discussed, contribute usefully to the diagnostic process. In keeping with general conventions, a diagnosis for ADHD is secured at the start of a course of therapy. Although it is widely accepted today that a diagnosis ultimately represents a clinical diagnosis, the results of psychological examination procedures can contribute important elements. This is especially the case with procedures developed in close association with a classification system. Depending on the procedure, individual diagnostic symptom criteria are recorded and in some cases quantified, as are aspects of the impairment.

No direct diagnoses can be derived from neuropsychological procedures as there are, so far, no specific procedures available for this, and the multifarious facets of the disorder are not specifiable solely by means of neuropsychological procedures. The results of a neuropsychological examination can, however, yield supplementary information (see the sections below). Specific deficits become recognisable and quantifiable. Following the establishment of a diagnosis for ADHD and before medical regulation of the disorder with stimulants or other suitable substances, a thorough clinical somatic examination is required. This consists of a somatic medical history, a physical medical examination as well as laboratory tests. In addition, further examinations may be undertaken as deemed necessary.

Especially with adult ADHD patients, consideration must be given to a wider spectrum of potential comorbid disorders. Some of these may develop as secondary disorders as a result of repeated and sustained experiences of frustration and failure over many years (e.g., depressions, disorders provoked through psychotropic substance abuse). Other mental disorders also typically have their onset in adolescence or in early adulthood. Noteworthy are e.g., personality disorders, especially borderline personality disorder, but also schizophrenia. These may be comorbid but must equally be considered as possible differential diagnoses for other disorders. Adults in particular are also prone to suffer from physical illnesses which display ADHD-like symptoms such as hypothyreosis or hyperthyreosis, diabetes or certain heart conditions.

3. ADHD and Other Psychiatric Disorders

3.1. ADHD and Autism Spectrum Disorders

3.1.1. Prevalence

In both ADHD and Autism Spectrum Disorder (ASD) cases the majority of children affected continue to fulfil the diagnostic criteria for these disorders also in adulthood. With ADHD, the percentage of cases where symptoms persist through adolescence and into adulthood lies between 50-70% (Rasmussen and Gillberg 2000; Biederman et al. 2007), with ASD at around 80% (Billstedt et al. 2005; McGovern and Sigman 2005), whereby the figures vary between studies and the development of individual cases depends on personal and environmental factors. Thus the probability of a reduction in the severity of autism symptoms during a lifespan in high-functioning autism or Asperger's syndrome patients respectively is markedly higher than in cases affected by other forms of autism (Kočovská et al. 2013; Helles et al. 2014; McGovern and Sigman 2005).

Prevalence rates of autism spectrum disorders (ASD) in children are estimated at 1% (Lehnhardt et al. 2013; Baron-Cohen et al. 2009) with no reliable estimates available so far for ASD in adulthood. ADHD with estimated rates of up to 7% (see Section above) is thus a more frequently occurring type of disorder than ASD. Among affected children both ASD as well as ADHD appear to be more commonly found in boys rather than in girls (Roy et al. 2009; Kohn and Esser 2008). Prevalence estimates for ASD conditions in childhood indicate that for every three diagnosed cases of children at primary school age two remain undetected (Baron-Cohen et al. 2009). This suggests that a large number of cases reach adulthood remaining undiagnosed. Especially autism sufferers with normal cognitive development can, on account of masking their difficulties through effective compensation strategies, remain clinically undetected over extended periods of time. It is frequently not until they face special life challenges beyond school age such as seeking employment or leaving the parental home that their limitations become evident. ASD, although a clinical condition, can, depending on symptom severity and level of cognitive ability, allow sufferers to successfully lead a largely clinically indifferent life. In DSM-IV and ICD-10, ASD and ADHD diagnoses remain mutually exclusive, as a result of which past literature largely ignored comorbidity with both these disorders. Only a small number of studies so far have investigated symptoms overlap and potential comorbidity of ADHD and ASD. The new DSM-5 permits both diagnoses simultaneously and thus also allows for possible comorbidity of both disorders.

3.1.2. Differential Diagnosis

Core symptoms of autistic disorders are 1) persistent impaired social communication and interaction in various contexts and 2) restricted, repetitive range of behaviour patterns, interests or activities. Concerning this point DSM-5 now also includes hyper- or hypo-reactive responses to sensory stimuli or unusually intense levels of interest in environmental stimuli. This stands in contrast to DSM-IV which, unlike DSM-5, attributes no significance to these issues. Additionally, DSM-5 treats autism as a spectrum disorder, which dispenses with the previously necessary differentiation between various subtypes such as Kanner's autism, atypical autism or Asperger's autism.

In diagnostic differentiation of ASD from ADHD, it is important to remember that with ASD, too, inattention remains an observed symptom (Roy et al. 2013; Lehnhardt et al. 2013). While with ADHD attention deficits occur predominantly as a result of increased distractibility in response to external stimuli, with ASD such symptoms occur as a manifestation of limited inner flexibility in adjusting to changed foci of attention. Equally, however, both cases may display an increased in-depth focus of attention in particular areas of interest which, in the case of ADHD, emerges as a hyperfocus on a specifically targeted interest area, whilst in ASD it manifests itself within the parameters of avidly pursued special interests. Impulsivity is a symptom observed in both ADHD and ASD. Whilst in ADHD impulsivity constitutes a core symptom, in ASD it may be explained as a result of previously experienced high levels of stress caused by, e.g., involuntary disruption to familiar patterns of behaviour or routine sequences of events. Difficulties at an interpersonal level of social interaction can be present in both ADHD and ASD, in the case of ADHD in the form of increased levels of impulsivity and attention deficits, in ASD through impaired cognitive empathy and social intuition. ASD may also lead to increased physical activity (such as rocking and shaking) which, as stereotypical and repetitive behaviour, may erroneously be interpreted as symptoms of hyperactivity attributable to ADHD. Sensory over-responsivity can be symptomatic of ADHD as well as ASD (in the case of ASD hyposensitivity is equally possible), whilst difficulties with motor coordination are further symptoms associated with both disorders (Roy et al. 2013; Lenhardt et al. 2013). An overview of symptoms particular to ASD and/or ADHD is provided in Table 2. Phenomenologically, ASD is distinguished from ADHD by the following symptoms (cf. Lehnhardt et al. 2013):

a) More severe problems at social and emotional interactional levels
b) More severely impaired verbal and non-verbal communication
c) Stereotypic or repetitive/ritualistic behaviours
d) Obsessive adherence to routines and rituals
e) Highly specific, fixated areas of interest, unusual in level of intensity or specificity of contents
f) Detail-focused perceptual processing
g) Compared to ADHD, in ADS more rarely observed higher levels of disorganisation as well as flightiness of thought and action

3.1.3. Comorbidity

In diagnosing ADHD or autism it is important to allow for the possibility that both these disorders may be comorbid, a fact which DSM-5 recognises. In 30-40% of adult ASD patients, diagnostic criteria for ADHD are fulfilled also (Hallerbäck et al. 2014; Rydén and Bejerot 2008; Rybakowski et al. 2014; Stahlberg et al. 2004). Amongst adult patients with a first-time ADHD diagnosis, too, a sub-group of patients is identified with comorbid ASD. In 15% of patients diagnosed with ADHD, Roy et al. (2013) found a comorbid occurrence of Asperger's syndrome. From a neurobiological viewpoint there clearly appear to be certain shared traits, although research findings in this area remain as yet vague and inconclusive (Gargaro et al. 2011).

Table 2. Symptoms in ADHD and Autism

Symptoms	ADHD		ASD	
	present?	reason	present?	reason
Deficits in social interaction	✓	Might be present in ADHD due to impatience, attentional problems, impulsivity. Empathy might be constrained by attentional problems.	✓	Core symptom of ASD Impaired cognitive empathy/Theory of Mind, deficits in non-verbal communication and socio-emotional interaction.
Repetitive or stereotypic behaviour	X		✓	Core symptoms of Autism Might be misinterpreted as ADHD symptoms.
Routines or rituals	X		✓	Core symptom of ASD
Special interests	✓	Possibly hyper-focusing on high-interest tasks	✓	Corc symptom of ASD Highly restricted interests, that are abnormal in intensity or focus.
Sensoric hypo- or hypersensitivity	✓	Heightened sensitivity, e.g., towards sounds, due to increased distractibility.	✓	Lack of/increased sensitivity to sensory stimuli such as sounds, touch, pain, light.
Attentional problems	✓	Core symptom of ADHD Distractibility, especially due to external cues	✓	Low flexibility when shifting attention, heightened distractibility due to sensory stimuli and stress intolerance.
Hyperactivity	✓	Core symptom of ADHD	✓	Increased bodily movements in the context of repetitive or stereotypic behavior might be misinterpreted as ADHD-hyperactivity.

Table 2. (Continued)

Symptoms	ADHD		ASD	
	present?	reason	present?	reason
Impulsivity	✓	Core symptom of ADHD	✓	Might occur in case of involuntary disruption of habitual courses of events. Deviation of the status quo might cause stress and anger, which appears as impulsive behaviour.
Detail-oriented perception	X		✓	Impairment of central coherence
Motoric abnormalities	✓	Motoric hyperactivity and clumsiness might be present.	✓	Clumsiness might be present.

✓: present; X: not present.

A further debatable aspect is whether ADHD-like symptoms in autism cases do in effect point to comorbidity or whether they are, instead, indicative of, e.g., a specific subtype of ASD with ADHD-like symptoms (Sinzig et al. 2009).

Various studies demonstrate that ASD and ADHD are highly heritable neurodevelopmental disorders. Around 80% of phenotypic variance is attributable to genetic factors (Lichtenstein et al. 2010; Taurines et al. 2012). Family studies with ADHD patients show a familial aggregation of ASD symptoms within ADHD families. Studies on twin pairs suggest that 50-70% of the covariance of ADHD and autism symptoms is attributable to common genetic factors (Rommelse et al. 2010; Taurines et al. 2012). However, despite this highly heritable component, ADHD and autism patients do not necessarily remain permanently afflicted, since the brain displays high levels of neural plasticity also in adulthood which, under the influence of appropriate treatment or particular environmental factors, can enable neurodevelopmental disturbances to be outgrown (Ehninger et al. 2008).

So far, only scant research into the comorbidity between ASD and ADHD exists, with inconclusive results. Thus the question remains whether a comorbidity between ADHD and ASD is representative of an additive symptoms overlap between the two disorders, or, indeed, of a new distinct clinical condition. The former assumption finds support in the results of a meta-study, albeit limited to childhood cases (Berenguer-Forner et al. 2015), where a combined disorder shows a more severe clinical profile than that found in patients diagnosed with either ASD or ADHD only, which indicates a symptoms overlap between ASD and ADHD. Research by Nydén et al. (2010) contradicts these findings, however, where of the three patient groups investigated (ASD, ADHD, ASD + ADHD), it was the ADHD group rather than the group with comorbid ASD + ADHD which emerged as the most severely affected.

3.1.4. Neuropsychology

ADHD and ASD are both characterised by deficits of executive function abilities. Executive functions comprise various mental operations such as switching focus of attention (set-switching), cognitive flexibility, initiation and choice of action, strategic action planning, self-monitoring and working knowledge (Leung et al. 2015). Such deficits result from dysfunctions in the frontostriatal circuit which impair goal-oriented behaviour (Gonzalez-Gadea et al. 2013; Gargaro et al. 2011). Abnormalities in frontostriatal brain regions and biochemical imbalances are thus suspected at the root of observed behavioural deficits in ADHD and ASD, which would explain the similarities between these disorders (Gargaro et al. 2011).

Differences in severity of symptoms become evident in so far as with autism, difficulties with cognitive flexibility and planning are most prominent, whilst the problem of impaired executive functioning tends to be absent (Gargaro et al. 2011; Ambery 2006). By contrast, an ADHD profile contains impaired executive functioning and working memory and not cognitive flexibility and planning as primary symptoms (Gargaro et al. 2011; Sinzig 2008). In the areas of social cognition and, in particular, Theory of Mind (ToM) the findings are contradictory. Some research points to impaired ToM in ASD patients, which appears less likely to be the case with ADHD (Gonzalez-Gadea et al. 2013; Lehnhardt et al. 2011). Other findings contradict this hypothesis (Nydén et al. 2010), albeit under caveat by those authors that a display of lack of empathy/affection in relation to ToM in the ASD group may have emerged as a result of flawed ToM test validity (Nydén et al. 2010). Further studies on ASD patients found deficits in visual memory functioning (Ambery et al. 2006), linguistic pragmatics and holistic perception (Lehnhardt et al. 2011).

3.2. ADHD and Substance Use Disorder

3.2.1. Prevalence

Psychotropic substance use disorders as defined in ICD-10, or substance-related and additive disorders as defined in DSM-5, form a heterogeneous group with widely differing estimates for prevalence rates. The variability in these rates partly stems from the differentiated sub-typification of the disorders according to substance type and respective complications associated with its use (e.g., in ICD-10 acute intoxication, substance abuse, substance dependence). Such worldwide variability disallows establishing standardised, reliable estimates for global prevalence. Problems related to alcohol use, however, are relatively consistently regarded as being of particular importance in the context of ADHD and comorbid substance use disorder. Alcohol use disorder is a common disorder on a worldwide scale. In the United States, for example, its prevalence rate amongst adults aged 18 and above is estimated at 8.5% (12-month prevalence; APA 2013). For other substances, prevalence rates are considerably lower, e.g., for cannabinoids 1.5% and opioids 0.37% (APA 2013). In comparison with figures for prevalence rates for ADHD, only estimates for the prevalence of alcohol use are higher, while all other substance-related and additive disorders rank decidedly lower. From a differential diagnostic viewpoint, however, consideration of disorders related to psychotropic substances is essential, particularly in view of ADHD and its potential comorbidity with such disorders, especially in the case of alcohol use.

3.2.2. Differential Diagnosis

There are several challenges involved in establishing a diagnosis for ADHD and comorbid substance use disorder (SUD). Firstly, there is an overlap between a number of symptoms common to both disorders, as illustrated in Table 3, which warrants careful consideration. In addition, a further diagnostic problem emerges from the fact that patients are often unable to recall substance-free periods, which renders their ability to differentiate between individual symptoms difficult, not least because ADHD-like symptoms present also during episodes of substance withdrawal and abstinence. A course of detoxification treatment can further contribute to enhanced manifestation of ADHD symptoms. Ideally, a precondition for an ADHD diagnosis should therefore, wherever possible, be a completed course of detoxification therapy followed by a supervised sustained period of abstinence of a recommended minimum of 1 month. Also Tuckman (2007) confirms that in cases of prolonged and complex substance abuse it can become diagnostically difficult to determine which type of disorder a set of particular symptoms is attributable to. It would therefore be sensible to prioritise treatment for substance disorder and subsequently, after a 5-month period of abstinence, conduct a renewed assessment of the patient for ADHD symptoms. However, the proposition to defer a firm ADHD diagnosis until such time as successful completion of a prolonged episode of supervised sustained abstinence is attained remains, in a clinical context, often unrealistic. A more pragmatic approach would be an attempt to identify those symptoms which were attributable to ADHD before the onset of substance use, for which purpose the gathering and evaluation of information from third parties may become necessary.

3.2.3. Comorbidity

With the generally high rate of comorbidity in ADHD, comorbidity with psychotropic substance disorders is of particular interest. According to Wilens et al. (2003), untreated ADHD cases run a 1.5-fold increased risk of proceeding to develop substance abuse-related disorders. The significance of the combination of ADHD with substance disorders has been conclusively confirmed in a series of empirical studies. As well as other substances, this is especially the case in relation to alcohol.

Prevalence rates for comorbidity of ADHD with SUD are high, although the literature fails to present an entirely coherent picture. The National Comorbidity Survey Replication (NCS-R, cited in Mariani and Levin 2007) established a rate of prevalence for ADHD of 44%. Of the cases diagnosed with ADHD, 15.2% additionally met criteria for a SUD diagnosis; conversely, 10.8% of patients diagnosed with SUD were additionally found to be suffering from ADHD. In clinical treatment settings, these figures appear to be markedly higher. Torrens et al. (2012) identified 33% of ADHD patients as suffering from SUD, while 17-50% of SUD patients were diagnosed with comorbid ADHD.

Table 3. Clinical characteristics and outcome of patients with ADHD and SUD in relation to patients with ADHD or SUD

Earlier onset of substance use and abuse
More likely to initiate smoking and at a younger age, as well as become dependent on nicotine, and have more difficulty quitting smoking
More severity and chronicity of the addictive disorder
A more severe course of illness of ADHD
Less likely to achieve abstinence
Higher rates of poly-substance abuse
Increased psychiatric comorbidity
Lower treatment retention rates

(See Martinez-Raga et al. 2013)

In a clinical context, an analysis and explanation of the mechanics of the association between ADHD and comorbid SUD is highly desirable. Figure 1 contains an example which serves to illustrate a possible scenario for the development of the association between these two disorders over time.

ADHD is essentially a psychiatric disorder triggered by neurobiological factors, the symptoms of which become of relevance on their first manifestation in childhood (phase 1).

ADHD symptoms, which frequently fail to be diagnosed at their earliest stage of onset can, through aggregation of deficits over time (phase 2), result in a depressive episode (phase 3) during which a patient may resort to inadequate self-help and coping strategies in the form of substance use (phase 4). Such self-medication assumes particular significance for the adult patient, which is characteristic of that stage in the temporal developmental trajectory of ADHD.

Inattention is one of the symptoms which persist into adulthood, while childhood impulsivity and hyperactivity tend to decline with increasing age. In many adult patients, impulsivity and hyperactivity are replaced by increasing inner tension which can act as the catalyst for self-medication in the form of substance use. This is merely a simple, yet sufficiently plausible scenario and, particularly in a clinical setting, representative of an often observed combination of overall symptoms. It is important to remember that the sequences of symptoms development described here as phases 3 and 4 can, of course, occur in reverse order as well.

A further point is that this course of development is likely to manifest only in cases where ADHD failed to be recognised at an early stage of onset. Experience indicates, however, that in the context of adult psychiatry in special outpatient units, up to 90% of recorded cases were never previously assessed for or diagnosed with ADHD and had, correspondingly, never received appropriate treatment.

Preconditions:			
	Biological/cognitive vulnerability		
	Hazards/life stressors, situational risk factors		
phase 1:		→	incidence ADHD symptomatology
phase 2:		→	continuous failure
phase 3:	demoralization	→	depressive episode
phase 4:	inadequate coping mechanisms	→	substance misuse /dependency
ICD-10 diagnoses	**F32.1→ moderate depressive episode** (= admission/ indication for treatment)		
	F10.2→ alcohol dependence		
	F90.0→ ADHD		

Figure 1. Example of the development of comorbidity in adult ADHD.

Studies on childhood patients (e.g., Biedermann et al. 2000) indicate that failure to recognise ADHD symptoms in children can already during childhood lead to severe complications, one of which is an especially early onset of alcohol use. According to Tuckman (2007), stimulant therapy for ADHD in children exercises a protective effect in relation to later substance abuse. The reasons for this are twofold in that, firstly, patients who benefited from stimulant therapy to treat their childhood ADHD are in a better position to master their adult lives and, secondly, as a result they are less likely to resort to self-help strategies in the form of self-medication and psychoactive substance use.

The various problems arising from a combination of ADHD and comorbid substance disorder, and their respective outcome variables, are summarised in Table 4. This overview demonstrates the significance of the various consequences resulting from this combination of disorders and the need for their inclusion in any considerations regarding possible courses of treatment.

It further emphasises the clearly enhanced complexity of the association between ADHD and substance disorder and the concomitant high demands put upon the clinician in the management and treatment of these.

In the context of establishing a clinical diagnosis, the following two possible scenarios are of relevance:

- a patient with suspected ADHD seeks clinical assessment with an additional requirement for screening for SUD;
- a patient suffering from SUD seeks treatment or, alternatively, is already in receipt of treatment, and has an additional requirement for screening for ADHD.

Given the high rate of comorbidity of ADHD and SUD, and the fact that ADHD symptoms manifest prior to substance use, a timely and accurate ADHD diagnosis is essential in order to initiate prompt treatment and prevent adverse developments. ADHD patients have a predisposition for early development of more severe instances of substance abuse and dependence disorders. Cases of alcohol dependence are often also accompanied by risk-related patterns and practices of substance use as well as a progression from legal to illegal drug use. In all treatment settings where clinicians are confronted with potential ADHD cases, diagnostic precision and accuracy are of the essence.

Table 4. Symptomatology: overlapping aspects between ADHD and addiction

Components	psychopathology	clinical fatures
Substance effect	Acute intoxication or withdrawal symptoms	Agitation, mood instability, anxiety, intolerance, prone to frustration, restlessness, impulsivity, concentration, and memory difficulties
Addictive process	Craving and loss of control	Impulsivity, poor decision making, planning difficulties, mood instability, dysphoria, anxiety, continued substance use in spite of adverse consequences
Preexisting neuropsychological conditions	Deficits in executive functioning	Impulsivity, risk-taking behavior, inattention, inability to inhibit responses
Psychiatric comorbidity	Mood and anxiety disorders, borderline and antisocial personality disorders	Mood instability, anxiety, impulsivity, risk-taking behavior, intolerance to frustration

(see Fatseas et al. 2012).

It is imperative that patients diagnosed with ADHD are also screened for potential psychotropic substance disorders, for which a number of relevant screening instruments for ADHD as well as substance disorders are now available (e.g., Stieglitz and Raes 2015).

The importance of accurate diagnosis has been confirmed in various studies. McAweeny et al. (2010) for example point out that treatment programmes for psychotropic disorders often overlook ADHD symptoms. In their own study, McAweeny et al. further found that a mere 3% of the clinical medical histories of patients from his study contained an ADHD diagnosis which, however, in a comprehensive follow-up study, rose to an astonishing 44%. From these findings it may be concluded that there is, indeed, a pronounced risk that against the background of psychotropic substance use ADHD symptoms remain underdiagnosed, which is largely on account of the fact that the initial clinical picture obtained is more strongly defined by the symptoms relating to psychotropic substance use than it is by ADHD symptoms. According to Bukstein (2011) the cause for this often lies in SUD patients failing to be screened for ADHD symptoms, and in diagnoses for disorders such as depression and hypomania which serve to further obfuscate the path to an ADHD diagnosis. As a result, van der Glind et al. (2013) postulate that in view of the high prevalence of adult ADHD, all patients seeking treatment for SUD should be screened for ADHD and, in the case of a confirmed diagnosis, receive treatment for ADHD in order to prevent unfavourable treatment outcomes which, as outlined in the literature, would otherwise be likely to follow.

3.2.4. Neuropsychology

In a clinical context, the various facets of executive functioning (EF) play an important role in ADHD (cf. also other sections). EF-related impairments such as organisation deficits are often the reason behind a first assessment for ADHD and are at the root of long-term problems that patients encounter in the workplace and in social relationships. Also of central significance are attention deficit related problems. In contrast to hyperactivity and impulsivity, these represent the most persistent phenomena over time in so far as hyperactivity and impulsivity tend to decline with age, while attention deficits persist. In addition, patients repeatedly mention numerous problems related to various memory processes such as general forgetfulness, forgetfulness in respect of received instructions, or forgetfulness in connection with task fulfilment requirements. Various meta-analyses confirm, in comparison with healthy controls, the presence of such deficits in ADHD patients (e.g., Schoechlin and Engel 2005).

A similar picture emerges in patients with psychotropic substance use disorders. It has been demonstrated repeatedly that one to two thirds of persons with chronic alcohol or other psychoactive substance use disorders show deficits in various cognitive areas such as memory, attention, executive functions, information processing and other cognitive abilities (Scheurich and Brokate 2009; Verdejo-García et al. 2004). As may be expected, most publications available on psychotropic substance disorders relate to alcohol use. As a result, the majority of studies on alcohol-dependent persons found memory tests to show either no impairments, or impairments of medium severity only. With regard to executive functions, most diagnoses in alcohol-dependent patients indicated impairment or limitations to at least parts of the areas of executive functions. Studies also found, however, that in some cases, after a given period of abstinence, it was possible for patients to go into remission (Pawlikoswki and Brand 2013).

In relation to other substances, Verdejo-García et al. (2004) showed that chronic heroin use leads to various cognitive impairments in the areas of executive functions (e.g., working memory), attention, impulse control and decision making behaviour. As concerns use of cocaine, their study contains few conclusive findings. They identified especially the areas of short-term memory, attention, inhibition control, abstract reasoning and psychomotor activity as being affected by chronic cocaine use. Concerning cannabis use, the available data remains inconclusive as well. Initial studies indicate minor impairments at the levels of executive functions, memory and attention. Whilst with most substances only chronic use leads to impairments, studies have shown that with MDMA (Ecstasy) cognitive impairments in the areas of memory and working memory become already evident with mere sporadic use. Further extensive studies are needed in order to arrive at conclusive results, yet it clearly transpires already now that the neurotoxicity of the various substances appears to lead to specific neuropsychological deficits, and that chronic substance use impairs cognitive functional abilities (Pawlikowski and Brand 2013). In summary, it is evident that both SUD and ADHD show impairments in various neuropsychological relevant domains which, in parts, share certain similarities (e.g., affected executive functions and, to some degree, memory).

On the one hand, the presence of neuropsychological symptoms underlines the relevance. On the other hand, however, on account of the similarities between the symptoms of ADHD and SUD, the application of neuropsychological assessment procedures for differential diagnostic purposes is called into question.

3.3. Schizophrenia

3.3.1. Prevalence

Compared to ADHD, the prevalence of schizophrenia is considerably lower. Lifespan prevalence rates are estimated at between 0.5% and 1.6%. The onset of schizophrenia is believed to occur between the ages of 15 – 35, with two thirds of patients showing first symptoms before the age of 30. According to recent studies, however, first indications of a possible onset of the disorder may show at a still younger age. Men tend to become affected three to four years earlier than women. The gender ratio between male and female patients is roughly even.

3.3.2. Differential Diagnosis

In daily clinical practice, the differential diagnosis for either ADHD or schizophrenia does not generally pose a significant challenge, although schizophrenia does explicitly feature as an exclusion criterion in DSM-5 (APA 2013) („symptoms do not occur exclusively during the course of schizophrenia," p. 60). There exist common features between both disorders, which, however, do not stand up to a more thorough exploration according to diagnostic criteria.

Initially, on first comparison of the two symptom areas, no overlap is recognisable (cf. Table 5). Whilst the symptoms of schizophrenia are primarily those of the classic psychopathological type such as delusions, hallucinations, ego disorders and thought disorders, the symptoms of ADHD tend to be more in the emotional and behavioural areas. This greatly simplifies the process of medical history taking.

Table 5. Symptomatology of ADHD and Schizophrenia

	ADHD	Schizophrenia
Core symptoms (diagnostic criteria)	Inattention	
	Hyperactivity	
	Impulsivity	
		Ego-disorders
		Delusions
		Hallucinations
		Thought disoders
		Catatonic behavior
		Negative Symptoms
Associated features (examples)	Inner restlesness	Cognitive deficits like memory problems, inattention

Problems are more likely to arise at the level of associated features of schizophrenia, where a symptoms overlap with ADHD becomes possible in the context of symptoms like attention deficits, inner tension and disorganised behaviour. Studies on the subject of ADHD and comorbid schizophrenia are rare, as the validity of the concept of comorbidity between the two disorders remains disputed.

3.3.3. Comorbidity

Brown's reader (2009), for instance, contains no section on ADHD and schizophrenia, and the term *schizophrenia* does not feature in the index. There is a small number of studies, however, which do point towards the existence of a possible comorbidity between schizophrenia and ADHD. Ross et al. (2006) conducted research focused on children and adolescents aged 4-15. In their sample of 82 schizophrenia patients, 84% also tested positive for ADHD. Unenge Hallerbäck et al. (2014), in their sample of 41 adult patients with schizophrenia, diagnosed 10% with additional ADHD. Differences in diagnostic approaches and methods in areas such as conceptual problems (e.g., analysis and evaluation) prevent conclusive answers in respect of comorbidity. However, there seems to be agreement that treatment of a potential comorbidity between these two disorders requires approaches to their management and treatment to be adapted accordingly. Thus, the treatment of ADHD symptoms with methylphenidate in the presence of potential comorbid schizophrenia is generally regarded as contraindicative (cf. Kraemer et al. 2010).

3.3.4. Neuropsychology

The perception of neuropsychological deficits in schizophrenic patients has been modified over the past few years. Whilst cognitive deficits were initially regarded as an epiphenomenon or associated with long-term pharmacological treatment, they are now considered as core deficits of the disorder, as endophenotypes of schizophrenic psychosis, and as such count as mediating factors between genotype and phenotype of the disorder (Pflüger et al. 2013).

Neuropsychological deficits are a frequent and characteristic feature of schizophrenic disorders. They are generally reliably assessed, as there is now an almost endless array of studies available on the various aspects of cognitive performance in schizophrenic patients.

Despite considerable heterogeneity in methodological approaches adopted in individual studies, and heterogeneity also in type and extent of cognitive deficits present in patient populations, the findings of existing meta-analyses are surprisingly consistant (Exner and Lincoln 2012). Across the whole spectrum of functional areas included in a variety of assessment instruments deployed for diagnostic purposes, the performance levels of schizophrenic patients are found to be roughly one standard deviation below the mean of that of healthy controls. It is questionable whether, against the background of such globally impaired cognitive functioning, it remains possible to identify areas which are selectively more heavily impaired. The discussion centres around whether, for example, verbal episodic memory, executive functions, and cognitive processing and encoding speeds respectively are especially heavily affected, and to what extent attention-related sub-areas such as those of selective, shared or sustained attention may be impaired (Exner and Lincoln 2012). Schaefer et al. (2013) have confirmed findings from past meta-analyses in a recent meta-analysis of their own. They were able to demonstrate that patients with schizophrenia showed considerably lower values than controls in all cognitive tests and all areas of cognitive functioning (grand mean effect size, g = -1.03). The situation is thus of similar complexity to that of ADHD, in which partly similar symptoms present, with the result that neuropsychological procedures are likely to be less suited for differential diagnostic purposes. Direct comparisons between the two disorders remain, however, rare. Gansner et al. (in preparation) compared the neuropsychological performance of 233 ADHD patients against the performance of 127 ARMS (at-risk mental state) patients. In the *Continuous Performance Test* and the *California Verbal Learning Test*, the ADHD group performed significantly worse than ARMS subjects. In the Tower of Hanoi task, ARMS patients were markedly slower but made fewer mistakes than ADHD subjects. These results indicate that patients with ADHD perform considerably worse in tasks of executive functions, sustained attention and verbal learning and memory than ARMS individuals.

3.4. ADHD and Affective Disorders

3.4.1. Prevalence

Like ADHD, affective disorders, too, count amongst the most common psychiatric disorders (Kessler et al. 2009) and with their lifetime prevalence rate of 12% slightly exceed that of ADHD, which is estimated at a figure of 7%. Depending on the subtype of disorder, prevalence rates for affective disorders vary between 7.6 and 17.9%. In particular, the following lifespan rates of prevalence emerge: depressive disorders 4.0-10.0%; bipolar disorders 0.8-1.5% (for an overview, see Kessler et al. 2009). In industrialised countries rates for depressive disorders are higher than in the developing world, with women being almost twice as likely to be affected than men (1.7:1) (Kessler et al. 1993; Kessler et al. 2009). In contrast to ADHD, no such marked gender differences are recorded with bipolar disorders (Merikangas et al. 2007).

3.4.2. Differential diagnosis

Against the background of a high symptom overlap between affective disorders, in particular bipolar disorders, and adult ADHD, diagnostic differentiation between the two types of disorders in each instance of ADHD assessment is essential. Establishing a differential diagnosis between the symptoms of these two disorders remains, however, challenging, as both show a large overlap between at times barely distinguishable symptoms (see Table 6). A differentiation based on symptom areas and level of symptom severity becomes therefore only partly realisable.

Only certain symptom areas are involved in a symptoms overlap between depressive disorders and ADHD (in particular attention-deficit disorders and, to some extent, inner restlessness). As a result, symptoms such as severe depressive mood swings and profound loss of interest and inner drive, symptomatic of a depressive disorder, remain relatively clearly distinguishable from persistent hyperactivity and impulsivity found in ADHD (Kooij et al. 2012). By contrast, differentiation between ADHD and bipolar disorders with manic/hypomanic episodes proves more difficult, as these disorders show an overlap in various symptom areas. A differentiation of disorders on the basis of a differentiation between their symptoms only proves thus difficult (Asherson et al. 2014; Perroud et al. 2014; Skirrow et al. 2012).

However, with bipolar disorders and ADHD, too, specific characteristics are present in their respective symptoms which enable differentiation between them: whilst a reduced need for sleep, the presence of additional psychotic symptoms, inflated self-esteem and a subjective feeling of racing thoughts are specific to bipolar disorders, in ADHD low self-esteem and an increased distractibility are often dominant (Asherson et al. 2014; Perroud et al. 2014).

Table 6. Symptoms of ADHD, Major Depression and Bipolar I/II Disorder according to DSM-5

ADHD	Major depressive disorder (criteria of a major depressive episode)	Bipolar I/II disorder (criteria of a (hypo-) manic episode)
Inattention • Fails to give close attention to details/makes careless mistakes • Difficulty sustaining attention • Does not seem to listen when spoken to directly • Not follow through on instructions and fails to finish schoolwork, chores, or duties in the workspace • Difficulty organizating tasks and activities • Avoids, dislikes, or is reluctant to engage in tasks that require sustained mental effort • Loses things necessary for tasks or activities • Easily distracted by extraneous stimuli • Forgetful in daily activities	A-criteria: 8. Diminished ability to think or concentrate, or indecisiveness	B-criteria: 4. Flight of ideas or subjective experience that thoughts are racing 5. Distractibility
Hyperactivity and impulsivity • Fidgets with or taps hands or feet or squirms in seat • Leaves seat in situations when remaining seated is expected • Runs about or climbs in situations where it is inappropiate • Unable to play or engage in leisure activities quietly • "On the go", acting as if "driven by a motor" • Talks excessively	5. Psychomotor agitation or retardation nearly every day	6. Increase in goal-directed activity or psychomotor agitation 3. More talkaktive than

ADHD	Major depressive disorder (criteria of a major depressive episode)	Bipolar I/II disorder (criteria of a (hypo-) manic episode)
• Blurts out an answer before question has been completed • Difficulty waiting his or her turn • Interrupts or intrudes on others		usual or pressure to keep talking
Additional symptoms • affective lability • Stress intolerance • Outbursts of rage • Sleeping disorders • Low self-esteem/low self-concept	1. Depressed mood most of the day 4. Insomnia or hypersomnia 7. feeling of worthlessness or excessive or inappropriate guilt 2. Markedly diminished interest or pleasure in activities 3. Significant weight loss	2. Decreased need to sleep 1. Inflated self-esteem or grandiosity 7. Excessive involvement in activities that have a high potential for painful consequences
	when not dieting or weight gain or decrease or increase in appetite 6. Fatigue or loss of energy 9. Recurrent thoughts of death, suicidal ideation, or a suicide attempt	
Progress • Several symptoms were present prior to age 12 years • Chronic progress: symptoms remain after onset (fluctuations in the severity of symptoms possible)	• Onset in childhood and adulthood possible • Incidence appears to peak in the 20s • Five or more symptoms have been present during the same 2-week-period • Change from previous functioning within a period	• Onset in childhood and adulthood possible • Mean age at onset of the first episode is approximately 18 years • Distinct periods of abnormally and persistently elevated, expansive, or irritable mood and abnormally and persistently increased goal-directed activity or energy, lasting at least 4 days/1 week

Note. Modified criteria of DSM-5 (APA; 2013).

In addition, consideration of temporal progression should also always form part of the differential diagnostic process: while affective disorders progress through clearly definable episodes of pronounced manifestation of symptoms, ADHD is a chronic developmental disorder with persistent symptoms (Asherson et al. 2014; Skirrow et al. 2012). Various researchers regard careful and precise application of this criterion in the differential diagnostic process as imperative in order to enable differentiation between the symptoms of these disorders (e.g., Asherson et al. 2014; Perroud et al. 2014; Skirrow et al. 2012).

Differential diagnostic assessment should thus occur during the course of a euthymic phase (i.e., an interval of a balanced state of mood between manic/depressive phases). This approach should serve to diminish the potential for confusion and lead to more effective discrimination between the two types of disorder.

3.4.3. Comorbidity

Consideration must be given not only to the need for clear clinical differentiation between affective disorders and ADHD but also to the potential for concurrence of affective disorders with ADHD. The prevalence rates for comorbidity between ADHD and an affective disorder lie between 19% and 37% (Stieglitz et al. 2012), whereby comorbidity with dysthymia is particularly frequent. Different studies put prevalence rates for comorbidity of ADHD with depressive disorders at between 9.7% and 40.7% (Biedermann et al. 2008; Kessler et al. 2006; Pineiro-Dieguez et al. 2014). Still larger variability in comorbidity rates appear to exist between ADHD and bipolar disorders. In their review, Frías et al. (2015) report comorbidity rates of between 4% and 94% (with a mean value of 48%), depending on respective studies. They attribute such variability inter alia to starkly differing random sampling methodology adopted in the studies reviewed (e.g., outpatient vs. inpatient sampling; sampling of childhood onset bipolar disorder vs. adult bipolar disorder). According to Wilens et al. (2003), around 10% of ADHD patients develop an additional bipolar disorder, and 15% of patients with a bipolar disorder also suffer from ADHD. Later studies, too, yield equally inconsistent results. Di Nicola et al. (2014), for example, recorded in persons with bipolar disorders a prevalence rate of comorbidity between ADHD and bipolar disorders of 15.7%, and between ADHD and depressive disorders of 7.5%; whereas Pineiro-Dieguez et al. (2014) found in persons with ADHD a comorbidity rate between depressive disorders and ADHD of 9.7% and between bipolar disorders and ADHD of 2.5%. Studies further demonstrate a correlation between ADHD and comorbid bipolar disorders and an early onset of the bipolar disorder, a higher number of depressive and mixed episodes, fewer asymptomatic periods, worse outcomes and increased negative reaction to treatment (Karaahmet et al. 2013; Tamam et al. 2008). Furthermore, it has been shown that also the severity of ADHD symptoms during manic/hypomanic and mixed episodes becomes enhanced. Also, an increased number of comorbid disorders, in particular anxiety, substance use and borderline personality disorders, were found in patients suffering from both ADHD and bipolar disorders.

3.4.4. Neuropsychology

From a neuropsychological viewpoint, symptoms of all three disorders contain impaired executive functions which in depressive disorders remain largely restricted to affective episodes, whilst in ADHD they are of a chronic nature. Attention deficit problems in patients with bipolar disorders were, however, also found outside acute phases (for an overview see Hegerl et al. 2010).

Patients with ADHD as well as patients with bipolar disorders show similar cognitive impairments in various areas. In both groups, visual and verbal working memory and response inhibition are affected, while control and planning deficits are more associated with bipolar disorders, and deficits in spatial working memory and language fluency are reported to be more specific to ADHD. Different studies arrive at partly contradictory results as to which areas of impairment are more likely attributable to which disorder, resulting in a disparate picture which serves to complicate rather than facilitate the application of neurobiological testing procedures in the differentiation between the two disorders (Skirrow et al. 2012). Over the past few years, research has begun to focus on the neuropathology of ADHD and bipolar disorders. Under discussion are, amongst other issues, a potential genetic, neuropsychological and brain structural overlap (Hegerl et al. 2010; Di Nicola et al. 2014; Skirrow et al. 2012). Present findings and results appear here, too, to project a rather heterogeneous picture; while some findings demonstrate agreement on neural correlates, others indicate differing neural correlates for the two disorders (for an overview, see Hegerl et al. 2010; Skirrow et al. 2012). Currently, depending on the type of disorder, an increasing number of findings seem to speak for the application of imaging technology in the detection of symptoms in different anatomical and functional regions of the brain (Biederman et al. 2008; Brown et al. 2012; Faraone et al. 2001). These findings lead to the conclusion that the pathogenesis of each of the two types of disorder tends to develop independently of each other. Nevertheless, above-average prevalence rates of comorbidity point at least partly to a common pathogenesis of the disorders.

3.5. ADHD and Anxiety Disorders

3.5.1. Prevalence

ADHD affects roughly 4-12% of school-age children and 2-6% of adults amongst the normal population. This incidence rates have found to be stable across different cultures (e.g., White and Shah 2006). While in certain cultures or occupations, a predisposition towards ADHD might not affect the individuals a lot and it might even be regarded as a gift, it usually clashes with the values and way of life in Western cultures. This is why many people with ADHD develop comorbid disorders over the life time, such as depression, low self-esteem and, last but not least, anxiety disorders.

The prevalence of anxiety disorders in the normal population lies between 5 to 15%, whereby the life time prevalence of the group of the disorder can be as high as 25%. Furthermore, they tend to be highly comorbid with each other as well as with other psychiatric disorders. In their review, Somers et al. (2006) calculated the pooled 1-year and lifetime prevalence rates for all anxiety disorders being between 10.6% and 16.6%, with an average life-time prevalence rate for panic disorder of 3.8%, agoraphobia of 3.4%, social phobia of 7.8%, specific phobia of 10.1%, Obsessive Compulsive Disorders (OCD) of 0.9%, General Anxiety Disorder (GAD) of 2.3% (Bijl et al. 1998, with a total life-time anxiety rate of 19.3%), and Post-Traumatic Stress Disorder (PTSD) of 7.8% (Kessler et al. 1994, with a total life-time anxiety rate of 24.9%).

3.5.2. Differential Diagnostics

The differentiation between ADHD and other disorders is not easy, as many psychiatric disorders result in symptoms of inattention, hyperactivity and/or impulsivity. A general rule of thumb in differentiating between ADHD and anxiety disorders are persistent fears and worries accompanied by somatic symptoms in people with anxiety disorders, whereas ADHD subjects tend to be anxious in relation to specific academic or social situations in which they fear failure due to inattention or impulsivity (Quintana et al. 2007). More accurate methods include EEG measures, neuropsychological tests and highly elaborated psychometric assessment instruments. Table 7 provides an overview for discriminating between ADHD and anxiety disorders.

Turning to Electroencephalography (EEG) the most accurate measure in order to discriminate between ADHD populations and normal controls is the EEG theta-beta ratio, with a specificity as high as 94-98% (Monastra et al. 2001). Barry et al. (2003) carved out three different EEG patterns in people with ADHD: a hypoarousal group, showing increased theta waves, but lowered beta waves; a hyperarousal group, with increased beta waves, but decreased theta waves; and, the biggest group with increased delta and theta waves, but lowered alpha and beta waves.

Although seemingly obvious, these three EEG groups have been found to not correspond to the three subtypes of ADHD. Rather, the three subtypes differ in the strengths of the EEG abnormalities, with the combined type showing the highest degree of abnormality, followed by the hyperactive type; the inattentive type displayed the lowest degree of abnormal EEG patterns. In anxiety disorders, EEG abnormalities highly differ from those in ADHD subjects. For panic disorders, for example, a low alpha wave with normally functioning beta, theta and delta waves seems to be typical (Enoch et al. 1995). In OCD patients, beta waves tend to be increased rather than decreased as in ADHD individuals (Hammond 2005). Moreover, anxious individuals tend to show a greater relative right frontal electroencephalographic (EEG) activity compared to normal controls (Blackhart et al. 2006). In contrast, an over-connectivity between the two hemispheres has been observed in ADHD (Murias et al. 2006). Often, ADHD subjects clearly show higher cerebellar and basal ganglia dysfunctions than subjects with anxiety disorders.

Besides, there exists a raw of assessment instruments for diagnosing ADHD. Hereby it is essential not only to examine ADHD specific symptoms in ADHD diagnostic procedures, but to ask for typical symptoms of other disorders, as well, for avoiding false-positives. In regards to anxiety disorders, one could include screening instruments such as the BAI Beck Anxiety Inventory (Beck and Steer 1993), the M.I.N.I. Mini International Neuropsychiatric Interview (Sheehan et al. 1998) or the K-SADS-PL Supplements for Anxiety Disorders and Affective Disorders (Quintana et al. 2007). Sensitivity and specificity for anxiety disorders have been found to be good or very good for the M.I.N.I., besides for generalized anxiety disorders; in the latter case, one might use the GAD-7 Generalized Anxiety Disorder (7 items) instead, with high sensitivity (89%) and specificity (82%) (Spitzer et al. 2007). For further investigation of all anxiety disorders, which is not too time-consuming, the anxiety section of the SCID I (structured clinical interview for DSM-IV, axis I) might be suitable, with high sensitivity and specificity.

3.5.3. Comorbidity

Schatz and Rostain (2006) speak of a 25% comorbidity rate of ADHD with anxiety disorder; hence, every fourth adult presenting with ADHD in our psychotherapeutic office is likely to have some kind of comorbid anxiety disorder. Anxiety disorders in general have been found to affect ADHD symptoms in specific ways, whereby:

Table 7. Differential features between ADHD and Anxiety disorders

ADHD	Anxiety disorders
• High impulsivity and low cognitive inhibition, esp. response inhibition	• problems with working memory and general cognition other than cognitive inhibition
• dysfunctional social behaviour: disrupted family and peer relationships	• socially phobics tend to focus on themselves and worry about embarrassment
• lack of planning and control of cognitive processes	• planning and attentional shifting normal; spatial recognition, working memory and motor initiation impaired (esp. OCD)
• disorganized general cognition as a result of lack of executive functioning (independent of external cues)	
• poor executive regulatory control	
• lower sustained attention	
• strong preference for immediate rather than future rewards	
• disruptive and inappropriate behaviour	
• anxious in relation to specific academic or social situations in which they fear failure due to inattention or impulsivity	• persistent fears and worries accompanied by somatic symptoms
• deficits in monitoring attentional resources	
• lower error monitoring; lower interference control	• no association between error monitoring and anxious behaviour
• attentional disengagement	• attentional hyper-focussing
• spontaneous, impulsive decision making; delay aversion	• slower decision making than normal controls
• emotional dysregulation, sudden mood swings, high moment-to-moment fluctuations	• serotonine dysregulation, more permanent mood
• lower inhibition of a pre-potent response	
• higher-than-average abilities in creativity	
• increased cerebellar dysfunction	
• Impaired basal ganglia higher motor speed, higher capability of motor fluency and accuracy and increased choreoform and athetoid movements	• lower verbal creativity in OCD than in normal control
	• spatial working memory and spatial recognition impaired, motor initiation and execution slower than in normal controls;
• an impaired nucleus accumbens-striatum-orbitofrontal cortex circuit	• lower visuo-constructional functioning
	• impaired *septo-hippocampal system, amygdala, hypothalamus and periaqueductal grey;* especially hyper-activation of the *hypothalamus–pituitary axis;*
• dopamine dysregulation	
• BAS system higher activated -> greater impulsivity and risk-seeking behaviour	• acetylcholine dysregulation
• general memory malfunctions due to storage and retrieval problems.	• avoidance of novelty seeking
	• Panic disorder with/without agoraphobia, social phobia, OCD: impairments in episodic memory.

See: Schatz and Rostain (2006); Quintana et al. (2007); Gupta and Kar (2010); Vance et al. (2006).

- impulsivity and response inhibition deficits are likely to decrease,
- working memory deficits and other cognitive problems usually get worse.

Therefore, although there is not a higher rate of anxiety amongst the inattentive subtype compared to the mixed or more hyperactive subtypes, anxiety does increase the symptoms in the inattentive subtype, rendering a tendency towards sluggish cognitive tempo even worse. This, in turn, feeds feelings of anxiety, insufficiency and depression, so that a vicious circle develops affecting many areas in life, which explains why comorbid anxiety in ADHD usually appears differently compared to more phobic types of anxiety seen in pure anxiety samples.

3.5.4. Neuropsychology

People with ADHD display specific deficits in monitoring attentional resources, which negatively influence response inhibition, error monitoring, attentional disengagement, decision making processes and emotion regulation (Gupta and Kar 2010).The core difficulty for ADHD patients has been proven to be sustained and selective attention, affecting the attentional subsystems of alerting, orienting and executive functioning. Especially, staying in an alert state without warning signals is almost impossible for individuals with ADHD. Deficits in attentional processes also involve higher-order processes such as inhibition of a pre-potent response, interference control and emotion regulation. Moreover, individuals with ADHD tend to show high moment-to-moment fluctuations, which not only explains their sudden, uncontrollable mood swings, but also signifies a considerable difficulty when assessing ADHD per psychometric assessment instruments. It is believed, that this deficiency is the result of abnormal error processing. Although delayed responses to errors have been suggested to be influenced by ADHD individuals' emotional states, there has been no association between error monitoring and anxious behaviour.

Neurophysiological, a central deficiency of ADHD lies in the under-activated anterior cingulate, which is the reason why neurofeedback therapy focusses on this brain area in particular (Drechsler 2011). This explains the vast amount of symptoms in ADHD, for example in the study of Wu et al. (2006) examining the differences between ADHD individuals and normal controls in delay aversion; here, it evolved that while in both groups the ventral and dorsolateral prefrontal cortices as well as the insula were activated, only the normal controls showed an activation of the anterior cingulate and the hippocampus. As a consequence, ADHD individuals not only have problems in decision making, but also in memory and emotional processes. ERP studies and experiments using the Attentional Network Task (ANT) or Go/NoGo tasks replicated abnormalities in alerting in terms of slower response times to abrupt visual cues as well as difficulties in prefrontal response regulation and dealing with conflicting stimuli (Müller et al. 2011). Moreover, recent research about ADHD focus on cerebellar deficits and its connections to the basal ganglia, thalamic nuclei, prefrontal cortex, primary motor cortex and varied brainstem structures. Vance et al. (2006) were able to provide evidence for an increased cerebellar dysfunction in ADHD (combined type) compared to anxiety disorders. In concordance with the observations that the linkage of the cerebellum to the basal ganglia is important to consider, the latter has been found to be stronger impaired in ADHD than in anxiety disorders, leading to a higher motor speed; this includes positive effects, as well, such as a higher capability of motor fluency and accuracy and increased choreoform and athetoid movements, which might hint to the bio-evolutionary suggestion that the predisposition to ADHD might allow for better hunting abilities, having been an evolutionary advantage in former times. This is in concordance to the observation that in ADHD subjects, the behavioural activation system (BAS) is often higher activated accompanied by a greater impulsivity measure and a tendency to risk-seeking behaviour. In anxiety disorders, cognitive dysfunctions are very different from ADHD. For example, in OCD, planning and even attention are functioning normally, whereas spatial recognition and working memory as well as motor initiation (rather than inhibition, as in ADHD) are impaired. Social phobia has some overlaps with ADHD in terms of attentional problems, whereby socially phobics tend to focus on themselves, a problem not shared by ADHD patients. They also differ from ADHD populations in visuo-constructional functions. Moreover, OCD individuals usually display lower verbal creativity, whereas ADHD is characterized by higher-than-average abilities in creativity. Panic disorder with and without agoraphobia, social phobias as well as OCD are linked to impairments in episodic memory; ADHD individuals rather have problems with working memory (e.g.: Holmes et al. 2010). One of the main neurotransmitter involved in anxiety disorders is known to be serotonin, which also strongly influences our mood. Three main systems are involved in fear and anxiety: the *septo-hippocampal system*, the *amygdala* and the *hypothalamus and periaqueductal grey* (McNaughton et al. 2004). Further neurotransmitters involved in anxiety are acetylcholine and adrenaline; especially acetylcholine is responsible for common chronic stress-diseases due to a permanent hyper-activation of the *hypothalamus–pituitary axis*. On the contrary to ADHD patients, which display a tendency to spontaneous, impulsive decisions due to delay aversion, socially phobic individuals have difficulties in quick decision making and need more time for decisions than normal controls (Kaplan et al. 2006).

There are also common neuropsychological features in ADHD and anxiety disorders. Schatz and Rostain (2006) pointed out that a state of nonspecific arousal provoked by the lack of rewarding signals in ADHD might increase the disposition towards anxious reactions. Likewise, when stronger focussing on threatening stimuli, the BIS (behavioural inhibition system) tends to be higher activated in ADHD patients due to the inability to focus on relevant input. Obviously, also people with anxiety disorders are strongly BIS-orientated. Moreover, anxiety can evoke ADHD like symptoms via the neurotransmitter acetylcholine, which plays an important role in a range of cognitive domains; across empirical methods, working memory, attention, episodic memory encoding, and spatial memory processing are repeatedly, found to depend upon acetylcholine for normal functioning (Newman et al. 2012). In concordance with these findings, children of anxious mothers have a higher risk for developing ADHD (Perrin et al. 1996).

3.6. ADHD and Personality Disorders

3.6.1. Prevalence

Information on prevalence rates for personality disorders (PD) is sparse. Epidemiological studies on the prevalence of PD in the general population arrive at prevalence rates of between 4.4% and 15.7% (Coid et al. 2006; Lenzenweger et al. 2007; Samuels et al. 2002; Torgersen et al. 2001). In the US, estimated prevalence rates for the various types of PD as subdivided into the three DSM-IV/-5 Clusters, were 5.7% for Cluster A, 1.5% for Cluster B and 6.0% for Cluster C (Lenzenweger et al. 2007). In the same study, 5.2% of the research population were found to meet diagnostic criteria for avoidant PD, 4.9% for schizoid, 3.3% for schizotypal, 2.4% for obsessive-compulsive, 2.3% for paranoid, 1.6% for borderline, 1% for anti-social, and 0% each for histrionic and narcissistic PD. With psychiatric patients, prevalence rates for PD of between 40% and 60% are markedly higher (Bohus et al. 2012; Newton-Howes et al. 2010). In a more recent study conducted in the United Kingdom, the following estimates of prevalence rates for PD in psychiatric patients were established: 16.5% for avoidant, 16.0% for dependent, 8.5% for borderline, 6.7% for obsessive-compulsive, 5.0% for paranoid, 3.2% each for anti-social and histrionic, and 2.8% for schizoid PD (Newton-Howes et al. 2010).

3.6.2. Differential Diagnosis

Viewed from a phenomenological perspective, borderline personality disorder (BPD) and anti-social personality disorder (ASPD) show a certain symptoms overlap with ADHD, particularly in respect of impulsivity and emotional dysregulation. For this reason, these two types of PD warrant special attention, as only a very limited amount of specific studies on remaining PDs in the context of ADHD is available to date. An overview of the symptoms overlap between BPD, ASPD and ADHD is contained in Table 8 below.

Similarly to BPD, adult ADHD, too, is characterised by impulsivity, extreme outbursts of rage or persistent inner tension, mood lability and emotional over-reactivity in stressful situations (Corbisiero et al. 2013; Matthies and Philipsen 2014; Prada et al. 2014; Wender 1995).

Additionally, low self-esteem and impaired social relationships are observed in both disorders (Matthies and Philipsen 2014; Newark et al. 2012). A marked difference between the symptoms of the two disorders is found predominantly in their respective onsets: whilst ADHD is a developmental disorder already diagnosable in childhood (before the age of 12), symptoms of BPD are first observed in adolescence, with a full diagnosis following in adulthood only (DSM-5). A further marked difference between the two disorders lies in a chronic suicidal tendency and a tendency to self-harm, both core symptoms of BPD (DSM-5). These symptoms play a minor role in relation to ADHD, where they are regarded as possible consequences of the disorder (e.g., within the context of a depressive disorder) rather than defining characteristics (Philipsen et al. 2006; Prada et al. 2014). In ADHD, the cardinal symptom is inattention, the presence of which is mandatory to establishing an ADHD diagnosis (DSM-5; Wender 1995).

A similar relationship is found between ADHD and ASPD in relation to symptoms of lack of impulse control, emotional dysregulation and impaired interpersonal relationship problems.

In addition, however, ADHD patients also show high-risk behaviour with a pronounced need to seek out novelty value (Philipsen et al. 2006), e.g., display of aggressive behaviour in road traffic (Barkley and Murphy 2010; Sobanski et al. 2013) and, in the case of prisoners with ADHD, delinquency (Gudjonsson et al. 2012; Moore et al. 2013; Storebø and Simonsen 2013) in the accompanying absence of any sense of guilt or remorse (DSM-IV/-5).

Table 8. Symptomatic overlap and shared features between ADHD, BPD and ASPD (DSM-5; Utah-Criteria by Wender 1995)

Symptom/feature	ADHD[1]	BPD[2]	ASPD[3]
Inattention	✓		
Hyperactivity	✓		
Inner restlessness	✓	✓	✓
Impulsivity	✓	✓	✓
Emotional dysregulation	✓	✓	✓
• Affective lability	✓	✓	✓
• Hot temper	✓	✓	✓
• Stress intolerance	✓	✓	✓
Disorganisation	✓		✓
Interpersonal deficits	✓	✓	✓
Low self-esteem	✓	✓	
Risk behaviour	✓	✓	✓
Non suicidal self-injuries		✓	
Chronic suicidality		✓	
Chronic emptiness		✓	
Dissociation		✓	
Absence of repentance			✓
Substance abuse	✓	✓	✓

Note. [1]Attention Deficit Hyperactivity Disorder; [2]Borderline Personality Disorder; [3]Antisocial Personality Disorder.
✓: present.

3.6.3. Comorbidity

Prevalence rates for PD in ADHD patients are as high as 64.3% (Miller et al. 2008). In their recent study, Vidal et al. (2014) found that 24.78% of ADHD patients also met the diagnostic criteria for a PD. Cumyn et al. (2009), in a larger study with 335 ADHD patients, identified an overall figure of 50.7% of patients with a PD, with breakdown percentages of 27.68% fulfilling the criteria for compulsive PD, 24.11% for BPD, 12.54% for avoidant PD, 12.50% for narcissistic PD, and 5.07% for ASPD. The remaining types of PD, however, were also found concurrent with ADHD. In Williams et al. (2010) for example, 11% of their small sample of 47 ADHD patients tested positive for depressive PD, 9% each for paranoid and passive-aggressive PD, 6% for dependent PD and 2% for histrionic PD. Matthies et al. (2011) also found schizoid PD in 6.6%, and schizotypal PD in 6.7% of their research population 0). In general, patients tested positive for more than one PD (cf. Matthies et al. 2010; Williams et al. 2010). This leads to the conclusion that it is predominantly PD types from DSM-IV/-5 Clusters B (dramatic-emotional) and C (anxious-avoidant) which tend to co-occur with ADHD (Matthies et al. 2011).

Two types of PD which are closely linked to adult ADHD are BPD and ASPD. These two disorders show considerable overlap with ADHD both in respect of symptoms as well as at a neurobiological level. The more consistent prevalence rates for comorbidity are found between BPD and ADHD and are estimated at between 18.3% - 38.1% (Cumyn et al. 2009;

Ferrer et al. 2010; Instanes et al. 2013; Matthies et al. 2011; Miller et al. 2008). The estimated prevalence rate for comorbid ASPD among ADHD patients of 40.3%, however, was even higher (Instanes et al. 2013). In criminal offenders with ADHD the estimated percentage rate is reported to be higher still (cf. Gudjonsson et al., 2012; Moore et al. 2013).

Philipsen et al. (2008), in their study on a clinical population, reported that 41.5% of women diagnosed with BPD had displayed ADHD symptoms in childhood, with 16.1% proceeding to meet the diagnostic criteria for ADHD. The study also suggested that the higher the number of current adult BPD symptoms patients were able to relate, the greater the likelihood of a former presence of childhood ADHD in these patients, and that, as a consequence, childhood ADHD might pose a possible risk for the development of BPD in later life. Compared to patients diagnosed with BPD only, ADHD patients with comorbid BPD were reported to be at an increased risk of developing suicidal tendencies and additional mental disorders such as anxiety and substance disorders as well as ASPD. ADHD patients with comorbid BPD also told of higher incidence rates of emotional abuse than did patients diagnosed with BPD only (cf. inter alia Storebø and Simonsen 2014). In comparison with BPD patients and a healthy control group, ADHD patients displayed more BPD symptoms than the healthy controls. Self-harming behaviour and emotional dysregulation were, however, less frequently observed in ADHD patients with comorbid BPD than in patients diagnosed with BPD only (Philipsen et al. 2008). Findings of further studies also indicated that ADHD patients with comorbid BPD showed higher levels of impulsivity and aggressive behaviour than patients diagnosed with either ADHD or BPD only, or healthy controls (Prada, et al. 2014). A connection between ADHD and BPD was also found at a genetic level (Distel et al. 2011) with an estimated phenotypic correlation between ADHD and BPD symptoms of $r = .59$, of which 49% were attributable to genetic factors.

The development of ASPD is an aspect under consideration in connection with ADHD and social conduct disorder (SCD). Childhood ADHD with or without comorbid SCD appears to enhance the overall clinical symptomatology and with greater probably leads to the development of a later ASPD (Retz et al. 2013; Storebø and Simonsen 2013). Children with ADHD and comorbid SCD run an additional enhanced risk of slipping into crime and delinquency at a later stage in their lives (Storebø and Simonsen 2013). Emotional neglect, parental divorce, early separation from primary carers or attachment figures as well as past suicide attempts appear to be more frequent in persons with ASPD and comorbid ADHD; especially the level of impulsivity appears to feature as a prominent factor in the dynamics of the association between these two disorders (Storebø and Simonsen 2013).

3.6.4. Neuropsychology

The described symptoms overlap between ADHD, BPD and ASPD also manifests itself in a neuropsychological context. The neuropsychological deficits common to all three disorders are located in the prefrontal cortex (the core region of attention mechanisms) and in the orbito-frontal cortex (the core region of impulsivity and emotional dysregulation) (Dolan 2012; Philipsen 2006). ADHD as well as BPD patients display impaired impulse control and appear to suffer also from response inhibition, particularly in stressful situations (Krause-Utz et al. 2013; Matthies and Philipsen 2014; van Dijk et al. 2014). Impulse control in BPD patients, however, becomes particularly impaired in the face of emotional and interpersonal relationship difficulties or in the presence of a comorbid ADHD (Sebastian, Jacob, Lieb and Tüscher 2013). While with BPD patients lack of impulse control indicates primarily prefrontal impaired functioning in orbito-frontal, dorsomedial and dorsolateral brain areas, impaired activity in ADHD patients tends to be more concentrated in ventrolateral and medial prefrontal regions (Sebastian et al. 2014). Only few studies so far have compared the neuropsychological mechanisms of ADHD and BPD. Krause-Utz et al. (2013), in their study of various groups (BPD, BPD with and without ADHD, ADHD, and healthy controls), found that response inhibition (assessed through the *Immediate and Delayed Memory Task*; Dougherty and Marsh 2003) was particularly impaired in patients with BPD and co-occurring ADHD. These findings, however, stand in contradiction to a study by van Dijk et al. (2014), who observed response inhibition (assessed through the *Expectancy AX-CPT Task*) in both ADHD as well as BPD patients (regardless of whether comorbid BPD or ADHD respectively was present or not).

Emotional dysregulation has, until now, been generally defined as core to BPD symptoms (Matthies and Philipsen 2010) and has only in the past few years become the subject of more intensive research in the context of ADHD (Corbisiero et al. 2013). In ADHD, inattention appears to play an important role in the regulation of emotions, yet the neuropsychological mechanisms of the correlation between inattention and emotional dysregulation remains still unclear (Shaw et al. 2014). In the case of BPD, however, it is assumed that in the regulation of emotions, attention deficits play a less decisive role (Lampe et al. 2007).

The neuropsychological deficits in persons with ASPD are, similarly to ADHD, present in executive functions, although empirical evidence to this effect remains scarce: in particular, difficulties with planning ability, behavioural inhibition and set shifting were observed (Dolan 2012). A recently published study on ASPD patients and ADHD with ASPD patients investigated their ability to recognise emotions (joy and happiness, sadness, fear, disgust, anger, surprise, and neutral facial expression), which was measured through the *Emotion Recognition Test* containing facial expressions from Ekman and Friesen's series (Ekman 1999). The two groups displayed significant differences only in respect of the ability to recognise the emotion of disgust (Bagcioglu et al. 2014).

Summary and Perspectives

The clinical diagnostics of ADHD represent a complex process. In contrast to most other mental disorders, establishing a differential diagnosis in ADHD cases necessitates consideration of a lifespan in its entirety (not dissimilar to personality disorders). There is therefore a plethora of information to be gathered, to which end an increasingly large variety of assessment tools have become available. As well as information from patients themselves and from third parties, various additional sources of data require consideration and evaluation in the process. The diagnostic criteria, which meanwhile have been adapted in DSM-5 to adulthood, are less difficult to explore than in other disorders, making hardly any psychopathological knowledge necessary. Yet, partially overlapping symptom areas and the potential comorbidity of ADHD with other disorders pose particular challenges in establishing a differential diagnosis. On the one hand, the results of a variety of studies containing comprehensive accounts of clinical experiences offer a foundation upon which to base a reliable diagnosis. Conversely, however, a host of questions still remains unanswered.

In particular with regard to the relationship between ADHD and schizophrenia, further empirical research is required to shed light on the many open issues involved.

References

Ambery F. Z., Russell A. J., Perry K., Morris R. and Murphy D. G. (2006) Neuropsychological functioning in adults with Asperger syndrome. *Autism,* 10(6): 551-564.

APA (2013) Diagnostic and statistical manual of mental disorders. Fifth edition (DSM-5). Washington, DC: APA

Asherson P., Young A. H., Eich-Höchli D., Moran P., Porsdal V. and Deberdt W. (2014) Differential diagnosis, comorbidity, and treatment of attention-deficit/hyperactivity disorder in relation to bipolar disorder or borderline personality disorder in adults. *Current Medical Research Opinion*, 30(8): 1657-1672.

Bagcioglu E., Isikli H., Demirel H., Sahin E., Kandemir E., Dursun P., Yuksek E. and Emul M. (2014) Facial emotion recognition in male antisocial personality disorders with or without adult attention deficit hyperactivity disorder. *Comprehensive Psychiatry*, 55: 1152-1156.

Barkley R. A. and Murphy K. R. (2010) Deficient emotional self-regulation in adults with attention-deficit/hyperactivity disorder (ADHD): The relative contributions of emotional impulsiveness and ADHD symptoms to adaptive impairments in major life activities, *Journal of ADHD and Related Disorders,* 1: 5-37.

Baron-Cohen S., Scott F. J., Allison C., Williams J., Bolton P., Matthews F. E. and Brayne C. (2009) Prevalence of autism-spectrum conditions: UK school-based population study. *British Journal of Psychiatry*, 194: 500-509.

Barry R., Clarke A. and Johnstone S. (2003) A review of electrophysiology in attention-deficit/hyperactivity disorder: I. Qualitative and quantitative electroencephalography. *Clinical Neurophysiology*, 114: 171-183.

Beck, A. and Steer R. (1993) Beck Anxiety Inventory Manual. San Antonio: Harcourt Brace and Company.

Berenguer-Forner C., Miranda_Casas A., Pastor-Cerezuela G. and Roselló-Miranda R. (2015) Comorbidity of autism spectrum disorder and attention deficit with hyperactivity. A review study. *Review of Neurology*, 60 Suppl.: S37-43.

Biederman J., Ball S. W., Monuteaux M. C., Mick E., Spencer T. J., McCreary M. and Faraone S. V. (2008) New insights into the comorbidity between ADHD and major depression in adolescent and young adult females. *Journal of the American Academy of Child and Adolescent Psychiatry,* 47(4): 426-434.

Biederman J., Mick E. and Farone S. V. (2000) Age-dependent decline of symptoms of attention deficit hyperactivity disorder: Impact of remission definition and symptom type. *American Journal of Psychiatry*, 157(5): 816-818.

Biederman J., Petty C. R., Fried R., Doyle A. E., Spencer T., Seidman L. J. and Faraone S. V. (2007) Stability of executive function deficits into young adult years: a prospective longitudinal follow- up study of grown up males with ADHD. *Acta Psychiatrica Scandinavica*, 116(2): 129-136.

Bijl R., Ravelli A. and van Zessen G. (1998) Prevalence of psychiatric disorder in the general population: results of the Netherlands Mental Health Survey and Incidence Study (NEMESIS). *Social Psychiatry Psychiatric Epidemiology,* 33: 587-95.

Billstedt E., Gillberg C., and Gillberg C. (2005) Autism after adolescence: population-based 13-to 22-year follow-up study of 120 individuals with autism diagnosed in childhood. *Journal of Autism and Developmental Disorders,* 35(3): 351-360.

Blackhart G., Minnix J. and Kline (2006) Can EEG asymmetry patterns predict future development of anxiety and depression?: A preliminary study. *Biological Psychology,* 27 (1): 46-50.

Bohus M., Stieglitz R. D., Fiedler P., Hecht H., Herpertz S. C., Müller-Isberner R. and Berger M (2012). Persönlichkeitsstörungen. In: Berger M. (ed) Psychische Erkrankungen. Klinik und Therapie. *München: Urban and Fischer,* 709-786.

Brown T. E. (2009) ADHD comorbidity. Washington DC: American Psychiatric Association.

Brown A., Biederman J., Valera E., Lomedico A., Aleardi M., Makris N. and Seidman, L. J. (2012). Working memory network alterations and associated symptoms in adults with ADHD and Bipolar Disorder. *Journal of Psychiatric Research,* 46(4): 476-483.

Bukstein G. (2011) Attention Deficit Hyperactivity Disorder and Substance Use Disorder. Behavioral Neurosciences of Attention Deficit Hyperactivity Disorder and Its Treatment. *Current Topics in Behavioral Sciences,* 9: 145-172.

Coid J., Yang M., Tyrer P., Roberts A. and Ullrich S. (2006) Prevalence and correlates of personality disorder in Great Britain. *British Journal of Psychiatry,* 188: 423-431.

Corbisiero S., Stieglitz R. D., Retz W. and Rösler M. (2013) Is emotional dysregulation part of the psychopathology of ADHD in adults? *ADHD Attention Deficit and Hyperactivity Disorders,* 5: 83-92.

Cumyn L., French L. and Hechtman L. (2009) Comorbidity in adults with attention-deficit hyperactivity disorder. *Canadian Journal of Psychiatry,* 54: 673-683.

De Zwaan M., Gruß B., Müller A., Graap H., Martin A., Glaesmer H. and Philipsen A. (2012) The estimated prevalence and correlates of adult ADHD in a German community sample. *European Archives of Psychiatry and Clinical Neuroscience,* 262(1): 79-86.

Di Nicola M., Sala L., Romo, L., Catalano V., Even C., Dubertret C. and Gorwood P. (2014) Adult attention-deficit/hyperactivity disorder in major depressed and bipolar subjects: role of personality traits and clinical implications. *European Archives of Psychiatry Clinical Neuroscience,* 264(5): 391-400.

Distel M. A., Carlier A., Middeldorp C. M., Derom C. A., Lubke G. H. and Boomsma D. I. (2011) Borderline personality traits and adult attention-deficit hyperactivity disorder symptoms: A genetic analysis of comorbidity. *American Journal of Medical Genetics Part B: Neuropsychiatric Genetics,* 156: 817-825.

Dolan M. (2012) The neuropsychology of prefrontal function in antisocial personality disordered offenders with varying degrees of psychopathy. *Psychological Medicine,* 42: 1715-1725.

Dougherty D. and Marsh D. M. (2003) Immediate and Delayed Memory Tasks (IMT/DMT 2.0): A research tool for studying attention, memory, and impulsive behavior. Houston: Neurobehavioral Research Laboratory and Clinic, University of Texas Health Science Center at Houston.

Drechsler R. (2011) Übersichtsartikel - Ist Neurofeedbacktraining eine wirksame Therapiemethode zur Behandlung von ADHS? Ein Überblick über aktuelle Befunde. *Zeitschrift für Neuropsychologie*, 22, 2, 131-146.

Ehninger D., Li W., Fox K., Stryker M. P. and Silva A. J. (2008) Reversing neurodevelopmental disorders in adults. *Neuron,* 60(6): 950-960.

Ekman P. (1999) Facial Expressions. In: Power T. and and Dalgelish M. (eds.) Handbook of Cognition and Emotions. *New York: Wiley and Sons*, 301-320.

Enoch M., Rohrbaugh J. and Davis E. (1995) Relationship of genetically transmitted alpha EEG traits to anxiety disorders and alcoholism. Wiley Online Library.

Exner C. and Lincoln T. (2012) Neuropsychologie schizophrener Störungen. Göttingen: Hogrefe.

Faraone S. V., Biederman J. and Monuteaux M. C. (2001) Attention deficit hyperactivity disorder with bipolar disorder in girls: further evidence for a familial subtype? *Journal of Affective Disorders*, 64(1): 19-26.

Fatseas M., Debrabant R. and Auriacombe M. (2012) The diagnostic accuracy of attention-deficit/hyperactivity disorder in adults with substance use disorders. *Current Opinion in Psychiatry*, 25: 219-225.

Fayyad J., De Graaf R., Kessler R., Alonso J., Angermeyer M., Demyttenaere K. and Jin R. (2007) Cross-national prevalence and correlates of adult attention-deficit hyperactivity disorder. *British Journal of Psychiatry*, 190: 402-409.

Ferrer M., Andión O., Matalí J., Valero S., Navarro J. A., Ramos-Quiroga J. A., Torrubia R. and Casas, M. (2010) Comorbidity attention-deficit hyperactivity disorder in borderline patients defines an impulsive subtype of borderline personality disorder. *Journal of Personality Disorders*, 24: 812-822.

Frías A., Palma C. and Farriols N. (2015) Comorbidity in pediatric bipolar disorder: Prevalence, clinical impact, etiology and treatment. *Journal of Affective Disorders,* 174: 378-389.

Gansner N., Studerus E., Stieglitz R. D. and Riecher Rössler A. (in preparation). Neuropsychological deficits in at-risk mental states for psychosis compared with attention-deficit/hyperactivity disorder: An approach to facilitate differential diagnosis.

Gargaro B. A., Rinehart N. J., Bradshaw J. L., Tonge B. J. and Sheppard D. M. (2011) Autism and ADHD: how far have we come in the comorbidity debate?. *Neuroscience and Biobehavioral Reviews*, 35(5): 1081-1088.

Gonzalez-Gadea M. L., Baez S., Torralva T., Castellanos F. X., Rattazzi A., Bein V. and Ibanez A. (2013) Cognitive variability in adults with ADHD and AS: disentangling the roles of executive functions and social cognition. *Research in Developmental Disabilities*, 34(2): 817-830.

Gudjonsson G. H., Wells J. and Young S. (2012) Personality disorders and clinical syndromes in ADHD prisoners. *Journals of Attention Disorders,* 16: 304-313.

Gupta R. and Kar B. R. (2010) Specific Cognitive Deficits in ADHD: A Diagnostic Concern in Differential Diagnosis. *Journal of Child and Family Studies,* 19, 778-786.

Hallerbäck M. U., Lugnegård T. and Gillberg C. (2014) ADHD and nicotine use in schizophrenia or asperger syndrome: A controlled study. *Journal of Attention Disorders,* 18(5): 425-433.

Hammond D. (2005): Neurofeedback with anxiety and affective disorders. *Child Adolescence Psychiatric Clinic of North America*, 14: 105-123.

Hegerl U., Himmerich H., Engmann B. and Hensch T. (2010). Mania and attention-deficit/hyperactivity disorder: common symptomatology, common pathophysiology and common treatment? *Current Opinion in Psychiatry*, 23(1): 1-7.

Helles A., Gillberg C. I., Gillberg C., and Billstedt E. (2014) Asperger syndrome in males over two decades: stability and predictors of diagnosis. *Journal of Child Psychology and Psychiatry*, Online First.

Holmes J. SE Gathercole S. and Place M. (2010) Working memory deficits can be overcome: Impacts of training and medication on working memory in children with ADHD. *Psychology*, 24: 827-836.

Instanes J. T., Haavik J. and Halmøy A. (2013) Personality Traits and comorbidity in adults with ADHD. *Journal of Attention Disorders*, Online First.

Kaplan J. S., Erickson K., Luckenbaugh D. A., Weiland-Fiedler P., Geraci M., Sahakian B. J., Charney D., Drevets W. C. and Neumeister A. (2006) Differential performance on tasks of affective processing and decision-making in patients with panic disorder and panic disorder with comorbid major depressive disorder. *Journal of Affective Disorders*, 95: 165–171.

Karaahmet E., Konuk N., Dalkilic A., Saracli O., Atasoy N., Kurçer M. A. and Atik L. (2013) The comorbidity of adult attention-deficit/hyperactivity disorder in bipolar disorder patients. *Comprehensive Psychiatry*, 54(5): 549-555.

Kessler R. C., Adler L., Barkley R., Biederman J., Conners C. K., Demler O. and Zaslavsky A. M. (2006) The prevalence and correlates of adult ADHD in the United States: Results from the National Comorbidity Survey replication. *American Journal of Psychiatry*, 163(4): 716-723.

Kessler R. C., Aguilar-Gaxiola S., Alonso J., Chatterji S., Lee S., Ormel J. and Wang P. S. (2009) The global burden of mental disorders: An update from the WHO World Mental Health (WMH) Surveys. *Epidemiologia e psichiatria sociale,* 18(1): 23-33.

Kessler R. C., McGonagle K. A., Swartz M., Blazer D. G. and Nelson C. B. (1993) Sex and depression in the National Comorbidity Survey I: Lifetime prevalence, chronicity and recurrence. *Journal of Affective Disorders,* 29(2–3): 85-96.

Kessler R., McGonagle K., Zhao S., Nelson C., Hughes M., Eshleman S., Wittchen H. U. and Kendler K. (1994) Lifetime and 12-month prevalence of DSM-III-R psychiatric disorders in the U.S.: Results from the National Comorbidity Survey. *Archives of General Psychiatry*, 51: 8-19.

Kočovská E., Billstedt E., Ellefsen A., Kampmann H., Gillberg I. C., Biskupstø R. and Gillberg C. (2013) Autism in the Faroe Islands: Diagnostic stability from childhood to early adult life. *The Scientific World Journal,* Online First

Kohn D. P. J. and Esser G. (2008) ADHS im Jugend-und Erwachsenenalter. *Monatsschrift Kinderheilkunde*, 156(8): 748-756.

Kooij J. J., Huss M., Asherson P., Akehurst R., Beusterien K., French A. and Hodgkins P. (2012) Distinguishing comorbidity and successful management of adult ADHD. *Journal of Attention Disorders*, 16(5 Suppl.): 3s-19s.

Kraemer M., Uekermann J. Wiltfang J. and Kis B. (2010) Methlyphenidate-induced psychosis in adult attention deficit/hyperactivity disorder: report of 3 new cases and review of the literature. *Clinical Neuropharmacology,* 33: 204-206.

Krause-Utz A., Sobanski E., Alm B., Valerius G., Kleindienst N., Bohus M. and Schmahl C. (2013) Impulsivity in relation to stress in patients with borderline personality disorder with and without co-occurring attention-deficit/hyperactivity disorder: an exploratory study. *Journal of Nervous Mental Disease,* 201: 116-123.

Lampe K., Konrad K., Kroener S., Fast K., Kunert H. J. and Herpertz S. C. (2007). Neuropsychological and behavioral disinhibition in adult ADHD compared to borderline personality disorder. *Psychological Medicine*, 37: 1717-1729.

Lehnhardt F. G., Gawronski A., Pfeiffer K., Kockler H., Schilbach L. and Vogeley K. (2013) The investigation and differential diagnosis of Asperger syndrome in adults. *Deutsches Ärzteblatt,* 110(45): 755-763.

Lenzenweger M. F., Lane M. C., Loranger A. W. and Kessler R. C. (2007) DSM-IV Personality Disorders in the National Comorbidity Survey Replication. *Biological Psychiatry*, 62, 553-564.

Leung R. C., Vogan V. M., Powell T. L., Anagnostou E. and Taylor M. J. (2015) The role of executive functions in social impairment in Autism Spectrum Disorder. *Child Neuropsychology Mar*., 3:1-9 (ahead of print).

Lichtenstein P., Carlström E., Råstam M., Gillberg C. and Anckarsäter H. (2010) The genetics of autism spectrum disorders and related neuropsychiatric disorders in childhood. *American Journal of Psychiatry,* 167(11): 1357-1363.

Mariani J. and Levin F. (2007) Treatment Strategies for Co-Occurring ADHD and Substance Use Disorders. *AM Journal Addiction, 16 Suppl.* 1:45-54.

Martinez-Raga J., Szerman N., Knecht C. and de Alvaro R. (2013) Attention deficit hyperactivity disorder and dual disorders. Educational needs for an underdiagnosed condition. *International Journal of Adolescence Medicine and Health*, 25: 231-243.

Matthies S. D. and Philipsen A. (2014) Common ground in Attention Deficit Hyperactivity Disorder (ADHD) and Borderline Personality Disorder (BPD) – review of recent findings. *Borderline Personality Disorder and Emotional Dysregulation,* 1: 1-13.

Matthies S., Tebartz van Elst L., Feige Bernd, Fischer D., Scheel C., Krogmann E., Perlov E., Ebert D. and Philipsen A. (2010) Severity of childhood attention-deficit hyperacitivity disorder – A risk factor for personality disorders in adult life? *Journal of Personality Disorders*, 25: 101-114.

McAweeney M., Rogers N. L., Huddleston C. (2010) Symptom prevalence of ADHD in a community residential substance abuse treatment program. *Journal of Attention Disorders*, 13: 601-608.

McGovern C. W. and Sigman M. (2005) Continuity and change from early childhood to adolescence in autism. *Journal of Child Psychology and Psychiatry,* 46(4): 401-408.

McNaughton N. and Corrb P. (2004) A two-dimensional neuropsychology of defense: fear/anxiety and defensive distance. *Neuroscience and Biobehavioral Reviews,* 28: 285-305.

Merikangas K. R., Akiskal H. S., Angst J., Greenberg P. E., Hirschfeld R. M. A., Petukhova M. and Kessler R. C. (2007) Lifetime and 12-month prevalence of bipolar spectrum disorder in the national comorbidity survey replication. *Archives of General Psychiatry,* 64(5): 543-552.

Miller C. J., Flory J. D., Miller S. R., Harty S. C., Newcorn J. H. and Halperin J. M. (2008) Childhood ADHD and the emergence of personality disorders in adolescence: A prospective follow-up study. *Journal of Clinical Psychiatry,* 69: 1477-1484.

Monastra V., Lubar J. and Linden M. (2001) The development of a quantitative electroencephalographic scanning process for attention deficit–hyperactivity disorder: reliability and validity studies. *Neuropsychology*, 15: 136-144.

Moore E., Sunjic S., Kaye S., Archer V. and Indig D. (2013) Adult ADHD among NSW prisoners: Prevalence and psychiatric comorbidity. *Journal of Attention Disorders*, Online First.

Müller A., Candrian G. and Kropotov J. (2011) ADHS - Neurodiagnostik in der Praxis. New York, Berlin, Springer.

Murias M., Swanson J. and Sriniwasan R. (2006) Functional Connectivity of Frontal Cortex in Healthy and ADHD Children Reflected in EEG Coherence. *Cerebral Cortex*, 17: 1788-1799.

Newark P. E., Elsässer M. and Stieglitz R. D. (2012) Self-esteem, self-efficacy, and resources in adults with ADHD. *Journal of Attention Disorders,* 16: 1-12.

Newman E., Gupta K., Climer J., Monaghan C. and Hasselmo M. (2012) Cholinergic modulation of cognitive processing: insights drawn from computational models. *Frontiers in Behavioural Neuroscience*, 6:4.

Newton-Howes G., Tyrer P., Anagnostakis K., Cooper S., Bowden-Jones O. and Weaver T. (2010) The prevalence of personality disorder, its comorbidity with mental state disorders, and its clinical significance in community mental health teams. *Social Psychiatry and Psychiatric Epidemiology*, 45, 453-460.

Nydén A., Niklasson L., Stahlberg O., Anckarsater H., Wentz E., Rastam M. and Gillberg C. (2010) Adults with autism spectrum disorders and ADHD neuropsychological aspects. *Research in Developmental Disabilities*, 31(6): 1659-1668.

Pawlikowski M. and Brand M. (2013) Alkohol und andere toxische Substanzen. In: P Calabrese and HJ Markowitsch, Kognitive Störungen in Neurologie und Psychiatrie. *Bad Honnef: Hippocampus*, 239-258.

Perrin S. and Last C. (1996) Relationship between ADHD and Anxiety in Boys: Results from a Family Study. *Journal of the American Academy of Child and Adolescent Psychiatry*, 35 (8): 988-996.

Perroud N., Cordera P., Zimmermann J., Michalopoulos G., Bancila V., Prada P. and Aubry J. M. (2014) Comorbidity between attention deficit hyperactivity disorder (ADHD) and bipolar disorder in a specialized mood disorders outpatient clinic. *Journal of Affective Disorders*, 168: 161-166.

Pflüger M., Riecher-Rössler and Calabrese P. (2013) Schizophrene Psychosen. In P Calabrese and HJ Markowitsch, Kognitive Störungen in Neurologie und Psychiatrie. *Bad Honnef: Hippocampus*, 165-185.

Philipsen A. (2006) Differential diagnosis and comorbidity of attention-deficit/hyperactivity disorder (ADHD) and borderline personality disorder (BPD) in adults. *European Archive of Psychiatry and Clinical Neuroscience,* 256, Suppl. 1, I/42-I/56.

Philipsen A., Limberger M. F., Lieb K., Feige B., Kleindienst N., Ebner-Priemer U., Barth J., Schmahl C. and Bohus M. (2008) Attention-deficit hyperactivity disorder as a potentially aggravating factor in borderline personality disorder. *British Journal of Psychiatry*, 192, 118-23.

Pineiro-Dieguez B., Balanza-Martinez V., Garcia-Garcia P. and Soler-Lopez B. (2014) Psychiatric comorbidity at the time of diagnosis in adults with ADHD: The CAT study. *Journal of Attention Disorders*, Online First

Prada P., Hasler R., Baud P., Bednarz G., Ardu S., Krejci I., Nicastro R., Aubry J. M. and Perroud N. (2014) Distinguishing borderline personality disorder from adult attention deficit/hyperactivity disorder: A clinical and dimensional perspective. *Psychiatry Research*, 217: 107-114.

Quintana H., Snyderb S., Purnella W., Apontea C. and Sitaa J. (2007) Comparison of a standard psychiatric evaluation to rating scales and EEG in the differential diagnosis of attention-deficit/hyperactivity disorder. *Psychiatry Research*, 152 (2): 211-222.

Rasmussen P. and Gillberg C. (2000) Natural outcome of ADHD with developmental coordination disorder at age 22 years: a controlled, longitudinal, community-based study. *Journal of the American Academy of Child and Adolescent Psychiatry,* 39(11): 1424-1431.

Retz W., Boureghda S. S. T., Retz-Junginger P., Philipp-Wiegmann F. and Rösler M. (2013) Clinical symptoms of ADHD and psychopathy in perpetrators. *ADHD Attention Deficit Hyperactivity Disorder*, 5: 47-57.

Rommelse N. N., Franke B., Geurts H. M., Hartman C. A. and Buitelaar J. K. (2010) Shared heritability of attention-deficit/hyperactivity disorder and autism spectrum disorder. *European Child and Adolescent Psychiatry,* 19(3): 281-295.

Ross R. G., Heinlein, S. and Tregellas H. (2006) High rates of comorbidity are found in childhood-onset schizophrenia. *Schizophrenia Research*, 88: 90-95.

Roy M., Dillo, W. Emrich H. M. and Ohlmeier M. D. (2009) Asperger's syndrome in adulthood. *Deutsches Ärzteblatt international*, 106(5): 59-64.

Roy M., Ohlmeier M. D., Osterhagen L., Prox-Vagedes and V. Dillo W. (2013) Asperger Syndrome: a frequent comorbidity in first diagnosed adult ADHD patients? *Psychiatria Danubina*, 25(2): 133-141.

Rybakowski F., Bialek A., Chojnicka I., Dziechciarz P., Horvath A., Janas-Kozik M., Jeziorek A., Pisula E., Piwowarczyk A., Slopien A., Sykut-Cegielska J., Szajewska H., Szczaluba K., Szymanska K., Urbanek K., Waligórska A., Wojciechowska A., Wroniszewski M. and Dunajska A. (2014) Autism spectrum disorders - epidemiology, symptoms, comorbidity and diagnosis. *Psychiatry Po*, 48(4): 653-665.

Rydén E. and Bejerot S. (2008). Autism spectrum disorder in an adult psychiatric population. A naturalistic cross-sectional controlled study. *Clinical Neuropsychiatry*, 5: 13-21.

Samuels J., Eaton W. W., Bienvenu I. L. L. O., Brown C. H., Costa P. T. and Nestadt J. (2002) Prevalence and correlates of personality disorders in a community sample. *British Journal of Psychiatry*, 188, 536-542.

Schaefer J., Giangrande E., Weinberger D. R. and Dickinson, D. (2013) The global cognitive impairment in schizophrenia: Consistent over decades and around the world. *Schizophrenia Research*, 150: 43-50.

Schatz D. and Rostain A. (2006) ADHD with comorbid anxiety: a review of the current literature. *Journal of Attention Disorders*, 10, 2, 141-149.

Scheurich A. and Brokate B. (2009). Neuropsychologie der Alkoholabhängigkeit. Göttingen: Hogrefe.

Schoechlin C. and Engel R. (2005) Neuropsycholocial performence in adult attention-deficit hyperactivity disorder: Meta-analysis of empirical data. *Archives Clinical Neuropsychology* 2005, 20: 727-744.

Sebastian A., Jacob G., Lieb K. and Tüscher O. (2013) Impulsivity in Borderline Personality Disorder: A Matter of Disturbed Impulse Control or a Facet of Emotional Dysregulation? *Current Psychiatry Reports*, 15: 1-8.

Sebastian A., Jung P., Krause-Utz A., Lieb K., Schmahl C. and Tüscher, O. (2014) Frontal dysfunctions of impulse control – a systematic review in borderline personlity disorder and attention-deficit/hyperactivity disorder. *Frontiers in Human Neuroscience*, 8: 1-17.

Shaw P., Stringaris A., Nigg J. and Leibenluft E. (2014) Emotion dysregulation in attention deficit hyperactivity disorder, *American Journal of Psychiatry,* 171: 276-293.

Sheehan D., Lecrubier Y., Sheehan K., Amorim P., Janavs J., Weiller E., Hergueta T., Baker R., Dunbar G. (1998) The Mini-International Neuropsychiatric Interview (M.I.N.I.): the development and validation of a structured diagnostic psychiatric interview for DSM-IV and ICD-10. *Journal of Clinical Psychiatry*, 59: 22-33.

Sinzig J., Morsch D., Bruning N., Schmidt M. H. and Lehmkuhl G. (2008) Inhibition, flexibility, working memory and planning in autism spectrum disorders with and without comorbid ADHD-symptoms. *Child and Adolescent Psychiatry and Mental Health,* 2 (1): 4.

Sinzig J., Walter D. and Doepfner M. (2009) Attention deficit/hyperactivity disorder in children and adolescents with autism spectrum disorder: symptom or syndrome? *Journal of Attention Disorders*, Online First

Skirrow C., Hosang G. M., Farmer A. E. and Asherson P. (2012) An update on the debated association between ADHD and bipolar disorder across the lifespan. *Journal of Affective Disorders*, 141(2–3): 143-159.

Sobanski E., Sabljic D., Alm B., Dittmann R. W., Wehmeier P. M., Skopp G. and Strohbeck-Kühner P. (2013) Driving performance in adults with ADHD: Results from a randomized, waiting list controlled trial with atomoxetine. *European Psychiatry*, 28: 379-385.

Somers J., Goldner E., Waraichj P. and Hsu L. (2006) Prevalence and Incidence Studies of Anxiety Disorders: A Systematic Review of the Literature. *Canadian Journal of Psychiatry*, 51: 100-113.

Spitzer R., Kroenke K., Williams J. and Löwe B. (2006) A Brief Measure for Assessing Generalized Anxiety Disorder. The GAD-7 FREE. *Archives of International Medicine,* 166,10: 1092-1097.

Stahlberg O., Soderstrom H., Rastam M., Gillberg C. (2004) Bipolar disorder, schizophrenia, and other psychotic disorders in adults with childhood onset AD/HD and/or autism spectrum disorders. *Journal of Neural Transmission,* 111: 891-902.

Stieglitz R. D., Nyberg E., and Hofecker-Fallahpour M. (2012) ADHS im Erwachsenenalter. Göttingen: Hogrefe.

Stieglitz R. D. and Raes V. (2015) Assessment strategies and instruments in DD. In: Dom, G. and Moggi, F. (eds.), Co-accuring addictive and psychiatric disorders. Berlin: Springer, 239-259.

Storebø O. J. and Simonsen E. (2013). The association between ADHD and Antisocial Personality Disorder (ASPD): *A Review Journal of Attention Disorders,* Online First.

Storebø O. J. and Simonsen E. (2014) Is ADHD an early stage in the development of borderline personality disorder? *Nordic Journal of Psychiatry,* 68: 289-295.

Tamam L., Karakus G. and Ozpoyraz N. (2008) Comorbidity of adult attention-deficit hyperactivity disorder and bipolar disorder: prevalence and clinical correlates. *European Archives Psychiatry Clinical Neuroscience,* 258(7): 385-393.

Taurines R., Schwenck C., Westerwald E., Sachse M., Siniatchkin M. and Freitag C. (2012) ADHD and autism: differential diagnosis or overlapping traits? A selective review. *ADHD Attention Deficit and Hyperactivity Journal,* 4: 115–139.

Torgersen S., Kringlen E. and Cramer V. (2001) The prevalence of personality disorders in a community sample. *Archives of General Psychiatry*, 58: 590-596.

Torrens M., Rossi P. C., Martinez-Riera R., Martinez-Sanvisens D. and Bulbena A. (2012) Psychiatric co-morbidity and substance use disorders: treatment in parallel systems or in one integrated system? *Substance Use and Misuse,* 47: 1005-1014.

Tuckman A. (2007) Integrative Treatment for Adult ADHD. Oakland CA: New Harbinger Publications.

Unenge Hallerbäck M., Lugnegard T. and Gillberg C. (2014) ADHD and nicotine use in schizophrenia or Asperger syndrome: A controlled study. *Journal of Attention Disorders*, 18: 425-433.

Vance A., Arduca Y., Sanders M., Karamitsios M., Hall N. and Hetrick S. (2006) Attention deficit hyperactivity disorder, combined type, dysthymic disorder and anxiety disorders: differential patterns of neurodevelopmental deficits. *Psychiatry Research*, 143(2-3): 213-22.

Van der Glind G., Konstenius M., Koeter M. W., van Emmerik-van Oortmerssen K., Carpentier P. J., Kaye S., Degenhardt L., Skutle A., Franck J., Bu E. T., Moggi F., Dom G., Verspreet S., Demetrovics Z., Kapitány-Fövény M., Fatséas M., Auriacombe M., Schillinger A., Møller M., Johnson B., Faraone S. V., Ramos-Quiroga J. A., Casas M., Allsop S., Carruthers S., Schoevers R. A., Wallhed S., Barta C., Alleman P. and Levin F. R. van den Brink W., IASP Research Group (2013) Variability in the prevalence of adult ADHD in treatment seeking substance use disorder patients: Results from an international multi-center study exploring DSM-IV and DSM-5 criteria. *Drug Alcohol Depend.*, 134: 158-166.

Van Dijk F., Schellekens A., van den Broek P., Kan C., Verkes R. J. and Buitelaar J. (2014) Do cognitive measures of response inhibition differentiate between attention deficit/hyperactivity disorder and borderline personality disorder? *Psychiatry Research*, 215: 733-739.

Verdejo-García A., López-Torrecillas F., Giménez C. O. and Pérez-García M. (2004). Clinical implications and methodological challenges in the study of neuropsychological correlates of cannabis, stimulant, and opiod abuse. *Neuropsychological Review*, 14: 1-41.

Vidal R., Valero S., Nogueira M., Palomar G., Corrales M., Richarte V., Bosch R., Gomez-Barros N., Corominas M., Casas, M. and Ramos-Quiroga J. A. (2014) Emotional lability: The discriminative value in the diagnosis of attention deficit/hyperactivity disorder in adults. *Comprehensive Psychiatry,* 55: 1714-1719.

Weiss M., Trockenberg Hechtman L. and Weiss G. (1999) ADHD in adulthood: A guide to current theory, diagnosis, and treatment. Baltimore: john Hopkins University.

Wender P. H. (1995). Attention deficit hyperactivity disorder in adults. University Press: Oxford.

White H. and Shah P. (2006) Uninhibited imaginations: Creativity in adults with Attention-Deficit/Hyperactivity Disorder. *Personality and Individual Differences,* 40 1121-1131.

Wilens T. E., Farone S. V., Biederman J. and Gunawardene S. (2003). Does stimulant therapy of attention-deficit/hyperactivity disorder beget later substance abuse? Meta-analytic review of the literature. *Pediatrics,* 111: 179-185.

Williams E. D., Reimherr F. W., Marchant B. K., Strong R. E., Halls C., Soni P., Gale P. D. and Robison R. J. (2010). Personality disorder in ADHD. Part 1: Assessment of personality disorder in adult ADHD using data from a clinical trial of OROS methylphenidate. *Annals of Clinical Psychiatry*, 22: 84-93.

Wu and Lee AS (2006) Identification of AP-2 as an interactive target of Rb and a regulator of the G1/S control element of the hamster histone H3.2 promoter. *Nucleic Acids Research* 26(21):4837-4845

In: New Developments in Clinical Psychology Research
Editors: D. St. Stoyanov and R.-D. Stieglitz
ISBN: 978-1-63483-223-6

Chapter 7

BURN OUT SYNDROME IN HEALTH CARE: STRATEGIES FOR COMPLEX DIAGNOSTIC ASSESSMENT

Drozdstoj Stoyanov, MD, PhD, PGCert, and Boris Tilov, PhD
Medical University, Plovdiv, Bulgaria

ABSTRACT

Health care occupations are considered high-risk jobs in terms of stress. A study conducted recently in Bulgaria has revealed the existence of a disturbingly large number of people having occupational burnout syndrome. The growing rate of problems associated with the global economic crisis and inefficient reforms in the health care system are undermining the successful implementation of the open public health mission and contribute to a change in the concept of the leading social responsibility in the health care system. This reinforces the need to introduce a new approach to human resources management in order to maintain organizational effectiveness.

The Burnout Syndrome (BS) and stress-related disorders are common among medical specialists, but it is more and more frequently suggested that some health care workers are more susceptible to BS than others. The purpose of this study is to determine BS intensity among several groups of physicians: psychiatrists, general practitioners, surgeons, etc. and to make an assessment of the correlation relationships of dependence between BS intensity, personality characteristics of physicians, as well as between the level of BS and the psychological climate in the workplace with a view to creating a burnout-related vulnerability profile.

MATERIAL AND METHODS

The sample includes 154 medical professionals from intensive care sectors (including surgical wards), psychiatry, general medicine, etc., as well as 69 physicians committed at the same time to teaching at a higher medical education institution.

The evaluation toolkit includes the Maslach Burnout Inventory (MBI), the Cloninger Temperament and Character Inventory in its revised version (TCI-R) and a test for psychological climate evaluation (IMPC). According to data available from previous studies, 5 risk groups of health care professionals have been identified, who are strongly influenced by the burnout syndrome – general practitioners, doctors and nurses in the field of palliative care, psychiatrists, oncologists and emergency care specialists. The distribution of the input of 154 medical specialists in the field of health care in the target groups specified above for this study is the following – general practitioners (n = 32), psychiatrists (n = 14), surgeons, specialists in emergency care (n = 71) and other (n = 37). The cases in the extract have been selected from the same region in Southern Bulgaria. We have analyzed the results of the forms for the three questionnaires – TCI-R, IMPC and MBI, by previously testing the hypothesis of analyzed variables normal distribution with the Kolmogorov-Smirnov test. In the conditions of normal distribution of variables, we have performed a comparison between the investigated groups by applying dispersion analysis (one-way ANOVA) and Bonferroni test for Post Hoc Multiple Comparisons. For the variables with a distribution which is different from the normal we have applied the Kruskal-Wallis test for comparison of more than two independent extracts.

RESULTS

Emotional exhaustion is most prominently expressed with general practitioners ($F = 55.546$, $DF1 = 2$, $df2 = 156$, $p < 0.01$), whereas the result from the depersonalization measurement is the highest with surgeons ($F = 15.314$, $DF1 = 2$, $df2 = 156$, $p < 0.01$), as well as the decline in personal accomplishments ($F = 16.079$, $DF1 = 2$, $df2 = 156$, $p < 0.01$). We have found out that the “Harm avoidance” dimension (caution) leads more obviously to a development of BS, while self-directedness and cooperativeness are prominent with physicians with a low rate of BS, i.e., they can play a protective factor role. Harm avoidance is in a correlation with the high level of depersonalization and lack of personal accomplishments (reduced work efficiency), whereas the self-control is prominent among physicians with a low BS level. Studies among doctors, concurrently working as teachers, have revealed pronounced depressiveness and manifestations from the anxiety spectrum (vegetative, obsessive-phobic, etc.), which are in an explicit correlation with emotional exhaustion and reduced work efficiency as burnout syndrome signs. This brings forward the conclusion that the occupational burnout is a more complex multi-dimension construct, which is different from the major depressive episode. A battery of questionnaires was used for the needs of the study of the psychobiological profile and psychosocial well-being of the participants: the revised version of the Cloninger Temperament and Character Inventory - TCI-R (provided courtesy of the author), the Maslach Burnout Inventory on the burnout syndrome and the Koysand DeCotiis IMPC questionnaire in the assessment of the factors of the organizational psychological climate. Administrative documentation and human resources department records (regarding registered absences due to incapacity, staff turnover rates, etc.) have also been analyzed for the organizations in which the persons surveyed are employed. These methods make possible the verification of the hypothesis of a connection of the burnout syndrome as a cause (independent variable) with the administrative indicators as resultant (dependent variables). Based on the data obtained we have identified the internal consistency, the average values for the individual scales, the statistical deviation rate and the coefficient of reliability rate. The Pierson correlation coefficient has been calculated for the extract of 35 people among the responses to the two tests. The correlation between the responses to the test and re-test, as well as the correlation between individual subscales, have been compared to data from other studies in compatible populations in the validation of translated versions of the tools used. The reliability of the battery has been analyzed by means of regression analysis and structural modelling. We have presented the results as a mean arithmetic value ± standard deviation. In order to confirm the correlations between the temperament and character determinants, the changes in the psychological climate and the burnout syndrome, we have conducted a correlation analysis by applying Spearman nonparametric test (2-tailed) and presented the rank correlation coefficient (ρ). It is a valuable tool which establishes an association and makes an assessment of its strength between two groups of usually paired initial data, which at first appear in a rank sequence. We have calculated the Spearman correlation coefficient in our study in order to evaluate the association between the TCI-R determinants, the IMPC dimensions and the MBI results, and at the same time to measure the strength and direction of each of these associations. As a level of significance of the zero hypothesis has been assumed $P < 0.05$. The results have been processed with a statistical package for the social studies (SPSS – v.17).

Statistical Analysis

The internal uniformity of the scales used has been assessed where as a general indicator of structural validity are presented the values of Cronbach α coefficients for the responses from the test and re-test conducted, which have been found to be within the range of 0.71 to 0.96 for the tools included in the battery, which indicates a high level of reliability in accordance with accepted criteria. The highest level of reliability is shown on the IMPC scales where α values are around 0.9 in both measurements, except for the tension scale. The results also confirm the reliability of TCI-R (α is within the range 0.75 – 0.91), and these values are about 0.8 for all of the scales, and 0.9 with SD.

The results obtained for the subscales are lower; however, they are within the range of acceptable values for internal uniformity. The pilot data obtained for 4 of the subscales with α < 0.50 (HA3 shyness, CO2 empathy, CO3 helpfulness and RD4 reward dependence, SD3 resourcefulness) are compatible with the data obtained in a study using TCI in another country – Serbia, which is also located on the Balkans and has a predominant population of Slavic origin. Cultural similarities and the common past can account for the differences in the TCI results and their determinants in comparison with the American population, for which a toolkit has been developed for that purpose. The analysis of items and their relationship with toolkit reliability performed during the study of the extended extract has showed that there are questions that do not meet the homogeneity requirements in some of the TCI-R and IMPC subscales. The identification of inconsistent items is done on the basis of the following criteria – increase by more than 0.10 of the total reliability of the scale (Cronbach α), if the question is excluded or the correlation coefficient is smaller than 0.25 between the question and the result obtained for the scale.

The largest number of such questions can be found in subscales RD, ST and CO of the TCI-R, whereas with IMPC this applies to single questions in the scales for tension and recognition. The results obtained in the pilot study for meaningful and strong correlation connections between the subscales in a test and retest (r = 0.63 to 0.89) have confirmed in cross-cultural applicability and constructive validity of the battery of instruments used and more specifically the translated TCI-R and IMPC versions. The scales with low α values are an exception. The overall evaluation of the internal consistency of the scales has showed acceptable TCI-R values, except for the several subscales already mentioned (CO3 helpfulness, RD4 reward dependence, SD3 resourcefulness).

Similar results have been obtained in cross-cultural studies carried out with this toolkit in Belgium, France, Serbia, etc., which significantly differs from the data gathered in studies in the US and allows to make the assumption that the conceptual model and the inherent characteristics of the scales account for these differences to a larger extent than cultural factors do. The results for temperament and character evaluation scales in TCI-R obtained in Bulgaria are comparable to those reported by Serbian researchers, and in part to those for the population in the US. It is possible that the differences established are determined by certain character features that occur naturally in different cultures, but are unusual in terms of temperament, given its steady independence from cultural models.

Mean arithmetic and standard deviation values for TCI-R (n = 73) IMPC (n = 73) and MBI (n = 70) are 777.74 (SD 39.85), 142.82 (SD 28.24) and 62.96 (SD 13.69) respectively. In the extract have been reported low/medium/high scores for the character and temperament questionnaire, low/medium/high scores for the psychological climate and low/medium/high scores for the burnout syndrome. Normative data for the TCI-R, the evaluation key of the Maslach test and 5 (the number of questions in each group for the psychological climate in the 8 categories) x 5 (five-point scale) IMPC products have been used.

We have conducted a more in-depth analysis of the results by using the Bonferroni test, comparing each group with each one of the others. From the point of view of statistical significance, the lowest is the evaluation of psychiatrists for the "Reward dependence" subscale, being different from the evaluation of all other health care specialists. Regarding the "Persistence" (PS) scale, the highest evaluation is from general practitioners, and the lowest from psychiatrists again. The "self-directedness" scale again is most highly rated by general practitioners, and receives the lowest evaluation from surgeons and emergency unit specialists. They in turn give the highest score for the "cooperativeness" scale, followed by general practitioners. Last on this scale and on the "self-improvement" come psychiatrists. Comparative analysis has showed absence of statistically significant difference between different groups of health care specialists on all IMPC subscales except for the "pressure" subscale, which has received a significantly lower evaluation from general practitioners. All tested groups of health care specialists give high evaluation ratings regarding trust, support, justice, innovation and autonomy as psychological climate characteristics.

In all three areas – emotional exhaustion, depersonalization and reduced work efficiency, no statistically significant difference between the groups has been found. Therefore, we have analyzed the results for the overall group, where subject to the score in the three subscales we have received the distribution of health care professionals surveyed in three levels – high, medium and low. The mean subscale values obtained by us for all of the studied groups have showed that the surveyed group has a medium level of burnout manifestation. The mean value for the emotional exhaustion subscale is 21.68±0.89, which is within the medium level limits (from 17 to 26 points); for depersonalization – 6.62±0.34 (respectively in the range between 7 and 12 points) and work efficiency – 33.02±0.45 (from 32 to 38 points). It is alarming that almost 40% of the respondent health care professionals have high levels of emotional exhaustion (39.0%) and reduced work efficiency (39.6%).

Empirical Findings in Medical Specialists Working in Emergency Units, Surgical Wards and Anesthesiology and Intensive Care Wards

The object of examination in the research is a heterogeneous group that consists of several subgroups: medical specialists in emergency medicine, surgery, anesthesiology and resuscitation; medical nurses with different specialization and qualification levels. A common factor of the target group under examination is their place of work: emergency medical care, surgery and intensive care wards. The extract distribution by gender shows that the women in this study are 80.88%, and men are 19.12% of the total number of 68 surveyed individuals. The age of the group varies in the range from 25 to 62 (average age 44.78±9.5).

No statistically significant difference has been established in the subscale score between men and women, except for the "cooperativeness" subscale, where women have a statistically significant higher score than men ($P < 0.05$). The study of personality temperament and character profile of anesthesiologists has shown that they have lower mean values for "cooperativeness" and "persistence" compared to other medical specialists. We have revealed differences between BS and personality dimensions of surgeons. A positive correlation is found between low "personal accomplishments" (PA) from MBI and "reward dependence," "persistence", self-directedness" and "cooperativeness", and negative correlation between PA and "harm avoidance" or "threat avoidance." The analysis of the results of the empirical self-study shows relatively low self-evaluation of health and job satisfaction, and poor self-evaluation of subjective well-being among the medical specialists included in our survey. The high scores of "cooperativeness" and "self-improvement" or "self-outgrowth" of medical specialists included in our survey compared to the same indicators from other studies reveal a tendency for social tolerance, empathy, social support and a tendency for experiencing the joy of life. In turn, they bear an indirect impact on subjective well-being and happiness of medical specialists. This solidifies the profile of medical specialists working in emergency, surgical and intensive care units, which increases the risk of burnout occurrence.

In such cases of low level of individual stress factor threshold, the risk of burnout developing is large. In conclusion, we could sum up that high HA and ST values from the temperament and characteristic features and of "pressure" from the organizational psychological climate play an important role for the high emotional exhaustion (EE) levels and the risk of burnout syndrome occurrence.

No statistically significant differences in the mean score between men and women have been found with the three subscales of Maslach burnout questionnaire. In the subscale analysis by level (weight) we have received the following distribution of relative shares: 29.41% of surveyed individuals have low levels; 33.82% of the same group are with medium levels and 36.76% with high levels of mental and emotional exhaustion. Just the opposite is the distribution of the scores on the "depersonalization" scale, where 7.35% of respondents have high levels, 25.0% are with medium and 67.65% are with low levels on this scale. Regarding the "work efficiency" or "personal accomplishments" scale, the scores of the test group of professionals are respectively: 29.41% are with high rates; 39.71% of the individuals are with medium levels of work efficiency and 30.88% with values closer to low levels.

This is an important fact which must be taken into account in the measurement and evaluation of mental potential of the medical specialists observed by us. On the one hand this speaks of a low level of subjective satisfaction with work and unsatisfactory results from the personal employment performance among respondents, and on the other hand, retained social tolerance, empathy and care for the patient, willingness and seeking innovations in medical science and practice. When comparing the mean values on the scales (MBI) of the target group, a curious fact is observed – medical professionals have kept their desire for work despite the medium levels of "emotional exhaustion." This proves the mental stability and preserved personality of the specialists working in the emergency, intensive care and surgical wards. The larger relative number of individuals with low levels of "depersonalization" suggests the existence of willingness for professional development and humane attitude towards patients. The results in table 4 and their interrelation with the "emotional exhaustion" scale of MBI help us find several important relationships for the examined group. In the first scale "emotional exhaustion" (EE), we observe a positive dependence with scale "harm avoidance" (HA) of the TCI-R questionnaire. This dependence can be accounted for, given the specific nature of the harm avoidance that measures the levels of adaptation of the personality in a stressful environment. The high levels of the "harm avoidance" scale suggests that the employees working in emergency and intensive care sectors and in surgical wards are more tentative, anxious and difficult to adjust to the existing environment. We have measured the relationship between PA and characteristics "reward", "persistence," "self-improvement" and "pressure," where the degrees of causal dependence range from weak to medium and significant. The analysis of the results has revealed that the "personal accomplishments" of the respondents depend on medium-strength "novelty seeking" and dependence on "persistence" expressed by strength. The other two characteristics – "reward dependence" and "self-improvement" have minimal effect on the PA.

Regarding the relationship between the scale measuring the feature "self-improvement" of the surveyed individuals of MBI, with the "pressure" scale of IMPC, we have found a moderate correlation dependence $r = .431$, where $P < 0.01$. High levels of the "self-improvement" scale suggest that in its nature a person is creative, patient and self-updating. Low levels are indicators of a personality which is readily reconcilable and humble. It is for this reason that the "pressure" scale has a positive interrelation. Pressure can be an own initiative and incentive for the employees of intensive care sectors or a managerial style of introducing efficiency and activeness in the process of group interaction.

Clearly regulated rules of group interaction in the work process are important, both for the constantly self-improving staff and for those who do not possess a clear course of action and a sense of team interaction. The analysis of the "work efficiency" scale of MBI shows evidence of a strong dependence with the individual scales of TCI-R and IMPC regarding individual and group characteristics of specialists employed in the intensive care and emergency sectors. In interaction with the TCI-R questionnaire measuring personality temperament and character features, we have found the following dependencies. The "reward dependence" and "cooperativeness" scales correlate poorly, respectively where we have $r = 0.257$ ($P < 0.05$) for the first one, and $r = 0.254$ ($P < 0.05$) for the second one.

The scales which are of interest for our analysis are "novelty seeking", "persistence" and "self-improvement". Existence of a moderate correlation with the "work efficiency" scale of MBI is observed for the "novelty seeking" scale, where r = 0.415 (P < 0.01). High levels on the "novelty seeking" scale imply temperament nature that defines personality as adventurous and impulsive, and just the opposite – lower levels suggest humbleness and indifference. In this case, we believe that high levels on this scale could serve as a basis for the assumption that employees in intensive care sectors have larger work efficiency when they are purposeful for subjective reasons for acknowledgement. We believe that employees who have lower levels on the "novelty seeking" scale will experience difficulties in adapting to the specific nature of the job, which is characterized by high levels of activity and function. Regarding the second scale "persistence", we have noted the presence of a high correlation, where r = 0.500 (P < 0.01). This scale describes the temperament nature of the individual, where with its high levels the individual is diligent and persistent, and more passive and unassuming where levels are lower. This suggests that employees in intensive care sectors are committed to their work, doing it with persistence and irreconciliation to constantly changing external conditions. Regarding the "self-improvement" scale, we have also found the presence of dependence on work efficiency of health care staff in emergency and intensive care sectors, where r = 0.381 (P < 0.01). This dependence shows that the pursuit of self-improvement as a character trait presupposes the high levels of work efficiency performance of the surveyed group.

The relationship of the group characteristics of the IMPC questionnaire with the "work efficiency" scale of MBI shows the presence of a moderate correlation with individual scales.

Accordingly, the "support," "pressure," "recognition", "innovativeness" scales correlate poorly with the "work efficiency" scale.

Moderate dependencies have been found with the "autonomy" scales, where r = 0.450 (P < 0.01) scale, and with the "trust" scale," where r = 0.316 (P < 0.01). This implies that employees in the intensive care or emergency unit need their independence in accordance with the group interaction. The feeling of independence is a prerequisite for the good work efficiency of the surveyed persons and the other way round – administrative pressure can be detrimental to efficiency, both at a group and individual level. With higher levels of trust between team members and the team leader and the individual employee, the examined group has stated willingness to increase the efficiency of its work efficiency and the timely prevention of professional exhaustion. People surveyed also declared that the presence of support and recognition for a well-done work in various situations is a factor for the level of professionalism and adequacy. With the single-factor dispersion analysis we have also proved dependency and consistency between the efficiency and credibility of the workplace in intensive care and emergency sectors (F = 2.92, P < 0.01).

Sample from Medical Specialists Working in Psychiatry and in Other Fields of Medicine

The second surveyed group consists of health care specialists working in psychiatric sectors and wards. The unification of the first group is based on an insufficient number of individuals in various health care areas, whereas the number of individuals in the second group is considered to be sufficient for this study.

The distribution of the respondents of the first group by gender has showed that women make up 75% and men 25%. Age distribution for the surveyed group is the following: individuals under the age of 30 – 11.1%, from 31 to 40, 41 to 50 and 51 to 60 years of age the percentage is equal – 27.8%, and those over 60 years old make up 5.6%.

In the distribution of the mean values between the two groups, we have noticed that employees in the psychiatric sector have higher scores on the "novelty seeking" scale. This finding has showed that these health care workers are more curious and impulsive in their work when it is a matter of ambition to get a stimulus. In all the other scales, the first group has higher mean scores when compared to the second group. In comparing the two groups, we have found higher mean scores on the seven scales for the first group in reference to the scores of the psychiatric group. The "pressure" scale is the only one with higher scores for the individuals working in psychiatric units. This finding is due to the subjective judgment that there is a clear framework for compliance with certain rules and regulations and reporting specific results in a precise temporal aspect. From the distribution of mean scores in the first and the second group regarding the level of professional exhaustion, we have noticed that the group of specialists working in psychiatric units have higher scores than their colleagues in oncology wards, palliative care wards, etc. In psychiatric wards and sectors, employees are more emotionally exhausted, depersonalized and having lower levels of work efficiency. During the analysis of individual scale scores regarding purity and strength, we have found that 36.1% of the persons surveyed in the first group have low scores on the emotional exhaustion scale, 33.3% of the individuals in the same group have average scores and 30.6% have high scores on the mental and emotional exhaustion scale. The distribution of surveyed individuals in the second group of specialists working in psychiatric units shows that low and high levels of emotional exhaustion have the same percentage of responses – 38.9%. Comparing the levels of emotional exhaustion, we have noticed higher scores for professionals working in psychiatric wards and sectors compared to health care specialists in oncology, palliative care wards and dentistry. Regarding the "depersonalization" scale, we have found a reverse correlation in the first group, where the percentage distribution of low levels are observed with 50% of the surveyed group. 41.7% fall within the medium level on the scale, and only 8.3% declare high levels of this indicator. The scores in the second group are approximate too, where 44.4% of the individuals surveyed fall within the low level range of depersonalization, 38.9% of the respondents are persons with average scores and 16.7% with high levels on this scale. The results obtained mark higher mean scores of the medium levels in the first group. High levels of the "depersonalization" scale have higher scores in the group of psychiatrists compared to the first group. The analysis of the third group – "work efficiency" with the first group has showed that the largest percentage is found in the high levels – 44.4%, compared to the lower levels – 19.4%. Interestingly, the scores of the second group, the individuals working in psychiatric units, show a higher percentage of work efficiency compared to the first group, where 50% of the respondents have identified themselves as such. In conclusion, we can say that specialists working in the psychiatric sector are more emotionally exhausted, depersonalized, but at the same time having better work efficiency than the employees in oncology, palliative care, dentistry and rehabilitation.

The results have revealed high levels of correlation between the "emotional exhaustion" scale of MBI, the "avoidance of harm" scale of the TCI-R questionnaire and reverse correlation with the IMPC scales. The correlation dependence in the first group of emotional exhaustion with the harm avoidance, where $r = .458$ ($P < 0.01$), can be accounted for with the low levels of adaptation mechanisms in stressful environment of the employees in oncology, palliative care and dentistry. The more anxious and hard to adapt these employees are, the sooner they will reach high levels of emotional exhaustion, which is a prerequisite for rapid professional exhaustion. Correlation analysis of the "emotional exhaustion" scale, comparable to the other questionnaire on psychosocial climate, shows a moderate and good reverse correlation with individual scales. We have found moderate reverse correlation with the "unity" scales r = -.413 ($P < 0.05$) and the "recognition" scale r = -.462 ($P < 0.01$). These data show that the more the individual employees in these sectors feel the lack of unity, the more likely it is for them to reach emotional exhaustion and the other way round, with the uniting of the actions the level of emotional exhaustion drops. Recognition for a well-done job also has an effect on reducing the levels of emotional exhaustion. With two other scales we have found a perfect reverse correlation, respectively the "trust" scale, r = -.609 ($P < 0.01$), and the "support" scale, r = -.670 ($P < 0.01$). Open communication and demonstration of tolerance of each other on the one hand, and management on the other also have an effect on reducing the levels of emotional exhaustion. The last two scales, "honesty," r =- .591 ($P < 0.01$), and "innovation", r = -.559 ($P < 0.01$), also correlate well with reverse correlation. This means that the more the rules in a unit, team or group are adhered to, regardless of the regulatory situation, at the same time promoting creativity and risk-taking, the more limited will be the development of emotional exhaustion among those employed in oncology, palliative care and dentistry. The analysis of the "work efficiency" of MBI shows evidence of a strong correlation with the individual scales of IMPC and the "persistence" scale of the TCI-R, r = .463 ($P < 0.01$). The more committed, diligent and hard-working the employees in these units are, the more their subjective experience of work efficiency increases. In the interaction with the IMPC questionnaire measuring psychosocial climate in the workplace, we have found a moderate and good correlation with individual scales. Moderate correlation is observed with "unity" scales, r = -.426 ($P < 0.01$), "trust," r = .453 ($P < 0.01$) and "innovation," r = .457 ($P < 0.01$). The sense of unity, open communication and the promotion of creativity increase the levels of work efficiency in the surveyed group. Good correlation is demonstrated by the scales "honesty" r = .460 ($P < 0.01$), "support" r = .480 ($P < 0.01$) and "autonomy" r = .569 ($P < 0.01$). Adherence to and application of the rules laid down for all employees, the demonstration of tolerance for mistakes are another major factor for increasing work efficiency. Accordingly, the respondents declare explicitly that their activeness and efficiency in the work process are affected by self-esteem and the sense of independence in certain procedures and rules. During the analysis of the second group of health care employees in psychiatric units we have found less dependence between the individual scales of TCI-R and IMPC in the emotionally exhaustion scale and work efficiency of MBI, comparable to the first group. What we have found as a significant difference between the two groups is that with the second group there is a good correlation in individual and group characteristics with the "depersonalization" scale. With the TCI-R questionnaire we have noticed two scales measuring character dispositions with good correlation with the "depersonalization" scale. These are the scales "cooperativeness" r = .493 ($P < 0.05$) and the "self-improvement" scale r =.488 ($P < 0.05$). The more unscrupulous and vindictive employees in the psychiatric sector are, with no striving for professional development, combined with lack of understanding and imagination, the more dehumanized in their daily contact with patients they become. During the analysis of the correlation between the scales of IMPC and the "depersonalization" scale we find high level of reverse correlation.

Accordingly, with the scales "unity," r = -.687 (P < 0.01), "trust," r = -.628 (P < 0.01) and "honesty, r = -.628 (P < 0.01) we find a high level of correlation. The lack of sharing, impaired communication and questioning of management practices as being unequal for all employees, drastically increases the possibility for depersonalization of employees in psychiatric units. Slightly higher are the coefficients on the "support" scale, r = -.747 (P < 0.01) and "innovation" scale, r = -.705 (P < 0.01). Respondents strongly support the suggestion that the more penalized mistakes are and their risk-taking abilities in areas that concern the entire team are not rewarded, the more these individuals tend to become dehumanized, both to each other and to individual patients. In the analysis of the "emotional exhaustion" scale we find moderate reverse correlation with the scales "trust," r = -.502 (P < 0.01), "support," r = -.510 (P < 0.01), "honesty," r = -.517 (P < 0.01) and "innovation", r = -.528 (P < 0.01). This correlation has shoved that the lack of open communication, fear of reprisal, the duality in the application of established rules and the lack of a positive evaluation of creativity are obvious predictor of occurrence of emotional exhaustion of individuals employed in psychiatric units. The analysis of the "work efficiency" scale has showed correlation in two scales only responsible for individual and group characteristics. This is the TCI-R "responsibility avoidance" scale, r =-.718 (P < 0.01), and the IMPC "autonomy" scale, r = .612 (P < 0.01).

The results thus obtained indicate that the more pessimistic, hesitant and anxious an employee from a psychiatric ward or sector is, the lower their levels of work efficiency will be, and conversely, the more confident and stable the individual is, the more prone to higher professional abilities they are. Accordingly, it becomes clear from the "autonomy" scale that those employees who have greater freedom of action regarding established rules and standards on the workplace are more likely to identify themselves as capable of working.

SAMPLE OF GENERAL PRACTITIONERS

The characteristic distribution of the group under survey is the following: 33 (thirty-three) GP, average age of participants 45.00±1.65, length of work experience – 20.10±1.83. The distribution by gender shows that 87.90% of the participants in the survey are women. The analysis by category has revealed that 21.88% of the individuals under survey are in a state of high-level emotional exhaustion, 15.63% have a medium level and the largest share consists of those with a low level of emotional exhaustion - 62.50%. With the category "depersonalization," it has been established that the highest relative share is again for GP with low level of expression – 59.38%, followed by those with medium level 34.38%, and the lowest relative share is for GP with high level of depersonalization - 6.25%. The analysis of the group for the category "work efficiency" has showed that … of GP have low levels, which is an unfavourable position. The larges relative share is made of GP with average level of work efficiency - 40.63%, and just a little over 1/3 have scores. The high level of "depersonalization" is in direct weak correlation with a high level of "emotional exhaustion" of GP (r = 0.416, p < 0.05). The correlation is negative on the "work efficiency" scale both in reference to the "depersonalization" scale (r = -0.486) and the "emotional exhaustion" scale (r = 0.628 p < 0.01). A moderate positive correlation has been revealed between the "emotional exhaustion" scale of MBI scale and the "pressure" scale of IMPC, r = 0.548 P < 0.01. High levels of the "emotional exhaustion" scale suggest that the individual is experiencing pressure from the patients, administrative units and the overall social and economic situation. The correlation allows for the use of appropriate strategies, which by reducing pressure will also diminish the burnout manifestations. It should be pointed out that the "depersonalization" category of MBI, i.e., high level of loss of humanity, lack of desire for work and development, although demonstrated in the low relative share of GP, is in a weak negative correlation both with the "reward dependence" scale of TCI-R and the "trust", "support" and "recognition" scales (IMPC). Such results also reveal the potential for the prevention of burnout syndrome by regulating factors such as "reward," "recognition", "support" and "trust". These results reflect the empirically collected impressions of the negative image of individuals working as GP. It becomes evident from the results that there exists weak negative correlation between the "work efficiency" scale of MBI and the "harm avoidance" scale of the TCI-R questionnaire. Low levels of the "harm avoidance" scale imply that GP are more optimistic, self-confident, and more active. Undoubtedly, with personality temperament traits such as anxiety, shyness and hesitancy, work efficiency will be negatively affected. Interestingly, a weak negative correlation has been established between the "unity" scale (IMPC) and the "novelty seeking" scale, and a weak positive correlation with the "persistence" scale (TCI-R). Low levels of the "novelty seeking" scale suggest temperament nature possessing qualities like modesty, temperance, even indifference and disinterestedness. GP with low levels on this scale would find it more difficult to adapt to activities requiring unity, which is characterized by high levels of activity. The category of "persistence" describes the temperament of ambitious people aspiring to high accomplishments, workaholics and professionals.

Regression and Factor Models of Burnout

A hierarchical stepwise method of regression has been adopted for the purposes of this study, to serve as a base for determination of the model predicting burnout component levels and their determinants, with serial inclusion of three groups of factors. On the basis of the conceptual model for the interaction of the three main groups of factors, they have been successively included in the three blocks of regression analysis as predictors, and the three burnout dimensions have been included as independent variables. Data show that the value of R2 after the introduction of the psychological climate variables range from 0.24 (for EE) to 0.14 (for DP) with level of significance $P < 0.01$. The inclusion of personality temperament and character features in the model contributes to the enhancement of the predictive power of the models (Δ R2 is from 0.3 to 0.15). The models obtained, describing the impact of significant predictors on the values of the burnout components, account for more than 30% of the responses received to emotional exhaustion and personal performance, like the importance of models. Here should be taken into account a number of other popular in literature non-psychological factors with a psychological effect on the individual, such as reward size, material and social occupational conditions, physical or chemical hazardous factors of the environment, which are likely to account for (predict) the remaining approximately 60%. These factors are situated outside the cause-and-effect configuration of our model, but they can be mediated by it. The results from the factor analysis confirm to a large extent the conceptual model hypotheses for the relationship between organizational factors and personality characteristics in terms of vulnerability to burnout.

Our study along with numerous other studies gives reason to assume that the character and temperament personality characteristics (TCI-R scales) have both a direct and indirect effect on burnout dimensions. Very often the complex correlations under survey have a non-linear nature, which requires the completion of another type of factor analysis in order to evaluate the actual role as mediators of the psychological climate characteristics. The models in our study, obtained through regression analysis, although not directly including dimensions of organizational culture such as management style, management decision-taking model, adaptability, etc., correspond to this concept, validating the action of "autonomy" and 'pressure". With the introduction of latent organizational and cultural factors, the predictability potential of models significantly increases, reaching 66% with EE and nearing 30% with DP. Such results clearly indicate that burnout levels are much more determined by organizational culture factors than by the personality characteristics, which are the focus of research in this study. The opportunities for effective management and prevention of the burnout syndrome are within the area of management decisions and policy of health care organizations. In order to achieve maximum efficiency, it is imperative to integrate in management practices approaches both for psychological profiling and organizational culture assessment.

CONCLUSION

BS affects personal well-being and professional performance. It is important to identify the individuals who are susceptible to its development in order to take preventive measures, such as stress management and improving coping strategies at organizational level. All correlations in our study all between personality characteristics, psychological climate and burnout syndrome are established in the theoretically anticipated directions. In this study we have focused our attention on a set of predictors on an individual level (TCI-R), combined with the dimension of the psychological climate, in order to show that they are powerful predictors of the burnout syndrome. Correlation dependencies in our study support the new notion that high level of "persistence," strong "caution" and poor character development increase the individual vulnerability to occupational burnout. In other words, the personality of the individual is a powerful predictor of the level of burnout to which they are exposed in the workplace. However, this personality profile is not sufficient to induce burnout on its own. According to our diathesis-stress model, if the vocational burnout is about to occur, the vulnerable individual is experiencing difficulty adapt to provocative psychological climate conditions. Therefore, the design of our battery of evaluation tools includes the KoysandDeCotiis test. As is shown in the correlation matrices, the correlation between the personality and the burnout syndrome confirm our theoretical model. This study identifies the main effects of temperament and personality characteristics on the burnout syndrome, taking into consideration the dimensions of the psychological climate as well. The cause-and-effect connection between the combination of "caution" and moderate levels of "pressure" and the occurrence of the burnout syndrome has been verified: a cautious person (high level of harm avoidance), subjected to pressure (stress), is more vulnerable to "emotional exhaustion."

Reducing "personal accomplishments" is in a positive correlation with the high level of "persistence," combined with a low level of "autonomy."

This means that an individual with a high level of "persistence," placed in a work environment that is characterized by a low level of "autonomy" and "innovation", is at risk of diminishing their "personal accomplishments" and the other way round. The high level of "cooperativeness" in combination with a high level of "unity" are in a negative correlation with "depersonalization".

"Depersonalization" in itself looks unlikely with health care employees, considering the fact that the specifics of their professional obligations is in direct opposition to distanced behavior towards patients and colleagues. Our results have showed solid connections between the combination "self-directedness" and "autonomy" and two of the burnout syndrome scales – "personal accomplishments" and "emotional exhaustion." The correlation directions are influenced by combinations of the values in the scales for both "self-directedness" and "autonomy". Specific correlations appear as follows: a high level of "self-directedness" and high level of "autonomy" are positively related to "personal accomplishments" and negatively related to "emotional exhaustion." In this correlation we recognize a potential protective factor. Our results confirm the theoretical assumption that for the occurrence of the burnout syndrome is needed a reciprocal interaction between personal vulnerability and the psychological climate of the organization. In this way, they create a vicious circle of cause-and-effect interaction. The results of this study emphasize the importance of the fact that personal characteristics and the psychological climate and the burnout syndrome are a triune multi-faceted phenomenon. Keeping in mind the fact that our findings show significant correlations among the scales, they create the foundation for further discussion and exploration. The theories of the personality and the psychological climate have set up conceptual frameworks in which we have defined our statement: the burnout type is specifically related to the internal associations between personality dimensions and psychological climate determinants. The results obtained support the alternative hypothesis and in addition, a number of notable findings have been made. This study has made significant contributions in the field because it has successfully demonstrated the importance of individual differences, especially the personality dimensions in combination with the factors of the psychological climate as a regulatory domain for the manifestation of burnout. This study provides empirical evidence in support of the important relations between the scales and more specifically - of the internal consistency between their subscales. Despite the small size of the extract (low degree of validity), the sufficient heterogeneity of the professional groups enables us to summarize the results of the pilot study. In the subsequent statistical processing of the final data (n = 154) the strength and direction of the associations between the subscales has been unequivocally confirmed. Further to that, we have ascertained some additional cause-and-effect relations, significantly important, proven and cited in other scientific studies. This study is built on a remarkable and unique three-dimensional structure – the domains of personality vulnerability, anomalies in the psychological climate and the occupational burnout syndrome. The recognition of predisposition factors is crucial for the prevention of emotional exhaustion and depersonalization in the workplace. We expect that the early identification of these cause-and-effect phenomena, rather than concentrating on the eventually appearing symptoms, will make possible the introduction of appropriate measures aimed at the prevention of the burnout syndrome among health care specialists. Unfortunately, the burnout syndrome is hard to prevent. However, the need to introduce preventive programmes aimed at reducing workplace stress and preserving the health of medical staff has been confirmed by the results obtained in our study.

The programmes must be implemented in the organizations in order to change the system of reward receiving, improve social relations between employees and employers, and between colleagues, reduce the workload and the sense of threat. It is necessary to communicate the particular importance of teamwork and to provide a positive psychological climate for the employee to achieve satisfaction from the job. A frequent change of positions and duties is required in order to maintain the interest of the individuals in their work. On the other hand, this change must not be repeatedly expressed and it necessarily requires observing the professional qualifications of the individual (i.e., it would be wrong to de facto reduce in rank someone just to diversify their position).

Early identification of depression and other concurrently existing conditions is also essential as it could lead to a full and timely recovery. The natural adaptation mechanism for the reduction of the enormous social damage as a result of the burnout lies in the development of strategies and models of behavior aimed at reducing stress and overcoming it. The fundamental approaches include two aspects: organizational (development and implementation of programmes for provision of assistance to employees to cope with stress, stress management training with the help of various intervention components for its mitigation) and individual (identification and elimination of individual factors that cause stress). Both approaches are considered to be positively influenced by public support. It is important that employees are aware of health impacts caused by stress and the burnout syndrome, to develop skills for overcoming them and for restoring their own energy resources. Corporate programmes prepare employees to cope with the negative effects of everyday stress, to regulate their emotional state and improve their competence in the field of interpersonal relationships. According to a survey conducted among American physicians, the best burnout prevention is the promotion of personal and professional well-being on all levels: physical, emotional, mental and spiritual. This should be done throughout the whole professional life cycle of health care professionals, from university academic studies to retirement. This is a challenge not only for every physician, but also for the medical profession and for organizations working with physicians.

References

Cloninger, C. R., Przybeck, T. R., Svrakic, D. M., Wetzel, R. D. *The Temperament and Character Inventory—Revised*. St. Louis: Washington University; 1999.

Cloninger, C. R., Svrakic, D. M., Przybeck, T. R. (1993) A Psychobiological Model of Temperament and Character. *Archives of General Psychiatry* 50: 975–990).

Koys, D. J. and DeCotiis, T. A. (2001). Inductive measures of psychological climate. *Human Relations* 44, 265–285.

Maslach, C., Jackson, S. C. and Leiter, M. P. (1996). *Maslach Burnout Inventory*. Palo Alto, California: Consulting Psychologists Press.

Maslach, C., Schaufeli, W. B. (1993). Historical and conceptual development of burnout. In: W. B. Schaufeli, C. Maslach and T. Marek (Eds.). *Professional Burnout: Recent Developments in Theory and Research*. Washington, DC: Taylor and Francis, 1–16.

Stoyanov, D. S. and Cloninger, C. R. (2012). Relation of People-centered public health and person-centered healthcare management: a case study to reduce burn-out. *International Journal of Person Centered Medicine*, 2(1), 90–95.

Stoyanov, D., Stoikova, M., Tornyova, B., Tilov, B. G., Turnovska, T., Mateva, N., and Hyusein, N. (2011) *Burn out syndrome in health care personnel: Ethical, psychological and methodological implications*. 5th Balkan Congress on the History and Ethics of Medicine 11-15. X. 2011, Istanbul, pp. 449–462. ISBN 978-975-420-871-9.

Stoyanov, D., Tilov, B. and Tornyova, B. (2014). Theoretical Model of Vulnerability to Burn Out: Personality and Psychological Climate in the Context of BOS. *New Model of Burn Out Syndrome: Towards early diagnosis and prevention*, 1, 7.

Tilov, B., Dimitrova, D., Stoykova, M., Tornjova, B., Foreva, G., and Stoyanov, D. (2012). Cross-cultural validation of the revised temperament and character inventory in the Bulgarian language. *Journal of evaluation in clinical practice*, 18(6), 1180-1185.

III. Clinical Psychology and Other Disciplines

In: New Developments in Clinical Psychology Research
Editors: D. St. Stoyanov and R.-D. Stieglitz
ISBN: 978-1-63483-223-6

Chapter 8

THE TRANSLATIONAL VALIDATION AS NOVEL APPROACH TO INTEGRATION OF NEUROSCIENCE AND PSYCHIATRY

Drozdstoj S. Stoyanov, MD, PhD, PGCert[1,*], Rolf-Dieter Stieglitz, PhD[2], Claudia Lenz, PhD[3], and Stefan J Borgwardt, MD[3]

[1]Medical University of Plovdiv, Department of Psychiatry and Medical Psychology and Research Complex for Translational Neuroscience, Plovdiv, Bulgaria
[2]University of Basel, Switzerland, University Clinic of Psychiatry, Basel, Switzerland
[3]University Clinic of Psychiatry, Basel, Switzerland, Neuropsychiatry and Brain Imaging Group, University of Basel, Basel, Switzerland

ABSTRACT

Introduction and Aim

Contemporary psychopathology has adopted various approaches to establish its validity, such as content, criteria, convergent, divergent etc. validation procedures.

However, regardless of the progress in neuroscience, it has not been incorporated yet in psychiatric diagnosis as a possible source of external validity. In this paper, we aim at defining the construct of translational validity, which may eventually bridge the two fields of inquiry separated by the explanatory gap.

* Corresponding author: Prof. Dr Drozdstoj Stoyanov. Medical University of Plovdiv, Department of Psychiatry and Medical Psychology and Research Complex for Translational Neuroscience. E-mail: stojanovpisevski@gmail.com.

Argument

Both modern clinical assessment tools and functional imaging are validated within their disciplinary domains: clinical inventories are validated with other clinical tests or interviews while neurobiological markers are validated against other biological measures. The currently employed experimental neuroimaging designs inert psychological visual stimuli and can serve only as *neutral in terms of diagnosis emotional stimuli.*

This is to say that such stimuli have no diagnostic value and hence cannot relate or be embodied into validity operations between neuro-biological markers of disease and psychopathology.

In the same way, most of the clinical psychopathological assessment tools are not underpinned with robust neuroimaging findings.

Whenever any connections between the two types of measures are established, they represent mere statistical *post hoc* correlations. Therefore, they are not regarded as translation validity operations. Yet, they need convergent translational cross-validation in order to be integrated into psychiatric diagnosis.

Translational validity, on the other hand, represents the kind of validation to relate the two domains by means of translation. We suggest that brain imaging should involve real-time rating with *disorder-relevant clinical scales* performed simultaneously with fMRI instead of the neutral picture stimuli.

Conclusion

The novel paradigm for translational cross-validation among methods of psychiatry and neuroscience can potentially contribute to the integration of the inter-disciplinary explanatory models in psychiatry.

Keywords: Translation, neuroimaging, psychiatry, multimodal assessment

1. Introduction. Multimodal Assessment

It is generally agreed that human behaviour and experience have to be recorded in a multimodal way (other terms occasionally used: multimethod, multimethodically). Thus, distinctions are made between the following aspects (Baumann et al. 1985): databases, sources of data and functional ranges (see Table 1).

On occasions, another aspect is added: the type of instruments which are used to assess the relevant aspects of interest (e.g., rating scales, achievement tests, and technical procedures). Multimodal assessment can be understood as a *general framework* which has to be specified for the concrete assessment of individual persons or groups of persons, making it necessary to select specific instruments.

The choice should be made according to specific criteria. On the one hand, methodological aspects should play a central role (e.g., high psychometric quality, especially reliability and validity). At the same time conceptual considerations should be of equal relevance. This means instruments should be used which allow the characterization of the important aspects of the construct in question.

A multimodal approach is generally required for basic research (e.g., aetiology of a disorder) and for evaluation (e.g., of psychotherapy and psychotropic drugs research) in order to cope with the complexity of the phenomena studied and to account for the variance as to the degree of exactness in databases and data providers as well as functional ranges.

Furthermore, the necessity of a multimodal approach arises from the need to reduce investigator dependent rating bias and results in the inclusion of different perspectives.

With regard to the self-rating scales, bias may include acquiescence, central tendency, or social desirability; on the level of observer-rating scales it may come from insufficient experience with the scale, response sets like generosity error or error of leniency. In planning a study, care has to be taken that it contains sufficient distinct measures to cover the domain of interest, but also that it does not include redundant measures (reduction of statistical power).

The question of the degree to which the different databases and data providers correspond has aroused particular interest. If different data bases are identical at the same time, it is referred to as *concordance*, if they are not; this is referred to as *discordance*. If there is a correlation of two depression rating scales in the range of 0.80, convergence can be assumed. If the correlation is 0.50, this is no longer the case, i.e., both instruments cover different aspects of the syndrome (only 25% common variance). If the course of different parameters is parallel over time, there is synchronicity (e.g., parallel changes of cognitions and somatic symptoms during anxiety therapy), if not there is desynchronicity (e.g., reduction of avoidance behaviour in the continuous presence of negative conditions). Each case of discordance or desynchronicity requires an explanation, in clinical routine as well as in research.

Example

For most psychiatric disorders, a multimodal approach is necessary for an adequate description because a gold standard is missing. An example is presented in Table 2. Depressive disorders in particular are characterized as disorders with different components such as subjective experiences, specific behavioural reactions, and a broad spectrum of somatic/vegetative symptoms.

Depending on the specific aim of a study (e.g., the natural course, efficacy of a therapeutic intervention), a broad range of aspects has to be considered.

This chapter will highlight a novel approach to multimodal assessment in psychiatry by means of trans-disciplinary (or translational) validation of different assessment methods.

Table 1. Multimodal assessment

Databases	Basic units of consideration (perspectives: e.g., biochemical, physiological, neurobiological, psychological, social, ecological)
Sources of data	Data provider (e.g., patient, therapist, nursing staff, reference person, neutral observer)
Functional ranges	Partial aspect within a database (e.g., psychological databases: experiences, behaviour, feeling, working capacity)

Table 2. Multimodal assessment of depressive disorders (examples)

Databases	Psychological, biological, social
Sources of data	Patient, therapist, independent/trained rater, relevant others (e.g., family members).
Functional ranges	• Psychological database: cognitions, emotional reactions, behaviour • Physiological database: physiological reactions • Neurobiological database: neuroimaging data • Social database: impairments and handicaps, social support
Assessment instruments	e.g., self- and observer-rating scales, structured or standardized interviews, diaries, behaviour observations, behavioural tests, self-monitoring, physiological assessment instruments, fMRI.

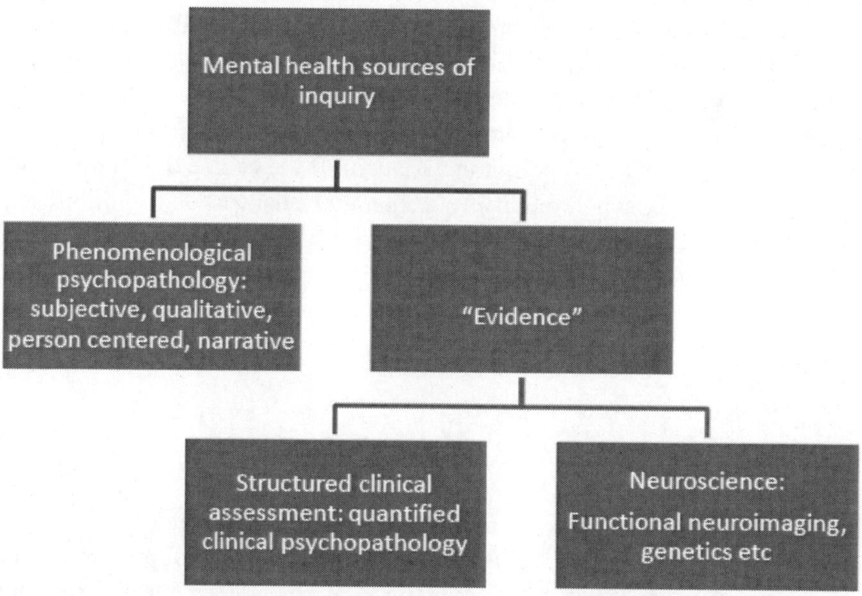

Figure 1. Sources of inquiry.

2. Validity and Validation Procedures in Disciplines Constituting Psychiatry

The explanatory gap separates two fundamentally divergent domains of scientific inquiry and respective operational languages. The *domain of phenomenology* is operating with qualitative, ideographic, subjective and person-centered narratives, as contrasted to the *domain of evidence*, which is operating with presumably objective quantitative nomothetic facts. Furthermore the domain of evidence is constituted from heterogenic disciplines in itself. As illustrated on Figure 1 it consists of two incommensurable kinds of quantitative methods.

The first kind is *clinical assessment methods*, structured interviews or inventories and the second kind are *neurobiological measures*, such as Blood Oxygenation Level Dependent (BOLD) functional magnetic resonance imaging (fMRI) (Stoyanov et al. 2011, 2012).

2.1. Disciplinary Structures and Validation Procedures

Clinical psychology is taken to represent the medical humanities domain and is therefore structured as ideographic discipline, concerned in the patients' narratives, the latter being studied with different interviews and inventories. Although the methods and data of contemporary clinical psychology claim to be scientific and nomothetic in some sense they remain decontextualized narratives as the items of the different assessment tools are in fact composed from excerpts of the patients and/or professional narratives (Stoyanov et al. 2012). Validation in clinical psychology is based on two levels of comparison. The first level is defined as item response, respectively score on the rating scale *under validation* with a rating scale which is already *assumed to be valid.* Usually the archaeology of the clinical rating scales is traced back to their prototype – Minesotta Multiphasic Personality Inventory (MMPI), designed in 1936 and published in 1937. The arguable query about the validity of that *prototype* clinical rating scale remains unresolved. Our analysis however demonstrated that the rationale behind the item selection and formulation of MMPI was nothing more but extraction of certain statements/questions from patients' narratives in a qualitative, virtually phenomenological psychiatric interview. Then the items are sorted into scales on the basis of their ability to distinguish given diagnostic groups where the diagnosis is practically *presumed to be correct* and uncontestable. If the measures between two instruments differ each from the other it is taken to be divergent or discriminant validity. When the two measures happen to overlap the result is regarded as indicator for convergent validity.

On the second level of comparison the clinical scales are administered under 'retest' procedure which means they are given to the same subjects after certain period of time. It is expected to deliver both information about reliability (retest stability of the subjects responses) and the internal consistency - or validity - of the test as measured with the statistical indicator alpha of Cronbach. Validity is regarded here as a property of language, i.e., the extent in which the subjects have mutual *understanding of the meaning of the items.*

Insofar validation procedures in clinical psychology are derived from predominantly statistical assumptions. Therefore the construct validity cannot be regarded as scientific, i.e., inherent to a nomothetic discipline, however quantitative, since the scores from rating scales and structured interviews are indeed quantitative measures.

Nonetheless clinical psychology remains to a greater extent ideographic knowledge, operating with different kinds of quantified narratives in first place, with primary source in phenomenological psychopathology. On the other hand contemporary neuroscience spanning from behavioral genetics to functional neuroimaging is a typical explanatory discipline. As robust natural science it claims to deliver the ultimate and objective scientific evidence about the mechanisms underlying mental disorders. Yet neuroscience suffers from many methodological limitations in terms of its validity and clinical utility (Borgwardt et al. 2012, 2013).

To address validation procedures magnetic resonance imaging (MRI) data acquisition parameters need to have demonstrated discriminative power at group or single-subject level. Moreover, MRI modalities have to be available across different MRI scanners, provide good test-retest, inter-subject and cross-scanner reliability. Especially for the case of psychiatric cross-centre imaging studies, where subtle changes in structural and functional brain imaging data sets are searched for, centre effects should not be underestimated and therefore have to be investigated in detail.

By conducting an MRI calibration study, the detection of centre bias effects becomes feasible and computation of voxel-wise intra-class correlation coefficients (ICC) can be used to quantify test-retest reliability. Also, ICC enables to calibrate MRI processing analyses steps while MRI data quality assurance procedures such as phantom measurements to monitor BOLD sensitivity, signal to noise ratio, signal to fluctuation noise ratio help to ensure reliability and assess scanner quality drifts. Psychopathology is the discipline supposed to occupy the very borderline area in-between psychology and neuroscience.

It is operating with *hybrid objects, called 'phenomena'* (Berrios 2008), which combine on instrumental level yet can be not be essentially identified in any of aforementioned conventional operational languages. Over the past decades after DSM III-R (1973) psychopathology has been operationalized with structured descriptive assessment tools like SCID, PANSS (for psychoses), MADRS (for depression) etc. Those standardized tools are derived also from narratives, however *professional*, i.e., including physician's observation record besides patient's responses to the items of the interview.

From epistemological point of view there is no substantial difference in terms of their cognitive content between clinical observation rating and self-assessment scales. This leads to certain *epistemic nonsense* in the era after DSM IV: current dimensional rating scale (like MMPI) is validated backwards to a structured clinical interview (SCID) which is validated forward to a similar if not the same clinical rating scale.

2.2. Meta-Language

Meta-language (Berrios 2009) is regarded to be methodological tool to integrate the divergent disciplinary languages, involved in psychiatry. To this end its construction is far out of reach.

The fundamental problem which exists before this integration is known as '*explanatory gap'* or Neo-Kantian dichotomy. It is defined as incommensurability of the nomothetic (explanatory) and ideographic (understanding) disciplinary languages (Broome 2008).

In pragmatic terms this means that the construct of 'depression' in clinical psychology, in psychopathology and in neuroscience is defined and measured in diverse and incompatible ways. All of them are equally estranged from the most significant and meaningful source of human subjectivity rooted back in phenomenological psychopathology.

There arise two conceptual worries in this sense. Firstly according to Nancy Andreasen (2007) the DSM and the relevant approach of 'quantitative' clinical evaluation caused the '*death of phenomenology*' and is one severe obstacle before genuine understanding of mental disorder as complex and qualitative experience.

Second, as it has already been noted in the preceding section, modern conventional classification of mental disorders in the relevant chapters of DSM and ICD have abandoned any explanatory background and thus tend to be mere observational constructs. The latter is in dissonance with the overall rationale of the medical taxonomy which is supposed to be essentially based on explanatory models of disease.

The above issues should be managed on both epistemological and empirical level.

3. Translational Validation As Epistemic Mediator between Phenomenological Psychiatry and Neuroscience

It has already been stated clinical and neurobiological measures are considered valid for different reasons inside their own divergent domains (disciplinary matrixes). All disciplines concerned with mental health establish virtually internal or *intra-correlative validity*, i.e., psychological measures are validated with other psychological measures, and neurobiological measures are validated with other neurobiological tests.

What is still missing is the *inter-correlative* or *inter-disciplinary validity* to connect neurobiology with phenomenological psychiatry and clinical psychology. Since there are involved not two but three domains of knowledge we would rather prefer the term '*trans-disciplinary*' which refers to the issue of translation.

Contemporary clinical assessment tools have borrowed over the past century "extracts" or "excerpts", artificially quantified fragments from phenomenological explorations to formulate their items. However the validity claim of the constructs, criteria, item selection is sustained exclusively inside the domain of quantitative clinical assessment. There hasn't been developed feedback link from structured clinical assessment to the original source of phenomenological psychopathology. This is why this connection is demonstrated with one way curve from phenomenology to clinical assessment on Figure 2. Besides this curve bypasses neuroscience which contributes to the poor evidence strength of the currently employed rating scales.

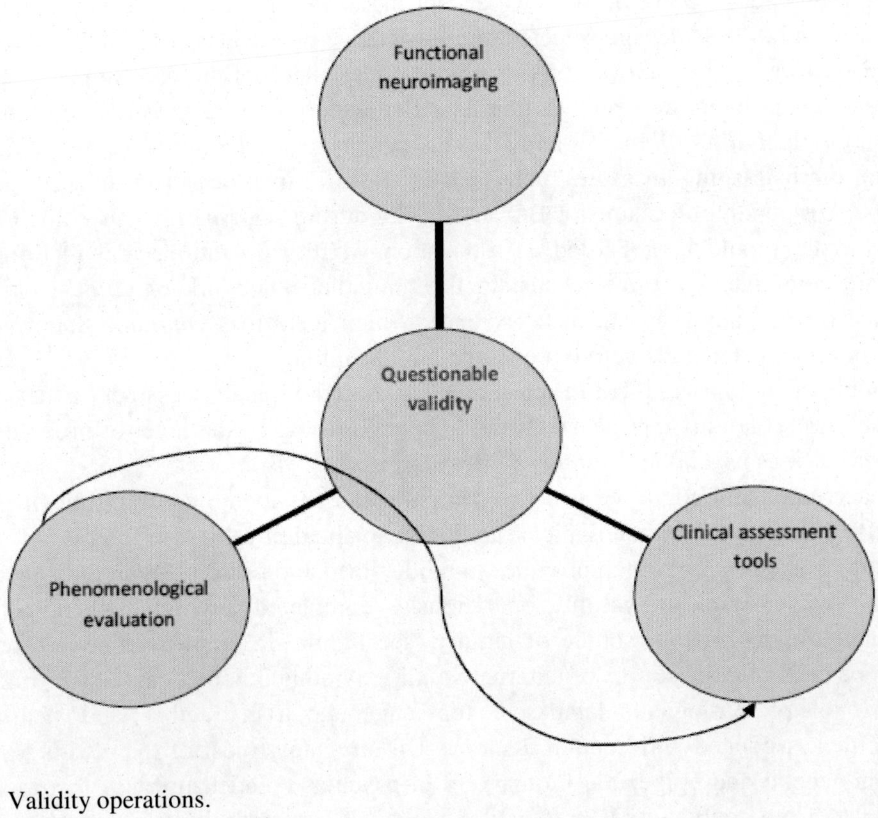

Figure 2. Validity operations.

T Neuroscience, functional brain imaging in particular remains discrete from the entire configuration of both qualitative and quantitative clinical evaluation due to lack of established convergent validity operations which may translate the neuroimaging evidence into clinical practice. This may be the explanation why the post hoc correlations between the two kinds of measures are found often to be inconsistent and contradictory.

Essentially the mediation between these domains should exist at the level of translation, similarly to disciplines in other field of human knowledge. As it has been exemplified elsewhere the literature and historical narrative is mediated through excavation archaeology facts; the judicial testimony is mediated through physical evidence and so forth.

However due to the lack of mutual understanding this is not the case in modern neuropsychiatry. To overcome this situation of epistemic discontinuity we have proposed the model of trans-disciplinary or translational validation. In our model phenomenological perspective is regarded as superstructure to a more robust nomothetic network, comprised from the terminology and methods of quantitative clinical psychology and functional brain imaging. In this configuration the items of the clinical rating scales are regarded as translation validity operations. This means that we investigate the real time correspondence of the self-assessment clinical measures (e.g., depression severity scores) and the measurement of brain activity during item response. The single item responses are then merged into overall BOLD activation in regions of interest to correlate with the total score. If the two values correspond to each other we take it as a convergent validity.

As it has been analyzed in previous publications rating scales (Stoyanov et al. 2012) may be constructed in either deductive (intuitive), or inductive or external (empirical) way.

From a procedural point of view we accept the *externalist* approach where the items of self-assessment rating scales are selected and formulated on the basis of non-structured, open-ended interviews, which allow comprehensive assessment of human subjectivity. Those phenomenological interviews provide the narrative excerpts to be incorporated into clinical assessment tools. Further both trait and state dependent scales should be cross-validated with functional brain imaging measure such as BOLD fMRI in order to establish translational validity. Corresponding measures of BOLD activity during scale performance and total score on rating scale should be regarded as translation validity operations and therefore as bi-conditional cognitive structures to sustain the nomothetic network of clinical psychology, descriptive psychopathology and neuroscience, which in turn is *condition sine qua non* to meet the normative demands before mental health disciplines.

It should be emphasized that in our model structured clinical assessment is designated to serve solely as screening approach to provide boundaries up to the level of broad diagnostic prototypes, such as psychotic disorder, depression, anxiety disorder etc.

The correspondent cognitive structures in clinical assessment and brain imaging are then validated forward to phenomenological qualitative evaluation as super-structure of the entire clinical diagnostic process which provides individualized and person centered diagnosis.

In this way a circle of validity operations is completed, involving phenomenological psychopathology as primary source of inquiry (see Figure 3). Neuroscience is taken in our model to be one potential source of external validity. Among others it can deliver information from two major biological databases: (epi-) genetic risk factors and neuroimaging abnormalities associated with mental disorder. Unfortunately most of the efforts to discover behavioral-genetic and epigenetic biomarkers in psychiatry ended up with inconsistent and unstable data from genome-wide association studies of susceptibility to schizophrenia and/or bipolar disorder, which can hardly underpin any translational validity (Yosifova 2009, Betcheva 2013). One critical consideration against the implications of genetic markers in psychiatric diagnosis is their '*state independence*'. The latter has been defined by protagonists of biological psychiatry (Hasler et al. 2006) as an advantage of the endophenotype strategy. Whilst it may be true assumption for some retest stable mental phenomena such as the traits in the psycho-biological model of personality (Cloninger et al. 1993) it is less relevant for clinical states like bipolar depression which are in fact determined by instability of emotional regulation.

In those cases 'state independence' would rather be a shortcoming then an advantage. On the contrary we argue that 'state dependence' should be rendered as an alternative and sounder approach to translation of the neurobiological mechanisms of mental disorders into clinical reality. We should take into consideration that structural and functional neuroimaging as potential external validator is also exposed to queries about their validity and clinical utility (Borgwardt 2012, Stoyanov 2013).

5. Functional Neuroimaging: Critical Reappraisal

This section is intended to present the advantages and methodological limitations of neuroimaging as translation validity operation.

Functional brain imaging methods such as fMRI, which allow the in vivo investigation of human brain function, have been increasingly employed to examine the neurophysiological substrate of cognitive processes and psychopathological features. As the signals of the human brain functions are universal in objective reality, fMRI studies that explore the neural substrates of psychopathology theoretically no longer rely on subjective measures, resulting in numerous publications of fMRI studies employing task and non-task related paradigms. However, despite the growing literature, the neural networks underlying the different psychopathological features are not clarified. Despite the impressive growth of functional and structural neuroimaging studies, neuroimaging has yet to become an established as diagnostic, let alone prognostic, instrument this area, partly as a result of significant heterogeneity across the findings from research studies. Interestingly, no consistent or reliable functional brain alterations have been univocally associated with any mental disorder and no clinical applications have been developed in psychiatric neuroimaging. Apart from exclusion of disorders due to another medical/neurological conditions (e.g., brain tumor) there is a gap between the use of psychiatric neuroimaging research and its translational relevance.

Methodological factors may account for the considerable heterogeneity in findings across fMRI studies. These factors include differences in relevant acquisition design, lack of statistical power due to small sample sizes, different methods of image analysis (i.e., parametric versus non-parametric), differences in the demographic and sociodemographic group characteristics, and confounding effects of medication or illness chronicity.

Analysis of the consistency and comparability of the results obtained using different fMRI acquisition and analysis methods on the same set of neuroimaging data is a crucial prerequisite for accurate localization of various brain functions. To reliably apply fMRI in clinical settings, stable and consistent results irrespective of particular image acquisition and analysis methods used are needed.

A number of methodological problems may underlie the inconsistencies across studies and the difficulty of identifying reliable results. Heterogeneity in psychiatric neuroimaging originates from multiple differences across studies: in conceptual issues underlying psychiatric diagnoses and psychopathology (Stoyanov et al. 2013), the clinical characteristics of psychiatric samples; the use of different paradigms and designs, and the use of different forms of image acquisition and image analysis. Because of multiple comparisons across different brain regions, reporting of region of interests (ROIs) can be guided by post-hoc significance of the results, with the whole brain results remaining unpublished (Fusar Poli and Broome 2006, Fusar Poli et al. 2009). These problems limit the *localization* of the potential brain abnormalities, which should be based on a *whole-brain* analysis of the differences between patients and controls. However, voxel-based meta-analyses have the potential to overcome the limited sample size of individual studies revealing functional abnormalities at specific brain coordinates rather than differences in volumes of pre-specified ROIs. A recent meta-analytic method, Signed Differential Mapping (Radua et al. 2010 2011), allows also for the consideration of null findings and mitigates the excessive influence of single study data sets.

In this context it has been suggested that imaging data contain information for predicting progression across different psychiatric disease stages. Multivariate pattern recognition methods as support vector machines (SVM) are able to categorize individual brain scans by separation of images from different groups taking into account the inter-regional dependencies of different pathologies. SVMs use information from all voxels to reflect differences between groups in order to create models that allow predictions of clinical outcomes in individual patients' i.e, prediction of subsequent conversion to psychosis with an accuracy of 82% (Radua et al. 2011).

In much of this neuroimaging field research, there is the implicit assumption that structural abnormalities are linked to functional abnormalities in the brain regions found so affected, or the functional circuits in which they take part. However, this is not necessarily the case since volumetric changes can occur without clear functional correlates, for example as a consequence of nutritional or hydration status or other confounds (23). To arrive at a reliable account for clinical applicability, it is therefore important to know which brain regions, show conjoint structural and functional abnormalities. In this context, voxel-based meta-analytical methods to *multimodally* examine (Radua et al. 2012) the relationship between structural and functional brain abnormalities were recently developed. This method may be useful to sustain multimodal imaging applications in broad fields of clinical psychiatry.

By overcoming some of the discussed issues, the results of psychiatric neuroimaging can become more reliable and have a translational impact on clinical practice. The following overview aims to provide practical guidelines to conduct or evaluate functional neuroimaging studies and ultimately help to improve reliability of psychiatric neuroimaging (Borgwardt 2012):

1. With an increasing number of ways of preprocessing the data becoming available;
2. ROIs studies (employing preselected masks or adopting Small Volume Corrections) should first report standard whole brain results and acknowledge if no significant clusters were detected at whole brain level before presenting the ROI findings;

3. Both ROIs and whole brain studies should first report the results significant at $p < 0.05$ corrected for multiple comparisons (i.e., FWE, FDR, Montecarlo) and then employ more liberal thresholds;
4. When several ROIs are used, correction for multiple comparisons should be based on a mask which includes all of them rather than considering each ROI separately;
5. Authors should be encouraged to blind the statistical analyses of the imaging datasets to avoid ROIs analyses be built post-hoc on the basis of the results;
6. All studies should report a statistical analysis modelling and agreed set of possible confounding variables; these could include, for instance, gender, age and handedness. In addition, studies would have the option of reporting further statistical analyses modelling additional study-specific confounding variables;
7. All studies should acknowledge the number of analyses or brain correlations performed, giving a clear rationale for each, to avoid conducting exploratory analyses and reporting the most significant result;
8. The potential overlapping of the patient and control group with previously published studies should be clearly acknowledged, and the spatial coordinates always reported, to assist future voxel-based meta-analyses in the field;
9. Peer-reviews should be as strict when assessing the methods of a study reporting abnormalities in expected brain regions, as when assessing the methods of a study not finding any expectable finding;
10. Acceptance or rejection of a manuscript should not depend on whether abnormalities are detected or not, or on the specific brain regions found to be abnormal.

To summarize fMRI may be considered in our perspective as translation validation tool because of the following reasons (Stoyanov et al. 2014):

- fMRI can capture very close to real time brain response to psychological stimuli of diagnostic significance (as compared to other imaging techniques);
- It can penetrate into the substrate of mental function - the oxygen metabolism of neurons
- Modern upgrades in fMRI designs facilitate multimodal imaging which can integrate further modalities like receptor expression and qEEG, the latter can substantially contribute to time resolution.

On the other hand we have identified so far several major shortcomings which seem to undermine the data translation from neuroimaging to psychiatry:

1. The psychological stimuli (such as emotional pictures processing) given during functional brain scans are specifically designed in the paradigm of neuroimaging and therefore have no relevance to the diagnosis in clinical psychiatry
2. Clinical assessment tools, both observational and self-assessment (such as MADRS, HAM-D) are given outside the brain scan procedure and are thus discrepant from the imaging findings. This argument concerns bipolar depression in first place since one of the cardinal features of bipolar disorder is the instability of the circadian rhythm of emotions.

3. Statistical correlations between neuroimaging measures and clinical assessment are performed *post-hoc*; are very often unstable (not replicated) in larger cohorts and have no validation objective. In this way no validity connections are traced across the explanatory and phenomenological knowledge in psychiatry.

Those shortcomings however can be managed with some modifications in the experimental paradigm, in particular with (i) simultaneous and (ii) *full length* administration of clinical measures with functional neuroimaging (see previous section). Should the two measures correspond they are regarded as convergent translational validity operations (Stoyanov at al. 2014).

The explicit objective of such protocol is aiming at cross-validation as complementary approach for the establishment of bi-conditional rules for translation of the data of neuroscience to psychopathology.

Those rules or '*manual for translation*' may provide synergistic explanation for the mechanism of production of the disorder and facilitate the inter-domain dialogue.

CONCLUSION

Neuroimaging methods may help to understand the pathogenesis of brain changes to clarify the onset and dynamic neurobiological processes underlying psychiatric disorders. However, for neuroimaging to be a clinically reliable tool, a methodological frame shift is necessary to link basic research and clinical assessment for people with psychiatric disorders.

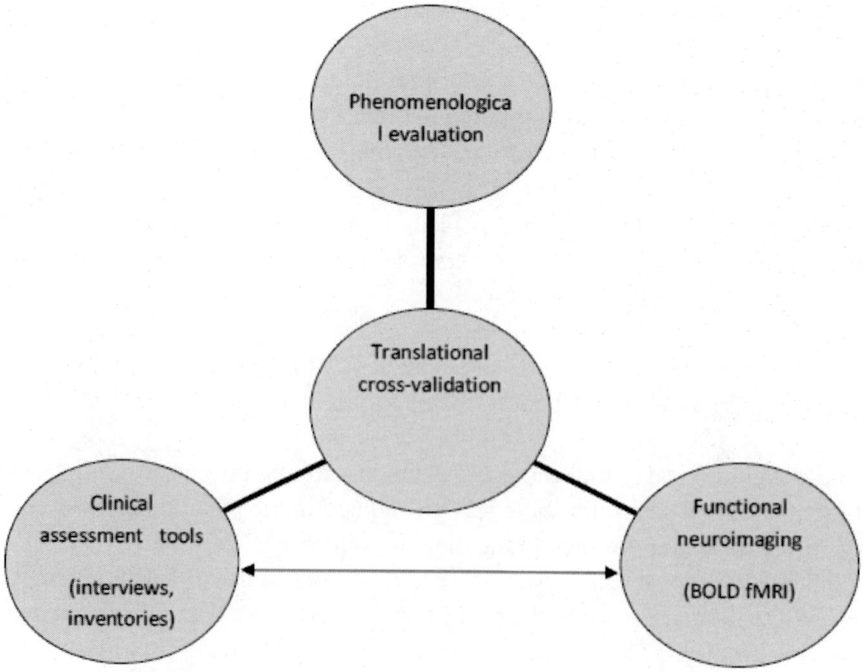

Figure 3. Validity operations revisited.

For state independent personality traits such as temper and character traits in the diagnosis of personality disorders, much progress has been achieved in relating functional imaging, genetic and psychological measures over the past decades especially in the psychobiological paradigm of C. Robert Cloninger.

Yet, the state dependent diagnostic methods still need to be revised under similar paradigms. Translational cross-validation provides a methodological toolkit to facilitate this revision, which may eventually change the configuration of mental health disciplines and thereby integrate phenomenological psychopathology, clinical psychology and neuroscience (Figure 3).

REFERENCES

Ambrosini, A. and Giovanni Stanghellini, The Concepts of 'Depressive Pathogenetic Situation' and 'Melancholic Type of Personality' as applied in the Case of Postpartum Depression, In: Stoyanov, D. ed. *Psychopathology: theory, perspectives and future approaches*. New York, NY Nova Science Publishers; 2013: 23-50.

Andreasen, N. C. DSM and the death of phenomenology in America: an example of unintended consequences. *Schizophrenia bulletin*. 2007; 33(1), 108-112.

Baumann, U., Eckmann, F. and Stieglitz, R.-D. Self-rating data as selecting factor in clinical trials of psychotropic drugs. *European Archive of Psychiatry and Neurological Science*. 1985; 235: 65-70.

Berrios, G. E. 'Mind in general'by Sir Alexander Crichton. *History of Psychiatry*. 2006; 17 (4), 469-486.

Betcheva, E., A. G. Yosifova, T. Mushiroda, M. Kubo, A. Takahashi, S. K. Karachanak, I. T. Zaharieva, S. P. Hadjidekova, I., I. Dimova, R. V. Vazharova, D. S. Stoyanov, V. K. Milanova, T. Tolev, G. Kirov, N. Kamatani, D. I. Toncheva, and Y. Nakamura. (2013). Whole genome association study in Bulgarian population reveals HHAT as schizophrenia susceptibility gene, *Psychiatric genetics*. 2013; 23(1): 11-19.

Borgwardt, S., Radua, J., Mechelli, A., and Fusar-Poli, P. Why are psychiatric imaging methods clinically unreliable? Conclusions and practical guidelines for authors, editors and reviewers. *Behav. Brain Funct*. 2012; 8(1): 46.

Broome, M. R. Philosophy as the science of value: neo-kantianism as a guide to psychiatric interviewing. *Philosophy, Psychiatry, and Psychology*. 2008; 15(2), 107-116.

Cloninger, C. R., Svrakic, D. M. and Przybeck, T. R. A psychobiological model of temperament and character. *Archives of general psychiatry*. 1993; 50(12), 975.

Fusar-Poli, P., Borgwardt, S., Valmaggia, L. Heterogeneity in the assessment of the at-risk mental state for psychosis. *Psychiatr. Serv*. 2008 Jul; 59(7): 813.

Fusar-Poli, P., Broome, M., Barale, F., Stanghellini, G. Why is psychiatric imaging clinically unreliable? Epistemological perspectives in clinical neuroscience, *Psychother. Psychosom*. 2009;78(5):320-1.

Fusar-Poli, P. and Broome, M. R. Conceptual issues in psychiatric neuroimaging. *Current Opinion in Psychiatry*. 2006; 19(6), 608-612.

Hasler, G., Drevets, W. C., Gould, T. D., Gottesman, I. I., and Manji, H. K. Toward constructing an endophenotype strategy for bipolar disorders. *Biological psychiatry*. 2006; 60(2), 93-105.

Ioannidis, J. P. Excess significance bias in the literature on brain volume abnormalities. *Arch. Gen. Psychiatry*. 2011; 68(8) 773-780.

Korf, J. and Gramsbergen, J. B. Timing of potential and metabolic brain energy. *Journal of neurochemistry*. 2007; 103(5): 1697-1708.

Koutsouleris, N., Borgwardt, S., Meisenzahl, E. M., Bottlender, R., Möller, H J., Riecher-Rössler, A. Disease prediction in the at-risk mental state for psychosis using neuroanatomical biomarkers: results from the FePsy study. *Schizophr. Bull.* 2012 Nov;38 (6):1234-46.

Marková, I. S. and Berrios, G. E. Epistemology of mental symptoms. *Psychopathology*. 2009; 42(6), 343-349.

Radua, J., Borgwardt, S., Crescini, A., Mataix-Cols, D., Meyer-Lindenberg, A., McGuire, P. K., Fusar-Poli, P., Multimodal meta-analysis of structural and functional brain changes in first episode psychosis and the effects of antipsychotic medication. *Neurosci. Biobehav. Rev.* 2012 Nov;36(10): 2325-33.

Radua, J., Mataix-Cols, D., Phillips, M. L., El-Hage, W., Kronhaus, D. M., Cardoner, N., Surguladze, S. A new meta-analytic method for neuroimaging studies that combines reported peak coordinates and statistical parametric maps. 2011; *Eur. Psychiatry*: Accessed online June 7.

Radua, J., van den Heuvel, O. A., Surguladze, S., Mataix-Cols, D. Meta-analytical comparison of voxel-based morphometry studies in obsessive-compulsive disorder vs. other anxiety disorders. *Arch. Gen. Psychiatry*. 2010; 67(7) 701-711.

Stojanov, D., Korf, J., de Jonge, P., and Popov, G. The possibility of evidence-based psychiatry: depression as a case. *Clinical epigenetics*. 2011; 2(1): 7-15.

Stoyanov, D., Borgwardt, S. J., Varga, S. The problem of translational validity across neuroscience and psychiatry. In: Zachar, P., Stoyanov, D., Aragona, M., Jablensky, A., eds. *Alternative perspectives of psychiatric validation*, Oxford: Oxford University Press; 2014:128-146.

Stoyanov, D., P. Machamer and K. Schaffner, A Fallacious forced choice: Cloninger and SMS are compatible, *Philosophy, Psychiatry and Psychology*, 2013: 261-273.

Stoyanov, D., P. Machamer and K. Schaffner, In Quest for Scientific Psychiatry: Towards Bridging the Explanatory Gap. *Philosophy, Psychiatry and Psychology*, 2013: 281-284.

Stoyanov, D., G. Stanghellini, M. Broome. Conceptual issues in psychiatric neuroimaging, *Current topics in medicinal chemistry*. 2012; 12(21): 2348-2356.

Stoyanov, D., Machamer, P. K. and Schaffner, K. F. Rendering clinical psychology an evidence-based scientific discipline: a case study. *Journal of Evaluation in Clinical Practice*, 2012; 18:149–154.

Weinberger, D. R., McClure, R. K. Neurotoxicity, neuroplasticity, and magnetic resonance imaging morphometry: what is happening in the schizophrenic brain? *Arch. Gen. Psychiatry*. 2002 Jun;59(6):553-8.

Yosifova, A., Mushiroda, T., Stoianov, D., Vazharova, R., Dimova, I., Karachanak, S., ... and Nakamura, Y. Case-control association study of 65 candidate genes revealed a possible association of a SNP of HTR5A to be a factor susceptible to bipolar disease in Bulgarian population. *Journal of affective disorders*. 2009; 117(1), 87-97.

In: New Developments in Clinical Psychology Research
Editors: D. St. Stoyanov and R.-D. Stieglitz
ISBN: 978-1-63483-223-6

Chapter 9

CLINICAL PSYCHOLOGY AND SPIRITUALITY

G. Gragnano[1], C. M. Bosma[2] and F. Pagnini[*,1,2,3]
[1]Department of Psychology, Catholic University of Milan, Italy
[2]Department of Psychology, Harvard University, Cambridge, MA, US
[3]Azienda Ospedaliera Niguarda Ca' Granda, Milan, Italy

ABSTRACT

Spirituality can be defined as the search for the sacred or divine through any life experience. Not to be confused with "religiousness," which implies a multifaceted concept including ethical and moral rules. Nevertheless, these two are not mutually exclusive concepts.

People who report to have spiritual and religious experiences during their lives are increasing, leading to a scene where spiritual and physical health are becoming almost equally important in defining the self (Mueller et al., 2001). Hence, spiritual needs during illness should not be underestimated when evaluating patients' quality of life: it has been demonstrated how religious involvement and spirituality are associated with better health outcomes (e.g., greater longevity, coping skills, together with less anxiety, depression, and suicide). These resources showed to have a crucial role among some disease-specific populations. For example, spiritual well-being was found to be related to the ability of enjoying life in oncology patients and HIV-positive patients. Furthermore, spirituality may influence health-related quality of life and subjective well-being, even during terminal and incurable diseases.

Nowadays, the well-known medical model – which focuses its aim on medicine, giving less importance to personal beliefs and faith – is viewed as too reductionist and mechanistic. Many scholars consider the medical model to not be comprehensive enough, as it generally does not address psychological well-being, such as spirituality, especially in terminal and incurable diseases. Among those patients, spiritual suffering is frequently ignored or dismissed, because of the difficulties in recognizing it (e.g., hopelessness and sense of meaninglessness might lead to a diagnosis of depression). Even in end-of-life situations, every patient often desires to give his life a meaning, making it possible to afford a peaceful death. Therefore, it is important to give more consideration to spiritual well-being in clinical interventions and palliative care.

What Does "Spirituality" Mean?

Just as it often happens when dealing with topics related to human experiences, to date, there is no consensus in finding an answer to the question: what does "spirituality" mean? The National Institute for Healthcare Research defines spirituality as "the search for the sacred or divine through any life experience" (1997). Spirituality is related to the spirit or soul as opposed to material or physical things. Another definition for a so-called "spiritual" person is someone who attempts to find meaning, purpose, and hope in relation to dimensions such as religion, philosophy, or even personal experience (Bussing et al. 2014).

Because of its nature i.e., searching for transcendent meaning, spirituality may be confused with "religiousness". Nevertheless, religion and spirituality are two different concepts: spirituality refers to an individual's or a group's relationship with the transcendent (Sulmasy 2002). Spirituality is often free of rules, regulations, and responsibilities (Nicastri 2014). For example, people can express their spirituality through arts, nature, philosophy, or in relationships (Sulmasy 2002).

On the other hand, religiousness implies a multifaceted concept including ethical and moral rules (Pagnini 2013). It is true that these concepts are not mutually exclusive (Pagnini et al. 2014), since most people express their spirituality in religious practice (Sulmasy 2002). Spirituality is, undoubtedly, a necessary part of religiousness, but one can be spiritual and not religious (Nicastri 2014). In other words, the car is not the road (Pagnini and Phillips 2015).

Aldwin and colleagues (2014) reviewed the literature on religiousness and spirituality with the aim of testing the different effects of the two concepts separately. Religiousness appeared to be associated with more prevalent healthy behavior habits (e.g., lower smoking and alcohol consumption and greater likelihood of medical screenings), but it was only weakly related to the attenuation of inflammatory processes underlying chronic illnesses.

Further, measures of spirituality were more strongly associated with better blood pressure, cardiac reactivity, immune factors, and attenuated disease progression (Aldwin et al. 2014). Human beings' existence is sometimes described as divided into two different realms: the outer, consisting of interactions with the world, and the inner, characterized by one's relationship with the transcendental (D'Souza 2007).

An interesting hypothesis by Shafrankse and Gorsuch assumed how, even among humanistic sciences, there is a substantial lack of connections between psychology and spirituality. Such a gap may be caused by the urgency by the field of psychology to dissociate itself from philosophy, aspiring to a personal and exclusive identity (Shafrankse and Gorsuch 1984).

To date, there is a growing desire from patients that spirituality should be addressed as an aspect of their care (Cook 2015). Attention in regard to the role of spirituality in determining quality of life is currently growing, especially in psychiatric practice (Cook 2015), together with the development of studies investigating how spirituality may alleviate burden and other issues in a condition of severe disease.

A dramatic increase in extant literature about the topic suffers from a lack of integrative theoretical models and well-defined constructs (Aldwin et al. 2014).

SPIRITUALITY, QUALITY OF LIFE, AND RESILIENCE

As previously mentioned, spiritual and transcendent habits have been shown to positively influence patients' healthy behavior as well as decision-making regarding healthcare (Bussing et al. 2014). That is to say, spiritual features are undoubtedly a benefit, not exclusively when dealing with an illness, but they are also useful in preventing unhealthy habits and promoting healthy ones. This happens on two different levels. First, in a more individual point of view, spirituality promotes the care of the self in every-day routines (e.g., through awareness, calmness, a healthy diet, a care of the body, etc.). Second, it can also lead to practices like voluntary work and socialization, with benefits for one's quality of life on a social level.

A study by Zullig and colleagues (2006) showed how college students who described themselves as spiritual were more likely to report greater self perceived health, supporting the contention that life satisfaction may be influenced by engagement in religiosity and spirituality (Zullig et al. 2006).

A similar descriptive survey found spirituality to be associated with the subjective perception of health workers' quality of life (Boero et al. 2005). Among the nine focus groups in a study conducted by O'Connell and colleagues (2010), spiritual strength, meaning in life, and inner peace were cited as relevant when assessing general health-related quality of life, whereas divine love, freedom to practice beliefs, and attachment (more related to religious practices) were less relevant. Additionally, coping strategies may be labeled as "spiritual," indicating those strategies which involve relationship with the self, others, a deity, or nature. The use of "spiritual coping strategies," however, is can be interpreted as being strongly related to religiosity, since it is often labeled as "religious coping" (Baldacchino and Draper 2001). Nevertheless, a study by Drutchas and Anandarajah (2014) on children and adolescents affected by chronic diseases (i.e., inflammatory bowel disease, asthma, and sickle cell disease) showed that such coping strategies in children markedly differ from the models seen in adults. Despite considerable interest in examining spirituality in health-related quality of life studies, there is a paucity of instruments that measure this construct (Daaleman et al. 2004). Although spirituality has been seen as irrelevant in the past, or at least difficult to measure, a growing body of articles point to a positive relationship between spiritual beliefs and other domains of quality of life (Pagnini et al. 2015).

Various efforts have been made to measure spirituality, in order to adequate capture its relationship with quality of life. In fact, despite the difficulty of measuring spirituality, several tools for the assessment of spirituality and existential issues exist. The McGill Quality of Life questionnaire, a tool that is widely used with people with terminal diseases, includes a spirituality and existential well-being subscale (Cohen et al. 1995). The Spiritual Well-Being Scale (Paloutzian et al. 1991) is a general indicator of perceived well-being which may be used for the assessment of congregational spiritual well-being (Ellison 2006): its subscales provide both scores for Religious Well-Being (assessing one's relationship with God), and for Existential Well-Being (assessing one's sense of life purpose and life satisfaction). An attempt of developing an index designed to measure the effect of spirituality on subjective well-being comes from Daaleman and Frey (2004), who postulated the Spirituality Index of Well-Being (SIWB). The instrument contains 12 items: 6 from a self-efficacy domain and 6 from a life scheme domain, and reports significant correlations with other quality-of-life instruments that measure well-being or spirituality (Daaleman and Frey 2004).

Spirituality in Facing an Illness

With the diagnosis of a chronic illness, there is a crisis of one's internal peace and sense of self (Drutchas and Anandarajah 2014). It is a crisis which has the ability to de-structure the self, and to modify one's every day life. A severe disease, especially when it entails a physical impairment and/or pain, often brings serious reflections about one's life, about which are the real priorities, about one's own fears, and about death itself.

Therefore, many people can discover their "spiritual features" only during such a difficult phase of the life cycle. During the Middle Ages, there was a strict link between illness and the inner world: every disease was considered as a cause of a sin committed by the suffering person, therefore it was treated with rituals intended to purify the spirit (D' Souza 2007).

Furthermore, ancients understood illness as a disturbance in relationships (Sulmasy 2002). As these people had a keen sense of relationship between human beings and the cosmos, the task of the shaman was to heal by restoring the relationship between the sick person and the cosmos. Thus, Sulmasy (2002) defines healing as a "religious act."

Since then, medical sciences have lost their "spiritual" and "inner" connotation in order to strive for more objectivity (D'Souza 2007). Following this mentality, a physician is not officially obliged to engage with the patient's spirituality, to the patient's hopes and beliefs, since such skills seem to be pertaining only to psychologists.

Objectivity and concreteness undoubtedly help during the diagnosis process and the selection of correct treatments; however, the verb "to cure" must not be confused with "to take care." Cassell, in his work "The Healer's heart," made this concept very clear: "Doctors and clinicians are healers through the caring relationships they form with patients" (Cassell et al. 1985). It has been shown spiritual practices have the power to alleviate, and sometimes even improve quality of life among different kinds of patients.

Among people with cardiovascular disease, greater levels of spiritual well-being, religiousness, and meaning or purpose in life experience greater quality of life and fewer depressive symptoms (Hooker et al. 2014).

This is also seen in families of children with disabilities (Poston and Turnbull 2004). In a qualitative study by Garssen and colleagues (2014), people with cancer mentioned emotion-focused roles of spirituality. More specifically, they felt supported by transcendental confidants, by acceptance, and by viewing problems from a distance.

Simmons and colleagues (2000) have assessed quality of life in patients with ALS: the construct did not correlate with strength or physical function, but it depended on psychological, existential and spiritual factors.

Spirituality represents a good support in a situation of cognitive impairment. A recent review of the literature about quality of life in older adults with dementia showed how the use of spirituality or faith in daily life enabled people to develop coping strategies to help in accepting their disease, maintaining their relationships, maintaining hope, and finding meaning in their lives, thereby improving their quality of life (Mackinlay 2015).

Moreover, it is interesting how such skills not only worked as coping strategies, but also servied as an active buffer towards cognitive disorders, with symptoms tending to reduce or stabilize in people who increasingly engaged in their spirituality or religion. Spirituality may influence health-related quality of life and subjective well-being even during terminal and incurable diseases (Brady et al. 2000; Pagnini, Bosma et al. 2014; Spinelli et al. 2014).

For example, in amyotrophic lateral sclerosis (ALS) patients, spiritual beliefs can provide an useful coping strategy with the merit of improving quality of life (Pagnini et al. 2011), despite the challenges posed by the illness in terms of depression (Pagnini, Manzoni et al., in press) and pain (Pagnini et al. 2012).

According to the work of Sulmasy (2002), in an end-of-life scenario, the focus should be also on the role of spiritual well-being for those who survive their loved, and on how they manage to give meaning to the bereavement. Sulmasy asserts that the end-of-life phase should be worthy of reflections also by clinicians, which can learn something from the spiritual lessons that the dying can teach them. Furthermore, Sulmasy (2012) maintains clinicians need to pay attention to their own spiritual histories and to be conscious of how this affects the care they give their patients.

It must be said that spiritual practice should not replace psychological and psychiatric help, but should instead integrate each other. Such practice cannot necessarily be prescribed, since it would lead to a total distortion of the real meaning of spirituality.

For this reason, a consensus panel of the American College of Physicians has suggested four simple questions that physicians could ask patients: 1.) Is faith important to you?; 2.) Has faith been important to you at other times in your life?; 3.) Do you have someone to talk to about religious matters?; and 4.) Would you like to explore religious, spiritual matters with someone? The last two questions listed above allow the clinician understand if someone's spiritual area is actually accessible.

Spirituality and the Biopsychosocial Model of Health

The Biopsychosocial model by George Engel (1977) asserts that "all three levels, biological, psycological, and social, must be taken into account in every health care task." During the 1950s, a neurologist and psychiatrist named Roy Grinker spread the concept of "biopsychosocial" by applying it to psychiatry to emphasise the "biology" against psychoanalytic orthodoxy (Grinker 1964).

Nevertheless, while Grinker recognized limits in the biopsychosocial approach, Engel claimed it as the best framework for both research and clinical practice in the world of health care (Ghaemi 2009).

The Biopsychosocial model laid out an alternative vision for health care, since it included affective, psychological, and social states of the patient as significant factors for his/her health. It represents a great step towards the understanding that health is actually affected by multiple levels of organization, from the societal to the molecular (Borrell-Carriò et al., 2004; Pagnini, Castelnuovo and Manzoni 2009).

The above framework is harmonious with the idea of spirituality acting as a mediator of quality of life (see Figure 1).

Nevertheless, the Biopsychosocial model does not yet consider spirituality separately from other subjective domains. Sulmasy recommend the so-called Biopsychosocial-Spiritual Model of Care (2002), which allows the consideration a person in his/her totality, including not simply the biological, psychological, and social aspects of the person, but also the spiritual aspects of the whole person as well.

As Froma Walsh et al. suggested (2008), "spirituality involves streams of experience that flow through all aspects of life, from family heritage to personal belief systems, rituals and practices, and shared faith communities." Indeed, her work focused more on a concept of "holistic biopsychosocial-spiritual orientation" rather than a standard "biopsychosocial model." In Walsh's opinion, "spiritual beliefs influence ways of dealing with adversity, the experience of suffering, and the meaning of symptoms, their cause, and their future course. They also influence how people communicate about their pain, their approach toward health and mental health professionals, and their preferred pathways in recovery" (Walsh et al. 2008).

AN EXAMPLE FROM A CLINICAL CASE

Dario is a 45-year-old man from Rome, Italy. He's been diagnosed with ALS in 2013. He has a wife, Carla, a son, Marco, and a daughter, Maria. Dario has always worked as an engineer in the civic sector. His job instilled in him a strong sense of concreteness and productivity, with emphasis on tangible outcomes. In the same way, Dario's personality and disposition have always been characterized by objectivity and calmness. Talking about himself before the diagnosis, Dario highlights how he often did not care about other people (sometimes even his next of kin), about their experience and their needs, saying how he has never paid attention to other's reactions to his own actions. Despite that, he says he has discovered his once-lost faith in God about ten years ago (eight before the diagnosis), but his nature never actually changed in a more sensitive or sociable manner.

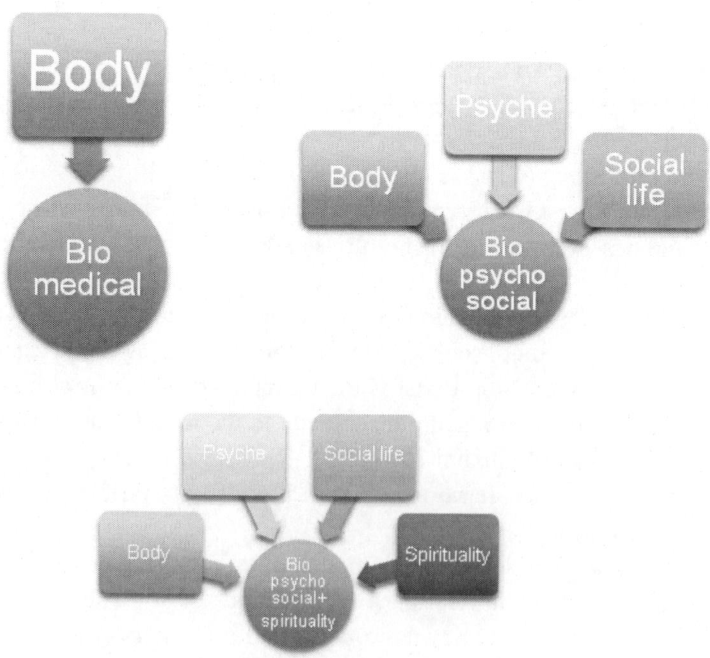

Figure 1. Different models of care.

The disease came into his life wiping out his foundations. Even his job, which had always been a source of certainty, was no longer an anchor.

A long period of crisis, depression and despair followed, in which Dario kept on asking why did it happen to him, and how long would it take to completely lose his faculties? His inability in introspections did not allow him to recognize the variability of his feelings towards the disease, bringing him feelings of distress and despair. His habit was to evaluate and calculate everything in his life, with the will of predicting facts and reactions of the surrounding world. He would report that, "I wasn't able to stay in the present-moment at all." The nature of such a diagnosis brought a lot of uncertainties. In ALS one cannot predict one's prognosis and what manner the progression the disease will take, and even searching for information on the internet may be misleading. As the disease progressed, Dario kept spending more and more time meditating on his existence, unable to continue avoiding the reality of his situation. He began meeting with psychologists.

Meanwhile, he came to recognize his social network as a support system. Not only his children and his wife, but also his friends and colleagues showed him support and encouragement. Such demonstrations of affection instilled in him considerations on how there were sources of joy, satisfaction, and solace, which are not related to his own individual success. This process led to a disinvestment towards those areas more devoted to practical productivity, without losing them completely (e.g., Dario decided to maintain his job as a part-time employee). Helped by faith, by his recovered network of peer support, and by psychotherapy, Dario stopped looking for a reason for his condition. His new will is now to find a reason everyday to push forward, becoming himself the one who relieves others' mood. His questions about "why is this happening to me?" have now been transformed into "what can I do now?" Now even his religious practices are felt as more genuine and meaningful. Dario has learned a lot more about himself, acquiring skills of self-exploration and assigning more value on things other than profit and personal success.

DISCUSSION

> "Helping, fixing, and serving represent three different ways of seeing life. When you help, you see life as weak. When you fix, you see life as broken. When you serve, you see life as whole. Fixing and helping may be the work of the ego, and service the work of the soul".
>
> (Remen, R. N. Kitchen Table Wisdom: Stories That Heal. New York: Riverhead Books; 1997)

Considering spirituality in health care often means to investigate patients' religiosity. This domain must not be underestimated, since religious convictions may affect decision making (Puchalski 2001). It should be the responsibility of the medical team to respect the family's sense of spirituality, helping the family during the delicate process of choosing (e.g., end of life decisions). Apart from decision making issues, patients themselves often want physicians to address their spirituality during an assessment. In the *US Weekend* Faith and Health Poll, 65% of patients felt that it was good for doctors to speak with them about their spiritual beliefs, yet only 10% said a doctor had had such a conversation with them (McNichol 1996).

However, most often, religious and spiritual issues are not discussed in psychotherapy, nor are they included in assessment or treatment planning (Vieten et al. 2013). One solution could be additional training for psychotherapists. As Vieten and colleagues suggest, "the field of psychology has already included religion and spirituality in most definitions of multiculturalism and requires training in multicultural competence, but most psychotherapists receive little or no training in religious and spiritual issues, in part because no agreed-on set of spiritual competencies or training guidelines exist" (Vieten et al. 2013).

Furthermore, we must not forget how, even within psychological practice, spiritual and religious matters are often seen under heterogeneous (and -sometimes- opposing) point of views. This is caused by substantial differences and gaps among theoretical frames in psychology. For instance, while existential-humanistic therapists regard religion as an important factor in the growth of personality and self-actualization, cognitive behavioral psychotherapists often define religion as a "cognitive error". Implicit in this statement is the stance of cognitivists that they do not consider religion as a conducive source for mental health (Hague 2000). Even Albert Ellis, a prominent cognitive psychologist, suggests that religious beliefs incorporate the concepts of sin and guilt, and are thus pathological for patients (Ellis himself later clarified his position, explaining that this idea was relevant only for devoutly religious people) (Hague 2000). Moving towards a completely different point of view, classical psychoanalysts did not recognize the importance of religion and spirituality, though with Jungians generally being an exception (Hague 2000). The acknowledgement of existential issues could also reduce the risk of a mindless diagnosis (Khoury, Langer, and Pagnini 2014). The attention on patients' spirituality lies in a framework in which care is declined in "compassionate care", where compassion is "more than just a natural response to suffering, rather that it is a moral choice" (Dietze et al. 2001).

What is the change clinicians are asked to pursue in their practice? What is involved in serving patients and providing compassionate care? Christina Puchalski (2001) in her study about the role of spirituality in health care, seeks to find an answer to those questions. Compassionate care needs listening and attention to the other person. That includes paying attention to the words and the sounds, but also to the body language. It means paying attention to the patient's needs, including those that are from the spiritual domain.

Lastly, it is proper to evaluate and contemplate even the "other side" of such phenomena. Puchalski describes a useful example of circumstances in which spiritual stances can lead to negative coping (2001). Patients may see a crisis (e.g., a disease) as a punishment from God, or may not resolve their anger when a cure does not occur after prayers. In relation to this, it is necessary to get back again to the distinction between "religious" and "spiritual", since the latter implies the act of acceptance and non-judgement more than devotion to an entity or a religious community.

Conclusion

To conciliate Middle Ages – where the link between the illness and the inner world was strict, where disturbances in relationships were considered as main causes of a disease (Sulmasy 2002) – with the heritage of ages of scientific progress may seem unrealistic, though ancients' thought should give clinicians a different and more spiritual point of view when dealing with patients. Skills such as being fully present, empathic, interested in one's spiritual history should distinguish clinicians who want to promote compassionate care. Such skills should go beyond any theoretical framework in clinical practice, since their effectiveness when dealing with severe disease is clear. Furthermore, those issues should pertain not only psychologists, but every member of a multidisciplinary care team.

It is important also for clinicians and physicians to distinguish spirituality from religiosity, knowing how the former may mean something more personal, inner, while the latter may bring also meanings related to devotion and social community.

To share the importance of spiritual issues in the process of healing is necessary to find the best way to evaluate their influences on patients' health and quality of life. Unfortunately, the substantial lack of instruments leads to the consequent lack of theoretical models and studies on the topic. What is essential for future growth in this area is the implementation of instruments (e.g., robust subscales of Quality of Life tools) which assess spiritual domains in patients. Given the development of new assessment methods, together with new research methodologies, including the attention of these domains could lead to a better understanding of those mechanisms, eventually resulting in in better psychological care.

REFERENCES

Agli, O., Bailly, N. and Ferrand, C. (2014). Spirituality and religion in older adults with dementia: a systematic review. *International Psychogeriatrics / IPA*, 1–11. doi:10.1017/S 1041610214001665.

Aldwin, C. M., Park, C. L., Jeong, Y.-J., and Nath, R. (n.d.). Differing pathways between religiousness, spirituality, and health: A self-regulation perspective.

Baldacchino, D. and Draper, P. (2001). Spiritual coping strategies: a review of the nursing research literature. *Journal of Advanced Nursing*, 34(6), 833–841. doi:10.1046/j.1365-2648.2001.01814.x.

Borrell-Carrió, F., Suchman, A. L. and Epstein, R. M. (2004). The biopsychosocial model 25 years later: principles, practice, and scientific inquiry. *Annals of Family Medicine*, 2(6), 576–82. doi:10.1370/afm.245.

Brunner, E. Promoting Hope and Resilience in Parkinson's Disease, *Master of Social Work Clinical Research Papers (2015)*. Retrieved from http://sophia.stkate.edu/msw_papers/297.

Bufford, R. K., Paloutzian, R. F. and Ellison, C. W. (n.d.). Norms for the Spiritual Well-Being Scale.

Büssing, A., Baumann, K., Hvidt, N. C., Koenig, H. G., Puchalski, C. M., and Swinton, J. (2014). Spirituality and health. *Evidence-Based Complementary and Alternative Medicine: eCAM, 2014*, 682817. doi:10.1155/2014/682817.

Cohen, A. B. and Koenig, H. G. (2003). Religion, religiosity and spirituality in the biopsychosocial model of health and ageing. *Ageing International*, 28(3), 215–241. doi: 10.1007/s12126-002-1005-1.

Cohen, S. R., Mount, B. M., Strobel, M. G., and Bui, F. (1995). The McGill Quality of Life Questionnaire: a measure of quality of life appropriate for people with advanced disease.

A preliminary study of validity and acceptability. *Palliative Medicine*, 9(3), 207–219. doi:10.1177/026921639500900306.

Daaleman, T. P. (2004). The Spirituality Index of Well-Being: A New Instrument for Health-Related Quality-of-Life Research. *The Annals of Family Medicine*, 2(5), 499–503. doi: 10.1370/afm.89.

Ellison, L. *The Spiritual Well-Being Scale, Counseling Faculty Research* (2006). Retrieved from http://mds.marshall.edu/co_faculty/9.

Engel, G. L. (1977). The need for a new medical model: a challenge for biomedicine. *Science (New York, N.Y.)*, 196(4286), 129–36. Retrieved from http://www.ncbi.nlm.nih.gov/pubmed/847460.

Garssen, B., Uwland-Sikkema, N. F. and Visser, A. (2014). How Spirituality Helps Cancer Patients with the Adjustment to their Disease. *Journal of Religion and Health*. doi:10.1007/s10943-014-9864-9.

Ghaemi, S. N. (2009). The rise and fall of the biopsychosocial model. *The British Journal of Psychiatry: The Journal of Mental Science*, 195(1), 3–4. doi:10.1192/bjp.bp.109.063859.

Grinker Sr, R. R. (1964). A struggle for eclecticism. *American Journal of Psychiatry*, 121(5), 451-457.

Khoury, B., Langer, E. J., & Pagnini, F. (2014). The DSM: Mindful Science or Mindless Power? *Frontiers in Psychology*, *5*, 602. doi: 10.3389/fpsyg.2014.00602.

Koenig, H. G. (2000). Religion, Spirituality, and Medicine: Application to Clinical Practice. *JAMA*, 284(13), 1708. doi:10.1001/jama.284.13.1708-JMS1004-5-1.

Lo, B., Quill, T. and Tulsky, J. (1999). Discussing Palliative Care with Patients. *Annals of Internal Medicine*, 130(9), 744. doi:10.7326/0003-4819-130-9-199905040-00015.

Mackinlay, E. (2015). Spirituality and religion in older adults: building knowledge in an emerging discipline. *International Psychogeriatrics*, 1–3. doi:10.1017/S 104161 0214002762.

More Than 9 in 10 Americans Continue to Believe in God. (n.d.). Retrieved January 19, 2015, from http://www.gallup.com/poll/147887/americans-continue-believe-god.aspx.

O'Connell, K. A. and Skevington, S. M. (2005). The relevance of spirituality, religion and personal beliefs to health-related quality of life: themes from focus groups in Britain. *British Journal of Health Psychology*, 10(Pt 3), 379–98. doi:10.1348/135910705X25471.

O'Connell, K. A. and Skevington, S. M. (2007). To measure or not to measure? Reviewing the assessment of spirituality and religion in health-related quality of life. *Chronic Illness*, 3(1), 77–87. doi:10.1177/1742395307079195.

Pagnini, F., Castelnuovo, G. and Manzoni, G. M. (2009). Towards an emotion-based medicine? *JAMA – The Journal of the American Medical Association*, 301(6), 600-601.

Pagnini, F., Lunetta, C., Banfi, P., Rossi, G., Fossati, F., Marconi, A., Castelnuovo, G., Corbo, M., and Molinari, E. (2012). Pain in Amyotrophic Lateral Sclerosis: a psychological perspective. *Neurological Sciences*, 3, 1193-1196.

Pagnini, F. (2013). Psychological well-being and quality of life in Amyotrophic Lateral Sclerosis: a review. *International Journal of Psychology*, 48(3), 194-205.

Pagnini, F., Bosma, C. M., Phillips, D., and Langer, E. (2014). Symptom changes in multiple sclerosis following psychological interventions: a systematic review. *BMC neurology*, 14 (1), 222.

Pagnini, F., Lunetta, C., Rossi, G., Castelnuovo, G., Corbo, M., and Molinari, E. (2011). Existential well-being of individuals with Amyotrophic Lateral Sclerosis is related to psychological well-being of their caregivers. *Amyotrophic Lateral Sclerosis*, 12(2), 105-108.

Pagnini, F., Di Credico, C., Gatto, R., Fabiani, V., Rossi, G., Lunetta, C., ... and Amadei, G. (2014). Meditation Training for People with Amyotrophic Lateral Sclerosis and Their Caregivers. *The Journal of Alternative and Complementary Medicine*, 20(4), 272-275.

Pagnini, F., Manzoni, G. M., Tagliaferri, A., and Gibbons, C. J. (accepted, in press). Depressive disorders in Amyotrophic Lateral Sclerosis: a meta-regression analysis of confounders. *Journal of Health Psychology*. doi: 10.1177/1359105314530453.

Pagnini, F. and Phillips, D. (2015). Being mindful about mindfulness. *The Lancet Psychiatry*, 2(4), 288-289. doi: S2215-0366(15)00041-3.

Pagnini, F., Phillips, D., Bosma, C., Reece, A., and Langer, E. (2015). Mindfulness, Physical Impairment and Psychological Well-Being in People with Amyotrophic Lateral Sclerosis. *Psychology and Health*, 30 (5), 503-517. DOI: 10.1080/08870446.2014.982652.

Poston, D. J. and Turnbull, A. P. (2004). Role of Spirituality and Religion in Family Quality of Life for Families of Children with Disabilities. *Education and Training in Developmental Disabilities*. Retrieved from http://kuscholarworks.ku.edu/handle/1808/6062.

Puchalski, C. M. (2001). The role of spirituality in health care. *Baylor University Medical Center Proceedings*, 14(4): 352-357.

Remen, R. N. (1997). *Kitchen Table Wisdom: Stories That Heal*. New York: Riverhead Books.

Simmons, Z., Bremer, B. A., Robbins, R. A., Walsh, S. M., and Fischer, S. (2000). Quality of life in ALS depends on factors other than strength and physical function. *Neurology*, 55(3), 388–392. doi:10.1212/WNL.55.3.388.

Spinelli, A., Carvello, M., D'Hoore, A., and Pagnini, F. (2014). Psychological Perspectives of Inflammatory Bowel Disease Patients Undergoing Surgery: Rightful Concerns and Preconceptions. *Current drug targets*, 15(11), 1074-1078.

Sulmasy, D. P. (2002). A Biopsychosocial-Spiritual Model for the Care of Patients at the End of Life. *The Gerontologist*, 42(Supplement 3), 24–33. doi:10.1093/geront/42.suppl_3.24.

The Healer's Art da Cassell, E J: Penguin Books, Harmondsworth - Anybook Ltd. (n.d.). Retrieved January 19, 2015, from http://www.abebooks.it/Healers-Art-Cassell-Penguin-Books-Harmondsworth/2756604157/bd.

Vieten, C., Scammell, S., Pilato, R., et al. (2013). Spiritual and religious competencies for psychologists. *Psychology of Religion and Spirituality*, 5(3) 129-144.

Von Dietze, E., Orb, A. (2001). Compassionate care: a moral dimension of nursing. *Nursing Inquiry*. 7(3), 166-174.

Walsh, F. (n.d.). Spirituality, healing, and resilience.

Zullig, K. J., Ward, R. M. and Horn, T. (2006). The Association Between Perceived Spirituality, Religiosity, and Life Satisfaction: The Mediating Role of Self-Rated Health. *Social Indicators Research*, 79(2), 255–274. doi:10.1007/s11205-005-4127-5.

In: New Developments in Clinical Psychology Research
Editors: D. St. Stoyanov and R.-D. Stieglitz
ISBN: 978-1-63483-223-6

Chapter 10

CONTINUING PROFESSIONAL DEVELOPMENT (CPD) PRACTICES AMONG CLINICAL PSYCHOLOGISTS AND SCHOOL PSYCHOLOGISTS

Jennifer M. Taylor[1,*], Greg J. Neimeyer[2] and Eric Rossen[3]
[1]West Virginia University, Morgantown, West Virginia, US
[2]University of Florida, Gainesville, FL, US
[3]National Association of School Psychologists, Bethesda, MD, US

ABSTRACT

A survey of 4130 North American clinical and school psychologists provided information regarding the nature of their participation in continuing professional development (CPD) activities and their perceptions of the outcomes related to those activities. Results revealed that clinical and school psychologists completed, on average, over 20 hours of CPD per year. The most common topics among clinical psychologists were ethics, anxiety disorders, and assessment; similarly, school psychologists most commonly completed CE in ethics, assessment and evaluation, and disorders and disabilities. Many of these CE areas were also nominated as the areas of greatest continuing need. The substantial majority of respondents in both groups reported that their CPD experiences were good or excellent, and most felt that they learned a great deal through their activities that translated into more informed, effective, and ethical service delivery. These results are interpreted in relation to the continuing movement towards developing ongoing professional competencies, and the directions for further research in this area.

* Corresponding author: Jennifer M. Taylor, Department Counseling, Rehabilitation Counseling, and Counseling Psychology, P.O. Box 6122, West Virginia University, Morgantown, WV 26506-6122.

INTRODUCTION

Continuing professional development (CPD) serves as a quality assurance measure that fulfills a range of functions. It is designed to promote lifelong learning, to maintain and enhance professional competencies, to remediate weaknesses or deficits in learning, and to protect the students and families who receive psychological services (Cohen and Dubin 1970; Hogg, Stratford, and Cameron 1989; Taylor and Neimeyer, in press; Taylor and Neimeyer 2015; Wnek, Klein, and Bracken 2008) through the delivery of more effective and ethical services (Neimeyer, Taylor, and Philip 2010). Taken further, engaging in high quality CPD opportunities can increase job satisfaction, mitigate stress and burnout, and increase commitment to the profession (see Armistead and Smallwood 2011). In this regard, many occupations consider CPD as both a requirement for ongoing practice and a professional and ethical responsibility. In this chapter we will explore CPD experiences among both clinical psychologists and school psychologists.

The critical roles that CPD are designed to fulfill are reflected in the mandates that surround it. In the specialty of clinical psychology 44 states plus the District of Columbia require continuing education for re-licensure. CE requirements vary quite drastically from state to state. Some states require as many as 60 formal CE credits over a two-year time span, whereas others require as few as 18 credits per cycle. States also vary with regard to topical requirements. The most common CE topical requirements are in ethics, cultural competence, and domestic violence. States also vary with regard to what qualifies as CPD for the purposes of re-licensure. Aside from formal CE, some states also allow a certain amount of informal, incidental, and non-formal forms of CE (e.g., consultation with colleagues, teaching a new course or workshop, independent reading).

In the specialty of school psychology, the National Association of School Psychologists (NASP) developed and administers the Nationally Certified School Psychologist (NCSP) credential. (For more information on NASP professional development and a list of NASP-approved providers of CPD, visit <http://www.nasponline.org/profdevel/index.aspx>.) In order to maintain this credential, individuals holding the NCSP must complete at least 75 hours of CPD every three years. States also individually set the requirements for the renewal of state credentials, both for independent practice and work within the school setting, which can vary considerably. Previous studies suggest that school psychologists generally meet or exceed the required number of hours, with NASP and non-NASP members showing similar patterns of CPD (Lewis, Truscott, and Vokker 2008). Fowler and Harrison (2001), for example, studied 235 school psychologists nationwide and found that that over one-quarter of them (28%) completed more than 41 hours of CPD per year. Among their sample, attending workshops and institutes, in service trainings, and self-study were the three most common types of CPD activities.

Although CPD programs are presented in many different formats, research suggests that certain learning methods may be more effective than others. Research on the effectiveness of continuing education for psychologists is still in its infancy, but research on the effectiveness of continuing medical education (CME) for physicians dates back several decades. A study of Iranian physicians found that CME is more effective when programs focus on outcome-based education rather than the traditional lecture-style approach to CME (Esmaily et al. 2009).

And just as the research suggests that there are differences in the effectiveness of certain CPD formats, the research also indicates particularly strong demand for CPD in selected topical areas. As one example, professional development in aspects of direct service and interventions, consultation, and to a lesser extent, assessment has ranked highly in relation to the needs of school psychologists (Fowler and Harrison 2001). As noted by Sullivan and Long, several areas pertaining to Response to Intervention (RtI) approaches also were areas of need, such as academic interventions, integrating assessments with intervention, and identifying student processing problems. In addition, Cleary, Gubi, and Prescott (2010) noted that school psychologists working in urban settings expressed greater need in select areas of CPD, such as responding to conduct-related problems, but otherwise showed similarity with the needs of their colleagues practicing in rural settings.

Interestingly, CPD needs in various parts of the world share some similarities. In both Quebec and the United States of America, for example, clinical and counseling psychologists have identified their greatest areas of CE needs in assessments, adult psychopathology, and various interventions (Bradley and Drapeau 2013; Taylor, Neimeyer, and Tate 2015). In the United States, the most frequently reported CE topical needs included anxiety disorders (e.g., OCD, PTSD, panic disorder), ethics, mood disorders (e.g., bipolar or unipolar depression), assessment, couples therapy, evaluation, disorders of children and adolescents (e.g., ADHD), cognitive therapy, trauma, and psychopharmacology (Taylor, Neimeyer, and Tate 2015).

Given the breadth of CPD needs, it is encouraging to find that psychologists tend to engage in lifelong learning and continuing professional development activities that directly relate to their CPD needs (see Neimeyer, Taylor, and Wear 2010). This finding suggests that the process of CPD selection is a rational, rather than random process. Neimeyer et al. (2010), for example, found that CPD activities varied by workplace settings, suggesting that psychologists are responsive to the distinctive demands of the workplace context. Fowler and Harrison (2001) likewise found that school psychologists reported personal interest and workplace needs as important factors in the selection of CPD activities. Still, other features, beyond curricular aspects, have been found to influence the selection of CPD activities for school psychologists, including the cost, convenience, and brevity of CPD activities (Mowder and Demartino 1979). And, of course, the growing demands associated with specialization within the field have also impacted the training needs and practices of clinical and school psychologists (Armistead, Castillo, Curtis, Chappel, and Cunningham 2013; Reynolds 2011), as has the movement towards competency-based training (Dally III, Doll, Schulte, and Fenning 2011; Noltemeyer and McLaughlin 2011).

While somewhat rare in the field of clinical psychology in the US, several tools are available to help school psychologists identify their strengths and CPD needs, including the Professional Development Needs Checklist (see Brown 2002), as well as the Self-Assessment for School Psychologists available on the NASP website <http://www.nasponline.org/standards/survey/self-assessment-intro.aspx>. The Self-Assessment for School Psychologists is a free web-based tool that is built around the framework of the 10 domains found in the NASP *Model for Comprehensive and Integrated School Psychological Services (NASP 2010).* It allows individuals to rate the extent to which they engage in various activities and the perceived importance of those activities to their overall effectiveness; in addition, individuals indicate their perceived areas of need for CPD based on the 10 domains.

A recent review of national data collected from the anonymous completion of this survey revealed student-level services (e.g., direct academic and social-emotional interventions) and systems-level services (e.g., school-wide practices to promote learning; preventive and responsive services) as the highest areas of perceived CPD needs (Rossen and Charvat 2011).

While individualized needs assessment programs for clinical psychologists are relatively uncommon in the US, in Ontario, clinical psychologists employ an innovative, personalized self-assessment program. This program invites psychologists to reflect on their strengths, weaknesses, and areas in need of remediation utilizing a Self-Assessment Guide and Professional Development Plan. After pinpointing areas in need of improvement and areas of specialization, psychologists develop their own professional development and lifelong learning plan, which is carried out in place of the traditional formal continuing education plan in the United States. Psychologists are asked to reflect on several areas of their professional identity: 1) legislation, standards of professional conduct, code of ethics and guidelines, 2) service to clients, 3) teaching/training and research activities, 4) supervisory activities, 5) current areas of practice and/or services provided, and 6) anticipated areas of future practice. From this self-assessment, they are then asked to devise a professional development plan, along with a reflection on that plan (as the plan may change over the two-year cycle).

The benefit of employing such personalized programs lies in the fact that psychologists wear many hats and may have many professional roles, which requires them to remain "current" in a wide variety of areas. The demand for CPD within psychology has been noted in the literature for over 30 years (Mowder 1978; Mowder and Demartino 1979; Ross 1974). It seems likely that the rapid increase of new knowledge, together with expanding roles and responsibilities, will increase the demands placed on psychologists to remain current within the field (e.g., Crespi and Rigazio-DiGilio 1992; Dubin 1972; Hynd, Pielstick, and Schakel 1981; Reynolds 2011). The shrinking "half-life" of professional knowledge reflects this growing profusion of knowledge and the related trends towards increased specialization, as well. The half-life of professional knowledge has been described as the time it takes, after initial licensure or certification, to become roughly half as knowledgeable or competent in a field in the absence of any new learning (Dubin 1972). Neimeyer, Taylor, Wear, and Linder-Crow (2012) found in their Delphi Poll of licensed psychologists that the overall half-life of knowledge in professional psychology was expected to decrease by more than 25% over the course of the next 10 years. For clinical psychologists, the current half-life of knowledge is approximately 11.45 years, but it is expected to decrease to about nine years by 2021. For school psychologists, the current half-life of knowledge was estimated to be approximately nine years, and is expected to continue to decline to less than eight years by 2021 (Neimeyer, Taylor, and Rozensky 2012; see also Neimeyer, Taylor, Rozensky, and Cox 2014).

The range of professional challenges confronting psychologists is substantial, requiring a diverse set of knowledge and skills for addressing these myriad challenges (see also Wnek et al. 2008). School psychologists, for example, routinely assess children for learning disabilities, behavioral problems, and emotional issues; they provide direct and indirect interventions aimed at improving academic, social, and emotional functioning; they conduct, interpret, and utilize research; they need to understand the evolving interplay between a child's school, family, and support systems; they act as consultants to school systems and guardians of children; they provide crisis response and offer preventive services at the student- and school-wide level; and they act as advocates and promote improvements in student and school performance and accountability (see also Gorin 2009; Sigmon 1986; Smith 1984). Continuing professional development serves as a key mechanism for ensuring the continuing competency of psychologists in relation to these and other critical areas of their service delivery (Dally III et al. 2011; Hogg et al. 1989; Jindal-Snape 2009; Kennedy, Cameron, and Monsen 2009; Wnek et al. 2008). Surprisingly, however, contemporary research is sparse concerning the current perceptions, practices and perceived outcomes associated with CPD activities among psychologists, even though CPD is mandated for most credentialed psychologists (see Lam and Yuen 2004).

In this chapter, we will explore the continuing professional development experiences of clinical psychologists and school psychologists in the United States of America, along with the psychologists' perceptions about continuing professional development. We will also explore the perceived impact of CPD for clinical and school psychologists.

METHOD

Clinical Psychology Participants

In cooperation with the State, Provincial and Territorial Psychological Associations (SPTAs), an Internet survey was conducted of licensed or registered psychologists across North America. A total of 3704 participants identified as clinical psychologists. Most of the participants identified as female (58.6%), which closely approximates the broader demographics among APA members, where 57.2% of members identify as women (APA 2012). The majority of respondents identified as Caucasian (89.6%), with 2.3% identifying as Spanish, Hispanic, or Latino, 1.6% African American, 1.5% Asian, 1.2% Biracial or Multiracial, 0.2% as American Indian or Alaskan, 0.2% as Native Hawaiian, 0.6% identified as Other, and 2.7% declined to say. Among the APA membership, 60.2% identify as Caucasian, 2.3% Asian, 2% Hispanic, 1.6% Black, 0.6% Multiracial/multi-ethnic, 0.2% American Indian, and 33.1% declined to say. In the current sample, ages ranged from 24 to 89, with a mean age of 52.5, compared with the mean age of 55 years for APA members.

Most clinical psychologists in the sample were seasoned professionals who received their degrees, on average, 19.5 years earlier (SD = 11.1 years). In addition, 72.1% carried a Ph.D., 22.2% had a Psy.D., 5.5% carried a M.S. or M.A, and 0.2% of the current participants carried an Ed.D. as their highest professional degree. This compares with 69.7% of APA members reported as having a Ph.D., 3.1% with an Ed.D., 15.1% with a Psy.D., 0.1 with a M.D., 1.9% with another doctorate that was not specified, 9.2% with a M.S., M.A., or M.Ed., and 0.1% with a baccalaureate or associate's degree.

Regarding their workplace settings, 58.6% of participants in the present study worked primarily in independent practice, 15.1% in a hospital or medical setting, 10.0% worked in other settings, including primary and secondary school settings, 7.3% in a community agency, 6.1% in a university academic department, and 2.9% in a university counseling center or mental health service. In comparison, the APA member survey reflected 31% of respondents working primarily in independent practice, 21.3% in university settings, 8.3% in hospitals, 7.1% in other human service, 5.1% in medical school/academic medical center, 4.7% in government, 4.2% in clinics, 3.2% working in school and other educational settings, 2.8% working for four-year colleges, 2.6% working in other academic settings, 1.6% in business and industry, 6.6% in other work settings, and 1.3% did not specify.

Thus, the overall demographics of the sample generally correspond to APA membership, and presumably the general field of clinical psychologists.

School Psychology Participants

A total of 426 individuals that responded to the survey identified themselves as school psychologists. The majority of the sample consisted of women (64.1%). Most respondents were Caucasian (91.5%), with 1.2% Bi-racial, 0.7% Hispanic/Latino, 0.7% African American, 0.5% Asian, 0.5% American Indian, and the remainder indicated Other or declined to respond. The percentages of ethnic minorities in the sample approximated the percentages of school psychologists represented in the membership of the National Association of School Psychologists, where 76.6% are female, and 90.7% are Caucasian, 3.4% are Hispanic, 3% are African American, 1.3% are Asian, 0.6% are American Indian or Native Alaskan, and 1% indicated "other" (Castillo, Curtis, Chappel, and Cunningham 2011). In the current sample, ages ranged from 24 to 79, with a mean age of 53.2, compared with the mean age of 47.4 years for NASP members (Castillo et al. 2011). Most school psychologists in the sample were experienced professionals who received their degrees, on average, 20.8 years earlier (SD = 10.0 years). In addition, 6.3% of the current participants carried an Ed.D. as their highest professional degree, 6.8% carried an M.Ed., 8.5% had an M.S. or M.A., 63.2% carried a Ph.D., and 15.1% had a Psy.D. This compares with 25.06% of NASP members reported as having a M.S., M.A., or M.Ed., 45.76% reported as having a specialist degree, and 24.17% reported as holding a doctorate degree (Castillo et al. 2011).

Regarding their workplace settings, 44.1% of participants in the present study worked primarily in independent practice, 9.4% in a university academic department, 8.7% in a hospital or medical setting, 6.1% in a community agency, 0.2% in a university counseling center or mental health service, and 31.5% worked in other settings, including primary and secondary school settings. In comparison, the NASP member survey reflected 80.6% of respondents working primarily in school settings, 7.5% university faculty, 4.5% administrators, 0.1% working for the state department, and 7.3% working in other settings (Castillo et al. 2011). Given that school psychologists are trained to provide services in a variety of settings (see Margison and Shore 2009) and very few studies have explored the CPD experiences of those in settings outside of traditional school settings, this subset of the professional community was chosen to target a diverse sample.

While the overall demographics of the sample generally correspond to NASP membership, and presumably the general field of school psychologists, the current sample drew relatively heavily from the subset of doctoral-level school psychologists working in independent practice contexts.

Materials

The survey solicited demographic information and examined participants' CPD participation and their perceptions of their CPD experience. Data concerning overall perceptions of licensed professional psychologists regarding their CPD experiences have been reported in Neimeyer et al. (2010); the current article reports findings from the 4130 clinical and school psychologists who participated in that larger sample. While this study is drawn from the larger sample reported in Neimeyer et al. (2010), both the specific sample of psychologists and the analyses conducted on their responses are unique to this study.

In the survey, participants were asked to note the overall amount of CPD (i.e., the number of hours) they completed over the past year. In addition, to assess the most popular CPD topics, participants were asked to specify which of 64 different CPD topics they completed over the course of the previous year (e.g., ethics, anxiety disorders, assessment). The 64 CPD topics used in this study were chosen based on a CPD needs assessment survey conducted by the American Psychological Association in 2007 (APA 2007). Participants were also asked to specify which of the 64 CPD areas would be of greatest need for them in relation to future CPD programming. A copy of the complete survey is available upon request.

In addition, participants were asked about their perceptions of CPD. Participants ranked their satisfaction with their CPD programs using a five-point rating scale, as well as the translation of their experiences into their practices, and the impact of the CPD on the outcomes of their service delivery.

Procedure

Executive Directors of the State, Provincial, and Territorial Psychology Associations (SPTAs) were solicited through the Council of Executives of State and Provincial Psychological Associations (CESPPA). Participating Executive Directors were provided with an email to forward to their memberships. The e-mail explained the nature of the study and included a link to the survey, which could be completed and submitted through a secured website.

RESULTS

Results revealed a number of important findings concerning the nature of clinical and school psychologists' CPD participation, their perceived needs for CPD, and their satisfaction with the CPD activities they engaged in.

Continuing Professional Development Participation

Overall, clinical psychologists reported completing on average over 20 hours of formal CPD within a given year (M = 21.92; SD = 15.19; N = 3603), in addition to a range of informal CPD activities (e.g., consultations with other clinical psychologists, watching professional videos, reading professional journals). Similar findings are noted among school psychologists, who reported completing on average over 20 hours of formal CPD within a given year (M = 21.40; SD = 17.56; N = 415), in addition to a range of informal CPD activities. This finding is broadly consistent with the earlier findings of Fowler and Harrison (2001) in their nationwide study of 235 school psychologists, although they noted that a substantial percentage of school psychologists completed significantly more CPD than this. The percentages of clinical and school psychologists who completed various amounts of CPD in the current study are shown in Tables 1 and 2 where the range and the nature of the distribution are also depicted.

In addition to exploring general levels of participation in CPD, respondents were also asked to specify the topics of the various CPD activities that they completed during the year. Among clinical psychologists, continuing professional development activities in ethics, anxiety disorders, and assessment were among the most common (see Table 3), a finding that is consistent with the professional responsibilities of most clinical psychologists. Among school psychologists, continuing professional development activities in assessment, evaluation, and diagnosis were among the most common, a finding that is also consistent with the professional responsibilities of many school psychologists (see Table 4). These results are broadly consistent with the findings of Fowler and Harrison (2001) who indicated that the largest proportion of the 235 school psychologists in their sample reported moderate to high levels of CPD activity in the area of direct service.

Table 1. Clinical Psychology Respondents' Amount (Clock Hours) of Formal Continuing Professional Development Activities in a One-Year Period

	N	%
< 5 hours	158	4.4
5-10 hours	437	12.1
11-15 hours	659	18.3
16-20 hours	1085	30.1
21-25 hours	456	12.7
26-30 hours	339	9.4
31-35 hours	65	1.8
36-40 hours	178	4.9
41+ hours	226	6.3

Table 2. School Psychology Respondents' Amount (Clock Hours) of Formal Continuing Professional Development Activities in a One-Year Period

	N	%
< 5 hours	33	8.0
5-10 hours	53	12.8
11-15 hours	96	23.1
16-20 hours	94	22.7
21-25 hours	45	10.9
26-30 hours	40	9.6
31-35 hours	3	0.7
36-40 hours	23	5.5
41+ hours	28	6.7

The fact that Fowler and Harrison (2001) also found that levels of perceived CPD need were correlated with levels of CPD activity in those identified areas of need supports the likelihood that CPD selection is a rational, instead of random, process (see Neimeyer et al. 2010). Among the school psychologist sample, this is an important point, because it suggests that despite the fact that school psychologists may not have as much flexibility to engage in certain CPD programs as do psychologists in private practice, for example (due to schools often bringing in professional development speakers on predetermined topics), school psychologists are still, for the most part, engaging in CPD related to topics commonly described as areas of greatest need.

Table 3. Clinical Psychology Respondents' Top Ten Most Commonly Completed Continuing Professional Development Topics

	N	%
Ethics		56.0
Anxiety Disorders (e.g., OCD, PTSD, Panic Disorder)	1246	33.6
Assessment	1081	29.2
Disorders of Children and Adolescents	884	23.9
Mood Disorders	802	21.7
Cognitive Therapy	445	19.0
Trauma	686	18.5
Psychopharmacology	616	16.6
Addiction	575	15.5
Law	570	15.4

Note: Percentages signify the proportion of clinical psychologists who noted participation in these areas.

Table 4. School Psychology Respondents' Top Ten Most Commonly Completed Continuing Professional Development Topics

	N	%
Ethics	208	48.9
Disorders of Children and Adolescents	197	46.2
Assessment	186	43.7
Anxiety Disorders (e.g., OCD, PTSD, Panic Disorder)	142	33.3
Evaluation	136	31.9
Disabilities/Special Abilities	97	22.8
Mood Disorders	86	20.2
Diagnosis	74	17.4
Law and Psychology	73	17.1
Cognitive Therapy	68	16.0

Note: Percentages signify the proportion of school psychologists who noted participation in these areas.

In addition to their participation in CPD activities, participants were also asked to indicate their greatest CPD needs. Among clinical psychologists, the greatest CPD needs reported were in the areas of anxiety disorders, ethics, mood disorders, couples therapy, trauma, clinical supervision, psychopharmacology, evaluation and assessment, disorders of children and adolescents, and cognitive therapy (see Table 5).

These needs closely align with many activities (e.g., supervision, couples counseling in private practice, evaluation and assessment) that clinical psychologists are engaged in during their professional lives. Over 30 years ago, school psychologists reported that they experienced the greatest continuing professional development needs in "learning disabilities/emotional disturbance, counseling and interviewing techniques, assessment techniques with various areas of exceptionality, neuropsychological assessment, group dynamics and counseling and preschool assessment" (Mowder and Demartino 1979, p. 831).

Some similarities in findings occurred in the present study. Current participants noted comparable needs in neuropsychology, assessment, and general disorders of children and adolescents (e.g., learning disabilities/emotional disturbance), and these findings build on the related findings of Cleary et al. (2010) and Lewis et al. (2008) (see Table 6).

However, findings in the present study differed from those in Rossen and Charvat (2011), likely because the studies involved different categories of CPD, with the current study containing more clinically-focused CPD topics.

Table 5. Clinical Psychology Respondents' Top Ten Greatest Continuing Professional Development Topical Needs

	N	%
Anxiety Disorders (e.g., OCD, PTSD, Panic Disorder)	1616	43.6
Ethics	1524	41.1
Mood Disorders (e.g., unipolar or bipolar depression)	1138	30.7
Couples Therapy	987	26.6
Trauma	964	26.0
Clinical Supervision	959	25.9
Psychopharmacology	948	25.6
Evaluation and Assessment	936	25.3
Disorders of children and adolescents (e.g., ADHD)	921	24.9
Cognitive Therapy	911	24.6

Note: Percentages signify the proportion of clinical psychologists who noted needs in these areas.

Table 6. School Psychology Respondents' Top Ten Greatest Continuing Professional Development Topical Needs

	N	%
Anxiety Disorders (e.g., OCD, PTSD, Panic Disorder)	192	45.1
Disorders of Children and Adolescents	185	43.4
Assessment	156	36.6
Evaluation	145	34.0
Ethics	136	31.9
Mood Disorders	132	31.0
Cognitive Therapy	117	27.5
Neuropsychology	115	27.0
Psychopharmacology	105	24.6
Brief/Short-Term Therapy	100	23.5

Note: Percentages signify the proportion of school psychologists who noted needs in these areas.

Continuing Professional Development Perceptions

Aside from studying CPD participation, respondents also reported their perceptions about their CPD and the outcomes associated with it. The majority of clinical and school psychologists reported positive attitudes towards their CPD experiences (see Tables 7 and 8). Most (76.6% of clinical psychologists and 75.2% of school psychologists) reported strong or agreement with the idea that CPD should be mandated.

Furthermore, when asked, "How would you rate the overall quality of your continuing education experiences during the last year", 77.7% of clinical psychologists and 80.2% of school psychologists reported their CPD experiences as either good or excellent (M = 2.16; SD = 0.87; N = 3624; M = 2.02; SD = 0.80; N = 409, respectively).

In addition, 62.2% of clinical psychologists and 63.1% of school psychologists reported that CPD translated to their professional practice either very often or often (M = 2.18; SD = 0.88; N = 3621; M = 2.21; SD = 0.87; N = 415, respectively).

The majority of clinical psychologists (61.9%) and school psychologists (64.4%) reported that they learned a great deal or quite a lot as a result of their CPD (M = 2.27; SD = .85; N = 3636; M = 2.24; SD = .82; N = 416, respectively), and 80.1% of clinical psychologists and 73.8% of school psychologists reported that CPD helped them become more effective in their professional work (M = 2.00; SD = 0.89; N = 3643; M = 1.95; SD = 0.82; N = 416, respectively). Clinical and school psychologists also reported that CPD has positively impacted their ethical behavior.

Table 7. Clinical Psychologist Responses to Questionnaire Scalar Items: Percentages and Means

Item	1	2	3	4	5	M	SD
1. How would you rate the overall quality of your CE experiences during the last year?[a]	18.1	59.6	11.4	9.9	1.1	2.16	0.87
2. How often does your CE activity translate into your professional practice?[b]	24.9	37.6	33.2	3.2	1.1	2.18	0.88
3. How much do you feel that you have learned from your CE experiences?[c]	17.5	44.4	29.9	5.0	1.3	2.27	0.85
4. Do you believe that CE has helped you become more effective as a psychologist?[d]	28.5	51.6	13.0	4.9	2.1	2.00	0.89
5. Do you believe that any ethics programs you have taken have improved your understanding of ethical issues in professional practice?[d]	21.0	51.2	19.6	6.1	2.0	2.17	0.90
6. Do you believe that any ethics program you have taken have translated into more informed and effective ethical practices on your part?[d]	18.1	47.5	24.4	7.7	2.3	2.29	0.93
7. Do you believe that any ethics programs you have taken have reduced your "exposure" or professional liability?[d]	13.7	46.0	30.0	8.3	2.0	2.39	0.89

Note: [a]1 = excellent, 5 = poor; [b]1 = very often, 5 = very rarely; [c]1 = a great deal, 5 = very little; [d]1 = strongly agree, 5 = strongly disagree. CE = continuing education.

Table 8. School Psychologist Responses to Questionnaire Scalar Items: Percentages and Means

Item	1	2	3	4	5	M	SD
1. How would you rate the overall quality of your CE experiences during the last year?[a]	17.4	62.8	10.3	9.0	0.5	2.02	0.80
2. How often does your CE activity translate into your professional practice?[b]	19.3	70.0	0.0	10.1	0.5	2.21	0.87
3. How much do you feel that you have learned from your CE experiences?[c]	17.3	47.1	30.5	4.1	1.0	2.24	0.82
4. Do you believe that CE has helped you become more effective as a psychologist?[d]	28.6	54.3	11.7	4.5	1.0	1.95	0.82
5. Do you believe that any ethics programs you have taken have improved your understanding of ethical issues in professional practice?[d]	20.3	53.5	21.7	2.5	1.9	2.12	0.83
6. Do you believe that any ethics program you have taken have translated into more informed and effective ethical practices on your part?[d]	18.0	48.8	27.7	3.0	2.5	2.23	0.87
7. Do you believe that any ethics programs you have taken have reduced your "exposure" or professional liability?[d]	11.0	48.2	33.1	6.3	1.4	2.39	0.82

Note: [a]1 = excellent, 5 = poor; [b]1 = very often, 5 = very rarely; [c]1 = a great deal, 5 = very little; [d]1 = strongly agree, 5 = strongly disagree. CE = continuing education.

Most clinical psychologists (72.2%) and school psychologists (73.8%) strongly agreed or agreed that CPD improved their understanding of ethical issues in professional practice (M = 2.17; SD = 0.90; N = 3421; M = 2.12; SD = 0.83; N = 359, respectively), 65.6% of clinical psychologists and 66.8% of school psychologists either strongly agreed or agreed that CPD programs translated into more informed and effective ethical practices on their part (M = 2.29; SD = 0.93; N = 3400; M = 2.23; SD = 0.87; N = 361, respectively), and 59.7% of clinical psychologists and 59.2% of school psychologists reported that CPD programs reduced their "exposure" or professional liability (M = 2.39; SD = 0.89; N = 3418; M = 2.39; SD = 0.82; N = 363, respectively). This finding supports the requirement for renewal of the NCSP to obtain a minimum of three CPD hours in ethics or legal regulation of school psychology during each three year renewal cycle.

DISCUSSION

The results from this study suggest that clinical and school psychologists are purposeful and rational in the selection of CPD and are generally satisfied with their CPD experiences and with the translation of their learning to professional contexts. These data build upon other studies that also suggest that CPD is effective and can promote or enhance ethical behavior (see Wise 2010). These data also support the American Psychological Association's Ethics Code which notes that the maintenance, enhancement, and remediation of professional competencies are crucial to ethical practice. Respondents perceived that their CPD activities enhanced their knowledge and skills and translated into more informed, effective, and ethical service delivery.

Applications to the Practice of School Psychologists

The findings from this study are encouraging, and also suggest some important CPD topics that are reported by school psychologists as necessary areas for further development. Wnek et al. (2008) note that often "hot topics" for CPD have been promoted through a "top-down" perspective, but those who are in the "front lines" of work, school psychologists, need to have greater say in what CPD topics are necessary. The present study works to bridge this gap and builds upon Wnek et al.'s earlier study, which found that many school psychologists reported that CPD in the areas of diagnosis and assessment or intervention linkage were most strongly perceived to be related to improvement in competence. Aside from the importance of offering CPD through a broad range of topics, some CPD topics may be linked to greater professional effectiveness. Wnek et al. found that CPD in assessment, for example, was perceived to be linked to greater competence, and the present study suggests that CPD in assessment is a common topic taken by school psychologists. However, further work should explore the connection between specific CPD programs and objective measures of professional competence in order to more definitively identify best practices in CPD programming.

In a recent study, Canadian school psychologists were surveyed and most reported spending the majority of their time conducting intellectual assessments and writing reports (Jordan, Hindes, and Saklofske 2009; see also Cole 1996 for information pertaining to school psychologists in the US and Corkum, French, and Dorey 2007 for a study pertaining to school psychologists in Nova Scotia). In the present study, over one-quarter of participants expressed a need for additional training in assessment, evaluation, and a specific intervention (Cognitive Therapy), consistent with the professional training needs proposed and outlined by Saklofske (1997). While many psychologists spend a significant amount of their time on assessments and evaluation, this study suggests that although many psychologists complete CPD in assessments, many also wish there were additional assessment trainings offered in this area. Other notable areas of interest included interests related to the field of medicine. Approximately one-quarter of participants expressed a need for greater training in psychopharmacology, consistent with the perspective of Margison and Shore (2009), who note the increased need for collaboration among the health and helping professions, particularly with regard to the movement toward interprofessional practice in the field and the rising demands of managed care among professionals.

The nature of the study's findings, while informative, must be interpreted within the context of its limitations. This study consisted of self-reported measures of CPD participation and perceptions and, as a result, is subject to many of the biases that are inherent in self-report. For example, although participants were asked to select their greatest CPD needs, not all participants may have a good grasp on what their needs are, given the literature that questions the accuracy of self-assessment (Davis et al. 2006). There are, however, some self-assessment measures, such as the one created by NASP, designed to help school psychologists better determine their own professional development needs (see also Cleary et al. 2010).

Additionally, it is worth noting that only North American, and primarily doctoral-level, clinical and school psychologists were included in this sample, with a strong representation of those in independent practice settings; thus, these data may have limited generalizability to majority of school-based school psychologists, for example, who hold a specialist-level degree and do not possess an independent practice license. And third, although the survey assessed 64 different continuing education topics, it is possible that some topics considered important for future CPD, or some topics that had already been taken, were omitted in the survey responses regarding further CPD needs. These limitations of the current study might be explored in relation to future studies of CPD and its various outcomes.

Notwithstanding its limitations, the present study provides a glimpse into the participation and perceptions of clinical and school psychologists in relation to their CPD activities. Supporting involvement in CPD and a culture of competence may entail inculcating clinical and school psychology students with the attitudes, knowledge, and skills necessary for lifelong learning (see Salofske 1997). There is also a need for greater self-assessment competency measures to support psychologists in choosing CPD topics that meet their needs. The importance of continuing professional development in psychology cannot be overstated. Brown (1994) notes that the effectiveness of continuing professional development activities will shape the future of the field.

Cole (1996) concurs, adding that psychologists are "...often motivated to participate [in CPD] when they perceive that the learning is related to their needs rather than an attack on their competence." (p. 120). Findings suggest that psychologists complete CPD on a wide variety of topics that likely relate to the areas of professional practice in which they are most active and express interest in CPD that best meets their workplace demands. In addition, they reported high levels of satisfaction with their continuing professional development programs, and perceived that those activities frequently translated into more effective and ethical practice. This study adds to the growing literature on CPD and is aimed at stimulating additional work that explores the relationship between ongoing professional development and continuing professional competencies.

REFERENCES

American Psychological Association (2012). *Demographic characteristics of APA members by membership status*. Washington, DC.

American Psychological Association. (2007). *Unpublished Education Directorate survey*. Washington, D.C.

Armistead, L. D., Castillo, J. M., Curtis, M. J., Chappel, A., and Cunningham, J. (2013). School psychologists' continuing professional development preferences and practices. *Psychology in the Schools*, 50, 415-432.

Armistead, L. D. and Smallwood, D. (2011). Making a career of school psychology. In: T. M. Lionetti, E. P. Snyder and R. W. Christner (Eds.), *A practical guide to building professional competencies in school psychology* (245-262). New York: Springer.

Bradley, S. and Drapeau, M. (2013). Quebec psychologists and continuing education. *Canadian Psychology*, 54, 153-159.

Brown, D. T. (1994). Will the real school psychologist please stand up: Is the past a prologue for the future of school psychology? *School Psychology Review*, 23, 589-600.

Brown, M. (2002). Best practices in professional development. In: A. Thomas and J. Grimes (Eds.), *Best practices in school psychology IV* (pp. 183-194). Bethesda, MD: National Association of School Psychologists.

Castillo, J. M., Curtis, M. J., Chappel, A., and Cunningham, J. (2011, February). School psychology 2010: Results of the national membership study. *Paper presented at the annual convention of the National Association of School Psychologists*, San Francisco, CA.

Cleary, T. J., Gubi, A. and Prescott, M. V. (2010). Motivation and self-regulation assessments: Professional practices and needs of school psychologists. *Psychology in the Schools*, 47, 985-1002.

Cohen, D. M. and Dubin, S. S. (1970). *Measuring professional updating in mathematical competence*. University Park: Department of Planning Studies, Continuing Education, Pennsylvania State University.

Cole, E. (1996). An integrative perspective on school psychology. *Canadian Journal of School Psychology*, 12, 115-121.

Corkum, P., French, F., Dorey, H. (2007). School psychology in Nova Scotia. *Canadian Journal of School Psychology*, 22, 108-120.

Crespi, T. D. and Rigazio-DiGilio, S. A. (1992). Professional development and continuing education: Implications for the school psychologist. *School Psychology International*, 13, 347-355.

Daly III., E. J., Doll, B., Schulte, A. C., and Finning, P. (2011). The competencies initiative in American professional psychology: Implications for school psychology preparation. *Psychology in the Schools*, 48, 872-886.

Davis, A. D., Mazmanian, P. E., Fordis, M., Harrison, R. V., Thorpe, K. E., and Perrier, L. (2006). Accuracy of physician self-assessment compared with observed measures of competence. *JAMA*, 296, 1094-1102.

Dubin, S. S. (1972). Obsolescence or lifelong education: A choice for the professional. *American Psychologist*, 27, 486-498.

Esmaily, H. M., Savage, C., Vahidi, R., Amini, A., Dastgiri, S., Hult, H., Dahlgren, L. O., and Wahlstrom, R. (2009). Does an outcome-based approach to continuing medical education improve physicians' competences in rational prescribing? *Medical Teacher*, 31, e500-e506.

Fowler, E. and Harrison, P. L. (2001). Continuing professional development needs and activities of school psychologists. *Psychology in the Schools*, 38, 75-88.

Gorin, S. (2009). *Positive school climate, student wellness, and improved academic outcomes: Bringing out the best in students and schools* [PDF document]. Retrieved from http://www.nasponline.org/advocacy/gorin_briefing_101009.pdf.

Hogg, D., Stratford, R. J. and Cameron, R. J. (1989). Professional training and development in educational psychology: An integrated approach. *School Psychology International*, 10, 57-67.

Hynd, G. W., Pielstick, N. L. and Schakel, J. A. (1981). Continuing professional development in school psychology: Current status. *School Psychology Review*, 10, 480-486.

Jordan, J. J., Hindes, Y. L. and Saklofske, D. H. (2009). School psychology in Canada: A survey of roles and functions, challenges and aspirations. *Canadian Journal of School Psychology*, 24, 245-264.

Kennedy, E. K., Cameron, R. J. and Monsen, J. (2009). Effective consultation in educational and child psychology practice: Professional training for both competence and capability. *School Psychology International*, 30, 603-625.

Lam, S. and Yuen, M. (2004). Continuing professional development in school psychology: Perspective from Hong Kong. *School Psychology International*, 25, 480-494.

Lewis, M. F, Truscott, S. D. and Volker, M. A. (2008). Demographics and professional practices of school psychologists: A comparison of NASP members and non-NAPS School psychologists by telephone survey. *Psychology in the Schools*, 45, 467-482.

Margison, J. A. and Shore, B. M. (2009). Interprofessional practice and education in health care: Their relevance to school psychology. *Canadian Journal of School Psychology*, 24, 125-139.

Mowder, B. A. (1978). Continuing education needs in school psychology. *NASP Communique*, 6, 7.

Mowder, B. A. and Demartino, R. A. (1979). Continuing education needs in school psychology. *Professional Psychology*, 10, 827-833.

National Association of School Psychologists. (2010). *Model for comprehensive and integrated school psychological services*. Bethesda, MD: Author.

National Association of School Psychologists. (n.d.). *New requirements to renew your NCSP*. Retrieved from http://www.nasponline.org/certification/renewing_NCSP.aspx.

Neimeyer, G. J., Taylor, J. M. and Philip, D. (2010). Continuing education in psychology: Patterns of perception and perceived outcomes among mandated and nonmandated psychologists. *Professional Psychology: Research and Practice*, 41, 435-441.

Neimeyer, G. J., Taylor, J. M. and Rozensky, R. (2012). The diminishing durability of knowledge in professional psychology: A Delphi poll of specialties and proficiencies. *Professional Psychology: Research and Practice*, 43, 364-371.

Neimeyer, G. J., Taylor, J. M., Rozensky, R., and Cox, D. (2014). The diminishing durability of knowledge in professional psychology: A second look at specializations. *Professional Psychology: Research and Practice*, 45, 92-98.

Neimeyer, G. J., Taylor, J. M. and Wear, D. M. (2010). Continuing education in psychology: Patterns of participation and aspects of selection. *Professional Psychology Research and Practice*, 41, 281-287.

Neimeyer, G. J., Taylor, J. M., Wear, D., and Linder-Crow, J. (2012b). Anticipating the future of CE in psychology: A Delphi poll. In: G. J. Neimeyer and J. M. Taylor (Eds.), *Continuing professional development and lifelong learning: Issues, impacts and outcomes* (pp. 371-388). Hauppauge, NY: Nova Science Publishers.

Noltemeyer, A. and McLaughlin, C. L. (2011). School psychology's Blueprint III: A survey of knowledge, use, and competence. *School Psychology Forum*, 5, 74-86.

Reynolds, C. R. (2011). Perspectives on specialization in school psychology training and practice, *Psychology in the Schools*, 48, 922-930.

Ross, A. O. (1974). Continuing professional development in psychology. *Professional Psychology*, 5, 122-128.

Rossen, E. and Charvat, J. (2011). Preliminary results from the NASP self-assessment tool. *Communiqué*, 40(4), 4.

Saklofske, D. H. (1997). Moving toward a core curriculum for training school psychologists. *Canadian Journal of School Psychology*, 12, 91-96.

Sigmon, S. B. (1986). Clients, roles, and functions of the school psychologist. *Professional Psychology: Research and Practice*, 17, 3-4.

Smith, D. K. (1984). Practicing school psychologists: Their characteristics, activities, and populations served. *Professional Psychology: Research and Practice*, 15, 798-810.

Sullivan, A. and Long, L. (2010). Examining the changing landscape of school psychology practice: A survey of school-based practitioners regarding Response to Intervention, *Psychology in the Schools*, 47, 1059-1070.

Taylor, J. M. and Neimeyer, G. J. (in press). Continuing education and lifelong learning. In: J. C. Norcross, G. R. VandenBos and D. K. Freedheim (Eds.). *APA Handbook of Clinical Psychology* (Vol. 5). Washington, DC: APA Books.

Taylor, J. M., & Neimeyer, G. J. (2015). Public perceptions of psychologists' professional development activities: The good, the bad, and the ugly. *Professional Psychology: Research and Practice, 46,* 140-146.

Taylor, J. M., Neimeyer, G. J. and Tate, K. (2015). A look at continuing professional development needs for clinical, counseling, and school psychologists. *Unpublished manuscript*, West Virginia University, Morgantown, WV.

Wise, E. H., Sturm, C. A., Nutt, R. L., Rodolfa, E., Schaffer, J. B., and Webb, C. (2010). Life-long learning for psychologists: Current status and a vision for the future. *Professional Psychology: Research and Practice*, 41, 288-297.

Wnek, A. C., Klein, G. and Bracken, B. A. (2008). Professional development issues for school psychologists: What's hot, what's not in the United States. *School Psychology International*, 29, 145-160.

INDEX

A

B

C

D

E

F

G

H

I

J

K

L

M

N

O

P

Q

R

S

T

U

V

W

Y